T0259554

Equine Colic

Editor

LOUISE L. SOUTHWOOD

VETERINARY CLINICS OF NORTH AMERICA: EQUINE PRACTICE

www.vetequine.theclinics.com

Consulting Editor
RAMIRO E. TORIBIO

August 2023 • Volume 39 • Number 2

ELSEVIER

1600 John F. Kennedy Boulevard • Suite 1800 • Philadelphia, Pennsylvania, 19103-2899

http://www.vetequine.theclinics.com

VETERINARY CLINICS OF NORTH AMERICA: EQUINE PRACTICE Volume 39, Number 2
August 2023 ISSN 0749-0739, ISBN-13: 978-0-323-97288-8

Editor: Taylor Hayes
Developmental Editor: Akshay Samson

Veterinary Clinics of North America: Equine Practice (ISSN 0749-0739) is published in April, August, and December by Elsevier Inc., 360 Park Avenue South, New York, NY 10010-1710. Business and Editorial Offices: 1600 John F. Kennedy Blvd., Suite 1800, Philadelphia, PA 19103-2899. Subscription prices are $308.00 per year (domestic individuals), $647.00 per year (domestic institutions), $100.00 per year (domestic students/residents), $351.00 per year (Canadian individuals), $814.00 per year (Canadian institutions), $383.00 per year (international individuals), $814.00 per year (international institutions), $100.00 per year (Canadian students/residents), and $180.00 per year (international students/residents). To receive student/resident rate, orders must be accompanied by name of affiliated institution, date of term, and the signature of program/residency coordinator on institution letterhead. Orders will be billed at individual rate until proof of status is received. Foreign air speed delivery is included in all *Clinics* subscription prices. All prices are subject to change without notice. **POSTMASTER:** Send address changes to *Veterinary Clinics of North America: Equine Practice*, 3251 Riverport Lane, Maryland Heights, MO 63043. Customer Service (orders, claims, online, change of address): Elsevier Health Sciences Division, Subscription **Customer Service, 3251 Riverport Lane, Maryland Heights, MO 63043. Tel: 1-800-654-2452 (U.S. and Canada); 314-447-8871 (outside U.S. and Canada). Fax: 314-447-8029. E-mail: journalscustomerservice-usa@elsevier.com (for print support);** E-mail: **journalsonlinesupport-usa@elsevier.com (for online support).**

Reprints. For copies of 100 or more of articles in this publication, please contact the Commercial Reprints Department, Elsevier Inc., 360 Park Avenue South, New York, NY 10010-1710. Tel.: 212-633-3874; Fax: 212-633-3820; E-mail: reprints@elsevier.com.

Veterinary Clinics of North America: Equine Practice is covered in *MEDLINE/PubMed (Index Medicus), Excerpta Medica, Current Contents/Agriculture, Biology and Environmental Sciences,* and *ISI.*

Contributors

CONSULTING EDITOR

RAMIRO E. TORIBIO, DVM, MS, PhD
Diplomate, American College of Veterinary Internal Medicine; Professor and Trueman Endowed Chair of Equine Medicine and Surgery, College of Veterinary Medicine, The Ohio State University, Columbus, Ohio, USA

EDITOR

LOUISE L. SOUTHWOOD, BVSc, PhD
Diplomate, American College of Veterinary Surgeons; Diplomate, American College of Veterinary Emergency and Critical Care; Professor of Large Animal Emergency and Critical Care, Department of Clinical Studies, New Bolton Center, University of Pennsylvania, School of Veterinary Medicine, Kennett Square, Pennsylvania, USA

AUTHORS

MAIA R. AITKEN, DVM
Diplomate, American College of Veterinary Surgeons–Large Animal; Diplomate, American College of Veterinary Emergency and Critical Care; Assistant Professor of Large Animal Emergency and Critical Care, Department of Clinical Studies, New Bolton Center, University of Pennsylvania, Kennett Square, Pennsylvania, USA

CAROLYN E. ARNOLD, DVM, PhD
Diplomate, American College of Veterinary Surgeons; School of Veterinary Medicine, Texas Tech University, Amarillo, Texas, USA

CHARLIE BARTON, DVM
Equine Surgery Resident, Department of Clinical Sciences, Colorado State University, College of Veterinary Medicine and Biological Sciences, Fort Collins, Colorado, USA

MICHELLE HENRY BARTON, DVM, PhD
Diplomate, American College of Veterinary Internal Medicine–Large Animal Internal Medicine; Fuller E. Callaway Endowed Professor, Josiah Meigs Distinguished Teaching Professor, College of Veterinary Medicine, University of Georgia, Athens, Georgia, USA

ANJE G. BAUCK, DVM, PhD
Diplomate, American College of Veterinary Surgeons–Large Animal; Clinical Assistant Professor, Department of Large Animal Clinical Sciences, University of Florida College of Veterinary Medicine, University of Florida, Gainesville, Florida, USA

LAUREN BOOKBINDER, DVM
Diplomate, American College of Veterinary Internal Medicine; Assistant Professor of Large Animal Internal Medicine, Michigan State University College of Veterinary Medicine, East Lansing, Michigan, USA

DEBRA CATHERINE ARCHER, BVMS, PhD
Diplomate, European College of Veterinary Surgeons, FRCVS; Professor of Equine Surgery, Department of Equine Clinical Science, Leahurst Campus, University of Liverpool, Wirral, United Kingdom

MICHELLE COLEMAN, DVM, PhD
Diplomate, American College of Veterinary Internal Medicine; Department of Large Animal Medicine, University of Georgia, Athens, Georgia, USA

CRISTOBAL NAVAS DE SOLIS, LV, PhD
Diplomate, American College of Veterinary Internal Medicine; Clinical Studies New Bolton Center, University of Pennsylvania, Kennett Square, Pennsylvania, USA

DAVID E. FREEMAN, MVB, PhD
Diplomate, American College of Veterinary Surgeons; University of Florida, College of Veterinary Medicine, Gainesville, Florida, USA

ALEXANDRA GILLEN, MA, MS, VetMB
Diplomate, American College of Veterinary Surgeons, MRCVS; Senior Lecturer in Equine Surgery, Department of Equine Clinical Science, Leahurst Campus, University of Liverpool, Wirral, United Kingdom

HANNA HAARDT, DVM
Department of Large Animal Surgery, Anaesthesia and Orthopaedics, Faculty of Veterinary Medicine, Ghent University, Merelbeke, Belgium

GAYLE D. HALLOWELL, MA, VetMB, PhD, CertVA, FRCVS
Diplomate, American College of Veterinary Internal Medicine–Large Animal Internal Medicine; Diplomate, American College of Veterinary Emergency and Critical Care; Diplomate, European College of Veterinary Sports Medicine and Rehabilitation; Principal Fellow of Higher Education Authority, Director of Veterinary Professional Development, IVC Evidensia, Upper Broughton, Nottinghamshire, United Kingdom

DIANA M. HASSEL, DVM, PhD
Diplomate, American College of Veterinary Surgeons; Diplomate, American College of Veterinary Emergency and Critical Care; Professor, Department of Clinical Sciences, Colorado State University, College of Veterinary Medicine and Biological Sciences, Fort Collins, Colorado, USA

LECI IRVIN, DVM
Hagyard Equine Medical Institute, McGee Medical Center, Lexington, Kentucky, USA

ISABELLE KILCOYNE, MVB
Diplomate, American College of Veterinary Surgeons; Associate Professor in Equine Emergency Surgery and Critical Care, Department of Surgical and Radiological Sciences, UC Davis School of Veterinary Medicine, Davis, California, USA

TIM MAIR, BVSc, PhD, DEIM, DESTS, AssocECVDI, FRCVS
Diplomate, European College of Equine Internal Medicine; CVS Ltd, Bell Equine Veterinary Clinic, Mereworth, Maidstone, Kent, United Kingdom

ANN MARTENS, DVM, PhD
Diplomate, European College of Veterinary Surgeons; Department of Large Animal Surgery, Anaesthesia and Orthopaedics, Faculty of Veterinary Medicine, Ghent University, Merelbeke, Belgium

RACHEL PILLA, DVM, PhD
Gastrointestinal Laboratory, Department of Small Animal Clinical Sciences, School of Veterinary Medicine, Texas A&M University, College Station, Texas, USA

AMANDA PRISK, VMD
Diplomate, American College of Veterinary Surgeons–Large Animal, Assistant Clinical Professor of Large Animal Surgery, Department of Clinical Sciences, Cummings School of Veterinary Medicine at Tufts University, North Grafton, Massachusetts, USA

CERI SHERLOCK, BVetMed, MS, MVetMed, MRCVS
Diplomate, American College of Veterinary Sports Medicine and Rehabilitation–Large Animal; Diplomate, European College of Veterinary Surgeons–Large Animal; Diplomate, European College of Veterinary Diagnostic Imaging–Large Animal; CVS Ltd, Bell Equine Veterinary Clinic, Mereworth, Maidstone, Kent, United Kingdom

NATHAN SLOVIS, DVM, CHT
Diplomate, American College of Veterinary Internal Medicine; Hagyard Equine Medical Institute, McGee Medical Center, Lexington, Kentucky, USA

LOUISE L. SOUTHWOOD, BVSc, PhD
Diplomate, American College of Veterinary Surgeons; Diplomate, American College of Veterinary Emergency and Critical Care; Professor of Large Animal Emergency and Critical Care, Department of Clinical Studies, New Bolton Center, University of Pennsylvania, School of Veterinary Medicine, Kennett Square, Pennsylvania, USA

Contents

Epidemiologic studies are essential for the generation of evidence-based, preventive health care strategies. This includes ways to minimize colic risk and assist informed decision making concerning diagnosis, treatment, and likely outcomes. It is important to consider that colic is not a simple "disease" but is a syndrome of abdominal pain that encompasses multiple different disease processes, and which is multifactorial in nature. This review focuses on prevention and diagnosis of colic, including specific forms of colic, communications with owners/carers concerning colic risk and management, and areas of future research.

Gastrointestinal colic is the most common primary care equine emergency and affects nearly one of four horses per year. Colic is a significant welfare concern for equine patients and a financial and emotional burden for owners. The primary care practitioner is instrumental in identifying critical cases quickly and making appropriate management recommendations to improve patient outcomes.

Abdominal sonography is currently a routine procedure in the evaluation of colic in the horse. This imaging technique is used in both the assessment of the horse presented in the emergency setting with acute colic and the assessment of the horse presented for chronic or recurrent colic in the nonemergency setting. Sonography for colic evaluation is used by specialists in different disciplines and by general practitioners in the ambulatory and hospital settings. In this review, we will focus on indications and clinical interpretation of findings as well as recent developments in abdominal sonography.

Horses with colic caused by intestinal strangulation can have an excellent outcome with early surgical correction of the obstruction. The expense associated with surgery is typically less with early lesion correction. The challenge is making an early diagnosis of intestinal strangulation. Although for some horses with a strangulating obstruction, the need for surgery is made based on severe colic signs or lack of response to analgesia, in other horses, it is less obvious. Signalment, history, and meticulous physical examination, combined with some targeted diagnostic procedures can help with early diagnosis of intestinal strangulation. Improving the outcome of these horses requires diligence and a team-based approach from the owner or caregiver, primary care veterinarian, and specialists.

The list of medical causes of acute or chronic colic in horses is extensive. The purpose of this article is to review 4 medical causes of equine colic with a focus on newer trends in treatment. The 4 topics selected include gastric impaction, gastric glandular disease, colon displacement, and inflammatory bowel disease.

The following article provides an overview of the last 5 years of research and innovation within the field of equine colic surgery, focusing on new techniques, new or recently described lesions, prevention of lesion recurrence or postoperative complications, and updates in prognoses. Early surgical intervention is an important factor in horse survival.

The 3 time periods around colic surgery (preoperative, operative, and postoperative) are all critical to successful outcomes. Although much focus is often paid to the first 2 time periods, the importance of sound clinical judgment and rational decision-making in the postoperative period cannot be overstated. This article will outline the basic principles of monitoring, fluid therapy, antimicrobial therapy, analgesia, nutrition, and other therapeutics routinely used in patients following colic surgery. Discussions of the economics of colic surgery and expectations for normal return to function will also be included.

A successful outcome to management of the critical colic patient is highly dependent on how the patient is monitored and treated, particularly, in the perioperative period. In this article, we will provide an update on monitoring techniques, advances in fluid therapy, nutrition management and pharmacotherapeutic agents, inclusive of pain monitoring and management, prokinetics, and management of systemic inflammatory response syndrome and the hypercoagulable state.

The fecal microbiome of the horse is reflective of the large colon and plays an important role in the health of the horse. The microbes of the gastrointestinal tract digest fiber and produce energy for the host. Healthy horses have Firmicutes, Bacteroidetes, and Verrucromicrobia as the most common phyla. During gastrointestinal disease such as colic or colitis, the microbiome shows less diversity and changes in bacterial community composition.

Most recurrent episodes of non-specific colic are self-limiting, and the results of clinical examinations are unremarkable. Differentiating these cases from serious diseases can be difficult, but repeated evaluations are warranted. Horses presenting with very frequent bouts of colic are more likely to have serious diseases and a higher mortality rate compared to horses presenting with less frequent bouts of transient colic. Horses with recurrent bouts of prolonged colic are more likely to have motility issues or partial intestinal obstruction. Non-gastrointestinal diseases can also cause recurrent bouts of pain ("false colic"). Adhesions are common causes of colic following abdominal surgery.

VETERINARY CLINICS OF
NORTH AMERICA: EQUINE PRACTICE

SERIES OF RELATED INTEREST

Veterinary Clinics of North America: Food Animal Practice
https://www.vetfood.theclinics.com/

THE CLINICS ARE NOW AVAILABLE ONLINE!
Access your subscription at:
www.theclinics.com

Preface

Equine Colic: Can We Do Better?

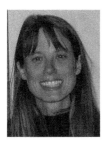

Louise L. Southwood, BVSc, PhD,
DACVS, DACVECC
Editor

Colic is often described in the lay literature as the "number one killer of horses." Successful outcome for horses with colic is dependent on a team approach between owners, caregivers, primary care veterinarians, specialists, and clinical researchers. This issue focuses on gastrointestinal causes of colic, covering a wide array of diagnostic, therapeutic, and research updates. The focus throughout is on early referral ("Updates on diagnosis and management of colic in the field and criteria for referral" by Bookbinder and Prisk), early recognition of intestinal strangulation ("Early identification of intestinal strangulation: why it is important and how to make an early diagnosis" by Southwood), prevention of complications ("When things don't go as planned: update on complications and impact on outcome" by Kilcoyne), and optimizing prognosis. A successful outcome is no longer defined as survival to hospital discharge. Rather, the expectations following colic surgery should be high with horses (and other equids) having a long, colic-free, and purposeful life. Decision making for euthanasia is addressed throughout this issue, underscoring the importance of communication and support for owners and caregivers. Economics is a critical component of veterinary medicine, and, as equine veterinarians, we must be fiscally responsible when making decisions to perform diagnostic and monitoring tests and avoid unnecessary treatment. Economics is discussed in several of the articles in this issue.

Much of the information that we have on the "causes" of colic and recurrent colic comes from epidemiologic studies. "By identifying modifiable risk-factors, epidemiological studies have enabled evidence-based strategies to be devised to reduce the

Vet Clin Equine 39 (2023) xiii–xv
https://doi.org/10.1016/j.cveq.2023.05.001
0749-0739/23/© 2023 Published by Elsevier Inc.

vetequine.theclinics.com

risk of colic"; the current knowledge and future directions for epidemiologic studies in equine colic are described in "Epidemiology of colic: current knowledge and future directions" by Archer and Gillen. Comprehensive details of current standards of care for management of horses with colic in the field, including decision making for referral ("Updates on diagnosis and management of colic in the field and criteria for referral" by Bookbinder and Prisk) and postoperative colic patients ("Basics of postoperative care of the equine colic patient" by Bauck and "Critical care of the colic patient: monitoring, fluid therapy, and more" by Barton and Hassel), are provided. Updates on diagnosing and managing gastric impaction and gastric glandular disease, inflammatory bowel disease, and medical management of colonic displacement ("Current topics in medical colic" by Barton and Hallowell), colic surgery ("Colic surgery: what's new?" by Aitken), and tips and tricks for diagnosis and management of mares and foals with colic ("Neonates, pregnant mares, and signalment-specific diseases and complications" by Slovis) are discussed. Recently, there has been research published on the equine intestinal microbiome, and "What is the microbiota and what is its role in colic?" by Arnold and Pilla explains the terminology used and interprets some of the findings of this research. Recurrent colic is a particularly frustrating problem for owners, caregivers, and veterinarians. A methodical approach to these horses is described in "Recurrent colic: diagnosis, management, and expectations" by Mair and Sherlock.

Considerable advances have been made over the past 15 years or so in transabdominal sonographic techniques, including accessibility and quality of available equipment, skill of the sonographer, and veterinary education on sonographic techniques, and interpretation of sonographic findings. Sonographic evaluation is mentioned throughout the issue, and "Abdominal sonographic evaluation: in the field, at the hospital, and after surgery" by Navas de Solis and Coleman provides information on progress in sonographic evaluation of the horse with colic and the potential of this diagnostic modality. Similarly, while laparoscopy in human surgery has replaced many invasive procedures, it is still somewhat in its infancy in equine abdominal surgery. There are, however, several reported laparoscopic procedures for diagnosis, treatment, and prevention of colic. "Role of laparoscopy in diagnosis and management of equine colic" by Martens and Haardt provides an update on these surgical procedures.

Horses with intestinal strangulation require emergency surgery. Recent reports in the literature show that, not surprisingly, a shorter colic duration leads to better long-term survival with fewer complications leading to less treatment-associated expense. In some instances, where the horse is persistently and moderately to markedly in pain, it is readily apparent that surgery is indicated. One the other hand, in other instances, it is less apparent. Similarly, early repeat celiotomy is essential for a successful outcome, for economic reasons, and for humane considerations in horses with certain types of complications particularly after small intestinal surgery and in horses with an initial diagnosis of a strangulating obstruction. "Early identification of intestinal strangulation: why it is important and how to make an early diagnosis" by Southwood describes tips for early identification of horses with intestinal strangulation, and "Repeat celiotomy: Current status" by Freeman and Bauck describes indications, technique, and outcome for repeat celiotomy.

Louise L. Southwood, BVSc, PhD, DACVS, DACVECC
Department of Clinical Studies
New Bolton Center
University of Pennsylvania
School of Veterinary Medicine
382 West Street Road
Kennett Square, PA 19348, USA

E-mail address:
southwoo@vet.upenn.edu

Epidemiology of Colic
Current Knowledge and Future Directions

Alexandra Gillen, MA, MS, VetMB DACVS,
Debra Catherine Archer, BVMS, PhD, DECVS*

KEYWORDS

- Colic • Epidemiology • Preventive strategies • Risk factors • Microbiome
- Biomarkers

KEY POINTS

- Colic continues to be a key health and welfare issue in horses, remaining a common concern for horse owners and a frequent reason for veterinary attendance with potential for death or euthanasia despite medical and/or surgical treatment.
- Education concerning colic prevention remains critical, taking into account the different perspectives that exist across different types of horse owners, including those with differing levels of education and with different perceptions and previous experiences concerning colic.
- Veterinary treatments, whether medical or surgical, should consider evidence of benefit, cost, and owner affordability.
- The use of "big data" through the generation of large patient medical databases, surveillance data, and research data sets across different equine populations and technological advances facilitating real-time clinic and stall-side data collection has great potential to add to the evidence base from the farm/clinic level to international studies, facilitating more accurate monitoring of colic prevalence, rapid assessment of the efficacy of new interventions, and generation of specific predictive models.

INTRODUCTION

Epidemiologic studies investigating colic provide important information that can be used to devise evidence-based preventive health care strategies to minimize the risk of colic and assist informed decision making concerning diagnosis, treatment options, and likely outcomes. Identification of risk factors for colic also provides further clues about cause, including potential pathophysiologic mechanisms that warrant further laboratory-based, fundamental research. Epidemiologic studies in this area are complicated by the fact that colic is not a simple "disease" but is a syndrome of

Department of Equine Clinical Science, School of Veterinary Sciences, Leahurst Campus, University of Liverpool, Leahurst, Neston, Wirral CH64 7TE, United Kingdom
* Corresponding author.
E-mail address: darcher@liverpool.ac.uk

abdominal pain that encompasses multiple different disease processes, and which is multifactorial in nature. Appraisal of such studies should consider study design, including the population being investigated and definition of colic used, and data analysis, including use of multivariable techniques. This is not an exhaustive review of the epidemiology of colic, which is beyond the scope of this article, but focuses on key aspects in relation to colic prevalence and impact, prevention, diagnosis, communications between veterinarians and owners/carers concerning colic risk and management, and areas of future research focus.

POPULATION STUDIES AND "BIG DATA"

Multiple epidemiologic studies conducted in the 1990s, mainly in the United States, demonstrated that colic has a significant impact on equine health and welfare, with a case fatality rate of 6.7% to 11%, accounting for up to 28% of equine deaths depending on the population studied.[1–3] In the US 2015 National Animal Health Monitoring System report,[4] colic continues to be one of the most common causes of morbidity, affecting 1.2% to 4.2% of horses based on age group. In the 12 months before the study,[4] the percentage of resident horses that developed colic was lowest in the less than 6-month age group (1.2%), and in the other groups was 2.2% (6 months to <1-year-olds), 3.1% (1 to <5-year-olds), 2.8% (5 to <20-year-olds), and 4.2% (horses aged 20 years old or more). Colic was the most common cause of mortality in horses aged between 1 and 20 years of age, accounting for 31.2% of deaths in this age category, and was the second most common cause of death in geriatric horses (13.4% of deaths in horses >20 years of age, second to "other causes," predominantly "old age").[4] These figures are consistent with morbidity and mortality data from other countries, based on equine insurance data sets.[5–8]

Colic is one of the most commonly cited equine medical concerns for veterinarians[9] and horse owners/carers,[10,11] including owners of working equids in developing countries.[12,13] Severe forms of colic, requiring surgery or euthanasia, have previously been considered to represent less than 10% of colic cases assessed by veterinarians in ambulatory practice.[2,14,15] However, a recent study reported that 23.5% of colic cases seen by veterinary practitioners in 2 UK ambulatory practices were classified as "critical" in nature (defined as cases that required intensive medical or surgical management, were euthanized, or died).[16] This difference was considered most likely because of a relatively greater proportion of aged horses in this ambulatory practice population compared with previous referral-center–based population data. In this age group, intestinal strangulation owing to pedunculated lipomas is more common, and euthanasia rather than referral for potential surgery may be more likely to be opted for by horse owners based on age alone and/or age-associated comorbidities. This figure may also reflect the increased availability and use of clinic-based, intensive medical treatments for management of some forms of colic compared with studies conducted greater than20 years previously. Colic is a common cause of out-of-hours (OOH) veterinary visits in equine ambulatory practice, being the most common equine emergency requiring veterinary attendance and accounting for 35% of OOH visits in 2 UK ambulatory equine practices,[17] and one of the most common causes of emergency admissions to large animal referral hospitals.[18] Colic, therefore, continues to be a key health issue for veterinarians and horse owners globally and remains an important focus for ongoing research.

By identifying modifiable risk factors, epidemiologic studies have enabled evidence-based strategies to be devised to reduce the risk of colic.[19,20] However, the degree to which colic incidence overall has changed since these risk factors started to be identified and quantified is difficult to determine. Very few studies have investigated the effect of interventions on the incidence of colic,[21] and this is an area for future research focus. Within managed equid populations, the incidence of colic has been estimated at between 4 and 26 episodes per 100-horse-years-at-risk.[15] Most studies have investigated colic incidence in specific equine populations and have been used to extrapolate likely incidence in the wider equid population. However, the true incidence of colic in the general equid population is unknown. These studies have traditionally been expensive and time-consuming to perform. However, technological advances may offer opportunities for more cost-effective, rapid collection, and reporting of data obtained from horse owners and veterinarians in field and hospital settings. These include data collection via mobile devices, such as phones and tablets, use of text-mining software to interrogate data records, and specifically designed computer programs and other electronic tools to facilitate real-time data collection and reporting.

Use of "big data" approaches is not a new concept for epidemiologic investigations of colic, using national survey data and insurance data sets as already outlined. Within the field of companion animal epidemiology, this is an area that has expanded rapidly, including development of large medical record data sets by veterinary corporate companies,[22] collaborations between epidemiologists, private and university-based veterinary practices, and hospitals (eg, SAVSNET,[23] VetCompass[24]), and development of research data sets (eg, Dogslife Project[25]). Although there are challenges concerning privacy, data security, and technical vulnerabilities, these large-scale data sets provide many opportunities for research and improvements in pet health.[26] Text-mining of large data sets to investigate the prevalence and survival of horses with chronic diseases[27] and antimicrobial prescribing practices in equine practice,[28] expansion of medical recording systems and surveillance data sets to include collection of equine data (eg, EVSNET[29]), and creation of colic audit and research data sets (INCISE[30]) all provide opportunities to enhance epidemiologic investigations into equine colic, including real-time reporting of data. However, it is important that such data are accurate and can be reliably collected and analyzed, including data collected outside clinic facilities, for example, ambulatory practice. For studies investigating colic, specific potential barriers to data collection, such as time constraints, concerns about confidentiality, and use of data, have already been identified.[31] Around a quarter of colic episodes may resolve spontaneously with no veterinary intervention,[15] so use of veterinary treatment records or direct veterinary reporting of colic episodes is likely to underestimate the true prevalence. Other limitations include biases in data collection, such as reporting bias owing to veterinarians only inputting data for selected cases (eg, more memorable cases or severe forms of colic) or observer bias, for example, veterinarian or horse owner misreporting colic cases.[32] Overall, although there are limitations and challenges, big-data approaches provide exciting new opportunities in colic epidemiologic research.

ECONOMICS AND AFFORDABILITY OF CARE

The current economic cost of colic to the global equine industry is unknown. In the 1990s, the economic impact of colic to the US equine industry was estimated at $115.3 million, with 66% of these costs associated with horse mortality.[1] These costs will now invariably be substantially greater given that colic remains a common cause of equine morbidity and mortality. The total world equid population has previously been estimated at 112 million, comprising 58.5 million horses and 53.5 million donkeys and mules, with working equids in low-income, net food-importing countries representing greater than one-third of all equids and greater than 50% of all donkeys.[33] In addition to direct economic costs of colic-related treatment and mortality, diseases such as colic have wider socioeconomic impacts in the latter populations.[34]

Economics also impact owner decision making and options for treatment. During periods of global economic recession, data from a US and a UK referral hospital population demonstrated a reduction in the proportion of horses presented for assessment of colic undergoing surgical treatment and increased proportion of horses being euthanized.[35] Increases in the cost of veterinary care owing to inflation and new therapies are not always associated with parallel increases in the cover provided by insurance companies,[36] and there are concerns that colic surgery may become unaffordable for some horse owners.[37] Therefore, the economics of treatment of colic and affordability for individual owners have to be considered. Similar to human health care, the costs of veterinary medical care have been increasing faster than inflation over the last 20 years.[38] The principle of value-based care has been used within human health care, where care is based on the principle of achieving the best patient-based outcomes for the lowest cost.[39] Development of a value-based veterinary care framework based on this principle has been proposed.[38] This concept focuses on ways to provide high-quality veterinary patient care while also considering outcomes and costs. Outcomes should not be limited to those that veterinary professionals (and those in other related fields, eg, experts in animal welfare/ethics) consider to be important, but must be developed in conjunction with owners/carers of veterinary patients. This would include development and use of observer (owner)-reported outcomes and owner-reported quality-of-life measures in addition to current standard outcome measures. Epidemiologic studies demonstrating efficacy of different treatments on colic outcomes, including well-designed interventional, multi-center studies and cost-benefit analyses of these are key areas for ongoing research. Such studies would assist veterinarians and owners in making informed decisions concerning treatment, particularly where economics are limited, and may constrain options, keeping treatment of colic (and in particular surgery) as affordable as possible for horse owners.

THE HUMAN ELEMENT

In addition to using an evidence-based approach to guide management of our patients, as veterinary professionals, we also must consider how we convey information from epidemiologic studies about preventive health care to animal owners. Horse owners/carers play a critical role in decisions about routine management of horses, which may impact on colic risk. These include recognition of signs of colic, decisions concerning seeking veterinary advice, and choice of treatment options, including potential surgical management. Social science approaches are widely used in the medical field to better understand the behavior of people, including barriers and motivators to improving human health, which can be used to develop tailored, educational strategies.[40] A UK study showed that multiple different owner typologies exist with variations not only between but within professional and nonprofessional (lay) horse owner groups in how they recognize and manage colic.[41] The motivation to contact a veterinarian and make decisions concerning treatment is related to the owner's primary attitude toward colic (for example, some owners choose to wait and see, some use lay treatments, and some choose to contact a veterinarian initially), as well as financial aspects. Owners' attitudes were also shown to be based on their previous experience of colic and the experiences of their friends and other horse owners. In a separate study, owner knowledge was also shown to have an impact on the speed of recognition of colic, as well as an estimation of severity.[42] Because of variations in horse owner attitudes toward colic and the disparity in knowledge between some, there is no "one-size-fits-all" approach, and veterinarians must tailor their approach to communication and education concerning colic prevention and care based on individual client knowledge and perceptions. This approach can help to develop educational campaigns concerning colic, such as the UK's British Horse Society "REACT Now to Beat Colic" campaign.[43] For working equid populations, in addition to conventional epidemiologic approaches,[44] use of participatory methods provides valuable and complementary information that can be used to inform interventions.[12,34] These approaches can be used to explore horse owners' understanding of colic and gaps in knowledge concerning colic[13] and subsequent development of interventional strategies to minimize colic risk.

Epidemiologic studies have also challenged some common perceptions held by horse owners and some veterinarians. One such example is surgical treatment of colic in geriatric horses and ponies. Epidemiologic studies have shown that horses and ponies older than 16 years of age are more likely to be euthanized before surgical intervention, compared with younger age groups.[45] However, there is no evidence of increased risk of postoperative mortality in geriatric patients treated for small intestinal strangulating disease.[46] Horse owners commonly cite perceived poor success rates of surgical treatment and concerns about horse's inability to return to athletic function (the authors' observations). However, in horses undergoing surgical treatment of colic that recover following anesthesia, although prognosis can vary dependent on a number of identified risk factors for nonsurvival, studies have demonstrated that overall 74% to 85% of horses survive to hospital discharge with 63% to 85% returning to athletic performance.[47] Therefore, it is important that veterinarians can present available evidence enabling horse owners to make informed decisions concerning colic management, including surgical treatment.

COLIC PREVENTION

Epidemiologic studies have demonstrated that there are various horse- and management-level risk factors for colic in general, and for specific forms of colic, which are often multiple and overlapping.[19,20,48] Factors, such as age, sex, and breed, cannot be modified but can assist identification of horses at higher risk of specific forms of colic, assisting decision making concerning likely diagnosis and treatment options (see next section). Where identified risk factors can be modified, this evidence can be used to devise preventive strategies to reduce the likelihood of colic developing, particularly in horses who have already had a colic episode. A longitudinal study performed in the United Kingdom demonstrated that of horses that required medical treatment for colic, 36.5% of horses had recurrence of colic in the following 12 months with a recurrence rate of 50 colic events per 100-horse-years-at-risk, which is much higher than the risk of colic in the general population.[49] Therefore, even when attending a horse that presents with colic for the first time and which resolves following medical treatment, veterinarians should provide advice concerning colic prevention. Most important in terms of identified modifiable risk factors are diet, time spent at pasture or stalled, parasite control, and dental prophylaxis, as outlined in the following sections.

Geography and season are known to play a role in colic risk, which likely reflect an interplay between various environmental- and management-related factors. Epidemiologic studies conducted at a more regional level can alert veterinary surgeons and owners to increased risk of specific forms of colic, in particular, geographic regions, such as those caused by enteroliths,[50,51] duodenitis-proximal jejunitis,[52] or more unusual forms of colic, such as idiopathic focal eosinophilic enteritis.[53] Anecdotal evidence of possible variation in colic incidence at specific times of the year (seasonality) has been suggested in various studies, but this is difficult to prove using conventional statistical methods. In the United Kingdom, this has been investigated using more complex mathematical models.[53,54] In a UK hospital population, consistent seasonal patterns for colic admissions of any type and specific forms of colic were identified and for others (pedunculated lipoma obstruction) where there was no evidence of seasonality (**Fig. 1**).[54] Cyclical patterns for all colic admissions, medical and surgical colic admissions, large colon displacements/volvulus coincided with spring and autumn (fall) months, coinciding with times of the year when horses are likely to undergo changes in diet, turnout, and other management-related factors, such as exercise. Other patterns, such as large colon impaction and epiploic foramen entrapment admissions, demonstrated a consistent cyclical increase in frequency over the winter months, times of the year when horses are more likely to be stalled, and where sudden changes in pasture turnout and feeding may occur.

Stalling, Pasture Turnout, and Exercise

These factors all have a degree of interplay, as a horse that is stalled for long periods of the day will also have reduced opportunity to graze at pasture and more limited ability for exercise. Epidemiologic studies demonstrate that, in general, colic risk is reduced by avoiding sudden changes in turnout and stalling, by avoiding long periods of time spent stalled, and by providing consistent pasture turnout.[55–57] Increasing time spent at pasture also reduced the likelihood of colic recurrence in horses subsequent to an episode of medical colic, making this an important intervention to consider in individual colic cases. For some groups of horses, such as those that display cribbing behavior, increased likelihood of colic has also been shown to be directly correlated with increased hours spent stalled per day and decreased hours of pasture turnout.[58] This is also an important risk factor for specific forms of colic, such as simple colonic obstruction/distention (SCOD), where risk is greatest in horses stalled for 24 hours per

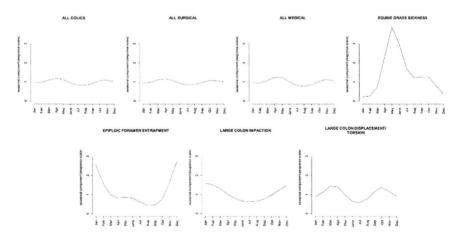

Fig. 1. Seasonal patterns of colic in cases presented to a UK referral hospital over a 10-year period, using estimates from a Bayesian regression model. (Reproduced with permission from Archer DC, Pinchbeck GL, Proudman CJ, Clough HE. Is equine colic seasonal? Novel application of a model based approach. *BMC Vet Res.* 2006;2. https://doi.org/10.1186/1746-6148-2-27.)

day[59] and where a recent decrease in exercise and transport less than 24 hours previously were also identified to increase SCOD risk, all factors that contribute to reduced gastrointestinal motility. Other examples of specific groups of horses where increased pasture turnout is protective include horses at risk of enterolithiasis.[51]

Diet

Epidemiologic studies have demonstrated that diet is a key element in colic risk and has been a focus of multiple investigations. Overall, colic risk in general is reduced by avoiding sudden (<2 weeks' duration) changes in forage type and batch and changes in concentrate type and quantity.[55–57,60,61] For horses in specific regions, such as those where enterolithiasis is more likely to occur or where specific feed types such as Coastal Bermuda hay are more likely to be fed, dietary interventions are important in reducing risk of enterolith-associated colic[50,51,62] or development of ileal impactions.[63] Diet is complex to assess, and in epidemiologic studies, it can be difficult to obtain detailed and reliable dietary data, even in prospective studies, and particularly on premises where multiple people may be involved in a horse's daily care. It is not currently clear why certain forage types or sugar beet pulp has been associated with increased risk of colic in specific groups of horses[58] or specific forms of colic.[64] Diet type, quantity, and dietary alterations may all be factors associated with changes at a more molecular level within the horse's gastrointestinal system.[65]

Technological developments have led to major advances in molecular gastrointestinal research, and increased availability and affordability have made these technologies accessible for equine intestinal research. A vast amount of research conducted in laboratory animals and people has demonstrated that the intestinal microbiome has effects on a range of host systems, including metabolism, immune system, and brain function.[66,67] Investigation of the equine microbiome in health and disease is an important and active area of current research.[68] In future epidemiologic studies, specific features of the equine microbiome may be important variables to include in multivariable models investigating colic risk. Studies have demonstrated that the microbiome of healthy horses varies with season, age, subsequent to parturition, and according to management-related factors, including changes in diet, access to pasture, gastrointestinal parasite status, and following administration of medications.[69–74] Microbiome alterations have been demonstrated in horses with colic,[75–77] but more studies are required to gain a greater understanding of specific features of the equine microbiome and association with colic risk across a range of different equine populations and different forms of colic. There is huge potential to conduct interventional studies to manipulate the microbiome through dietary supplementation, such as administration of probiotics,[78] particularly in horses that develop recurrent episodes of colic where there is no identifiable cause. Fungi are also key components of the microbial gut population,[79] and mycobiome studies are in their relative infancy in current equine gastrointestinal research. One recent study identified mycobiome alterations in the gastrointestinal tract of horses with grass sickness (equine dysautonomia),[80] providing important, new insights into this disease. It is important that such studies, including the effects of interventions to manipulate microbial populations of the equine gut, are well designed and use statistical models that take into account the normal differences between individual horses and effects of other potentially confounding factors, such as pasture turnout and concurrent administration of medications.

Parasite Prophylaxis

Epidemiologic studies provide evidence that minimizing gastrointestinal parasite burdens through administration of anthelmintics is associated with reduced risk of colic[44,55,59,81] and that high gastrointestinal burdens of the equine tapeworm, *Anoplo-cephala perfoliata*, is an important risk factor for spasmodic colic and ileal impaction, accounting for 81% of ileal impactions in one study.[82] However, frequent administration of anthelmintics increases selection pressure for anthelmintic resistance (AHR) and failure to be able to effectively minimize equine gastrointestinal parasite burdens owing to development of AHR could increase colic risk. There is evidence of AHR in strongyle populations in different geographic regions to different classes of anthelmintics used in horses,[83,84] and evidence that effects of climate change may also accelerate AHR.[85] Lack of development of any new classes of anthelmintics means that judicious, best practice in parasite control is critical.[84] Educational strategies in this area will become increasingly important, including use of targeted worming strategies and avoidance of anthelmintic administration as a sole means of parasite prophylaxis.

Dental Prophylaxis

Severe orodental disease is a risk factor for colic,[44] and known dental issues have been identified to increase the risk of colic recurrence[86] and impaction colic in donkeys.[87] Dental prophylaxis has also been shown to be associated with reduced risk of SCOD colic[59] and identification of quidding behavior, frequently associated with orodental pathologic condition, increases the risk of large colon volvulus.[64] Therefore, horse owners should be aware of the importance of regular (6–12 monthly), thorough dental assessment and appropriate treatment as a way to reduce colic risk.

Stereotypic Behavior

Horses that display oral stereotypic behaviors, including cribbing, have been shown to be at increased risk of colic,[44] recurrent colic,[86] and specific forms of colic, including SCOD[59] and epiploic foramen entrapment.[88,89] Once established, cribbing behavior is difficult to stop, making it important to try to prevent this behavior from developing during a horse's early life.[90] Interventions to physically prevent horses from cribbing are likely to severely compromise welfare,[91] and there is no evidence that such interventions reduce the risk of colic in these horses. Severity of cribbing behavior has also been shown to be associated with increased likelihood of a history of previous colic.[58] This is an area that requires more research to better understand the relationship between the gut-brain axis in horses that display oral stereotypic behaviors. Current evidence suggests that avoiding feeding of haylage and maximizing pasture turnout in the autumn (fall) months may help to reduce the likelihood of colic in these horses.[58]

Surgical Interventions to Prevent Colic

Specific forms of colic, including left and right dorsal displacement of the large (ascending) colon, large colon volvulus, epiploic foramen entrapment, and inguinal hernias, have more potential to recur compared with other forms of colic. This has resulted in the development of several surgical procedures to reduce the risk of recurrence of these specific forms of colic, including laparoscopic methods to close or ablate the nephrosplenic space,[92,93] epiploic foramen[94,95] and inguinal rings,[96–98] and colopexy or resection of the large colon.[99] From an epidemiologic viewpoint, the optimal way to demonstrate efficacy of an intervention is to assign these randomly. However, in practical terms, this is unlikely to be achievable, as these procedures are more likely to be biased toward horses who are considered good candidates for a specific surgical procedure, or horse owners who have the financial means/emotional investment in that horse. Demonstrating efficacy of any surgical intervention is essential, but when appraising studies where interventions are not randomly assigned, it is important to consider the potential for selection bias. Assessment of outcome following such procedures is important, and although it is important to consider the potential for bias, there is evidence to support their use in reducing recurrence of these specific forms of colic.[93,95,100]

DECISION MAKING CONCERNING LIKELY DIAGNOSIS AND TREATMENT

Early identification and surgical intervention for those forms of colic that cannot be managed medically are critical for optimal survival and reduction in postoperative morbidities. Multiple studies have demonstrated that reduced survival and increased incidence of postoperative complications are more likely in horses with severe cardio-vascular derangements before surgery, including elevations in heart rate, systemic packed cell volume, plasma, and peritoneal lactate.[101–103] However, in the early stages, many different pathologic lesions that cause abdominal pain, and which may or may not require surgery, present with similar signs. This makes the veterinarian's task challenging, particularly in the early stages of colic and where use of additional tests may not be feasible to perform outside of clinic facilities.

Epidemiologic studies have shown that different risk factors exist for specific forms of colic, some of which may overlap with other forms of colic. These studies also quantify the increase or decrease in risk associated with these different colic types (**Table 1**). Veterinarians can use a risk-based approach to consider how likely a horse is to have a particular form of colic (or not) by using information about horse signalment, prior colic history, current management, and knowledge of local geographic information about colic risk, in conjunction with the results of clinical examination and response to analgesia. An exact diagnosis is not essential before referral to a suitable facility for potential surgical intervention. Increasing certainty of a specific diagnosis by waiting for additional or worsening clinical signs to develop risks deteriorations in the horse's systemic status and potential requirement for intestinal resection, with consequent reduction in the chance of an optimal postoperative outcome. However, for horses that are at high risk for specific forms of colic that require surgical intervention, the decision for early referral and surgery may be facilitated through application of epidemiologic information and use of this in discussions with horse owners.

Identification of other risk factors that could increase the certainty of the need for surgical intervention at the earliest possible stages, particularly if this information can be used stall side, is a key area of ongoing research and could have major potential benefits for equine health and welfare. In recent years, research has focused on identification of biomarkers in blood or peritoneal fluid that can be detected in the earliest stages of the disease process. Alterations in lactate, serum amyloid A, haptoglobin, and creatinine kinase in peripheral blood and peritoneal fluid have all been identified as biomarkers for more severe forms of gastrointestinal disease.[104–107] However, there is a current lack of evidence concerning their ability to reliably detect surgical lesions using multivariable models and, apart from use of portable lactate meters, many of these biomarkers can only be measured in suitably equipped clinics.

Metabolomic and proteomic approaches have been widely used in the human medical field to assist identification and prognostication of human patients with a variety of disease conditions. Biomarkers, including L-histidine, pyruvic acid, and stearic acid, have been demonstrated to have clinical application in improving prediction of patient survival, as well as the likelihood of morbidities.[108,109] Nuclear magnetic resonance and mass spectroscopy are screening tools that can be used to assess large numbers of biomarkers in both tissues and biofluids. Although this approach is at a relatively early stage in equine colic research, it has been applied to analysis of blood and peritoneal fluid samples of horses with different forms of colic.[105–107,110] If one or more

Table 1
Horse and management level risk factors for specific forms of colic identified from epidemiologic studies selected on the basis of a suitable control population

Specific Colic Type	Risk factors	References
Epiploic foramen entrapment	↑ Risk: Cribbing behavior, history of colic in the prior 12 mo, increased stabling in the prior 28 d, increased height, person responsible for daily care, winter months ↓ Risk: Access to mineral/salt lick, behavioral features, not fed at the same time as other horses	54,88,89
Pedunculated lipoma obstruction	↑ Risk: Increasing age, geldings, and breed (Arabians, quarter horses, saddlebred, pony breeds)	117–119
Ileal impaction	↑ Risk: *A perfoliata* infection, feeding Coastal Bermuda hay, failure to administer a pyrantel salt in prior 3 mo	63,82,101
Idiopathic focal eosinophilic enteritis	↑ Risk: Younger age, geographic location, months between July and November	53
Large colon volvulus	↑ Risk: Increasing height, multiple colic episodes in the previous 12 mo, mares, mares that had previously foaled, quidding behavior, receiving medication (other than anthelmintics) in the previous 7 d, increase in the hours of stabling in the previous 14 d, greater number of horses on the premises, 3 or more people involved in horse's daily care, feeding of hay, feeding of sugar beet, a change in pasture in the previous 28 d, an alteration in amount of forage in the previous 7 d	64
Simple colonic obstruction and distention	↑ Risk: Cribbing behavior, increased hours stabled, recent reduction in exercise, transport in the previous 24 h, absence of administration of ivermectin or moxidectin in prior 12 mo, resident on premises <6 mo, history of previous colic, reduced frequency of dental prophylaxis	59
Impaction colic in donkeys	↑ Risk: Increasing age, receiving extra feed rations, previous history of colic, paper bedding, feeding of concentrates, limited pasture access, increasing number of carers, recent weight loss, recent vaccination, dental pathologic condition	87,120
Enterolithiasis	↑ Risk: Feeding alfalfa hay, feeding > or = 50% of the diet as alfalfa, feeding <50% of diet as oat hay or grass hay, lack of daily access to pasture grazing, ≤50% time spent outdoors, Arabian/Arabian x, miniature, Morgan, American saddlebred horse breeds, donkeys, dry climates, magnesium, ammonium phosphorus in diet ↓ Risk: Thoroughbred, standardbred, and warmblood breeds, stallions	50,51,62

novel biomarkers that can be easily assessed at one point or sequentially are identified, these will require testing in multivariable models to determine if this information improves the ability to better predict which horses may need surgical intervention and likely operative outcomes.

Multiple epidemiologic studies have been undertaken to determine factors that are associated with postoperative survival and likelihood of development of postoperative complications.[47] Evidence from these studies is important in assisting informed decision making in the primary care and referral hospital setting and can aid discussions with owners before, during, and following surgery regarding likely outcome and associated costs. A recent study demonstrated that previously developed single and multivariable predictive models[111–115] were poor predictors of patient survival in populations different from the population used to develop a specific model.[116] This highlights the importance of generating and maintaining large patient data sets, including pooling of data from multiple clinics. This would assist generation of additional multivariable models, some of which are based on more localized data, and updating of models using data obtained from larger populations of horses with colic.

SUMMARY

Colic continues to be a key health and welfare issue in horses, remaining a common concern for horse owners and a frequent reason for veterinary attendance with potential for death or euthanasia despite medical and/or surgical treatment. Education concerning colic prevention remains critical, taking into account the different perspectives that exist across different types of horse owners, including those with differing levels of education and with different perceptions and previous experiences concerning colic. Veterinary treatments, whether medical or surgical, should consider evidence of benefit, cost, and owner affordability. Development of large computer data sets across different equine populations and technological advances facilitating real-time clinic and stall-side data collection have great potential to add to the evidence base from farm/clinic level to international studies, facilitating more accurate monitoring of colic prevalence, rapid assessment of the efficacy of new interventions, and generation of specific predictive models. Concurrently, ongoing, and future equine gastrointestinal research using metabolomics, proteomics, and further studies of the equine gut microbiome and mycobiome is key in helping to better understand the pathophysiology of different forms of colic, improved methods of prevention, earlier detection of cases requiring potential surgical intervention, and more accurate prognostication.

CLINICS CARE POINTS

- Equine colic continues to be a frequent reason for veterinary attendance and veterinarians play an important role in educating horse owners about colic, taking into consideration the perspectives that different types of horse owners may have when formulating advice.

- Knowledge of modifiable risk factors for colic in general and for specific forms of colic enables veterinarians to provide evidence-based advice on ways to minimize colic development, particularly in high-risk horses.

- Whilst horse-level risk factors cannot be modified, knowledge of these can assist veterinarians when evaluating cases of colic, enabling potentially more serious forms of colic that may require surgical intervention to be identified at the earliest possible stage.

DISCLOSURE

Neither author has any commercial or financial conflicts of interests or funding sources related to the writing of this article.

FUNDING

We gratefully acknowledge Arden and Claudia Sims for funding Alexandra Gillen's PhD research studies.

REFERENCES

1. Traub-Dargatz JL, Kopral CA, Seitzinger AH, et al. Estimate of the national incidence of and operation-level risk factors for colic among horses in the United States, spring 1998 to spring 1999. J Am Vet Med Assoc 2001;219(1):67–71.
2. Tinker MK, White NA, Lessard P, et al. Prospective study of equine colic incidence and mortality. Equine Vet J 1997;29(6):448–53.
3. Cohen ND. The John Hickman memorial lecture: Colic by numbers. Equine Vet J 2003;35(4):343–9.
4. Baseline Reference of Equine Health and Management in the United States, 2015. National Animal Health Monitoring System December 2016 Report 1. Available at: https://www.aphis.usda.gov/animal_health/nahms/equine/downloads/equine15/Eq2015_Rept1.pdf.
5. Leblond A, Villard I, Leblond L, et al. A Retrospective Evaluation of the Causes of Death of 448 Insured French Horses in 1995. Vet Res Commun 2000;24(2):85–102.
6. Penell JC, Egenvall A, Bonnett BN, et al. Specific causes of morbidity among Swedish horses insured for veterinary care between 1997 and 2000. Vet Rec 2005;157(16):470–7.
7. Egenvall A, Penell J, Bonnett BN, et al. Demographics and costs of colic in Swedish horses. J Vet Intern Med 2008;22(4):1029–37.
8. Higuchi T. A retrospective survey of equine acute abdomen in a breeding region of Japan based on agricultural mutual relief insurance data. J Equine Sci 2006; 17(1):17–22.
9. Traub-Dargatz JL, Salman MD, Voss JL. Medical problems of adult horses, as ranked by equine practitioners. J Am Vet Med Assoc 1991;198(10):1745–7.
10. Mellor DJ, Love S, Walker R, et al. Sentinel practice-based survey of the management and health of horses in northern Britain. Vet Rec 2001;149(14):417–23.
11. Buckley P, Dunn T, More SJ. Owners' perceptions of the health and performance of Pony Club horses in Australia. Prev Vet Med 2004;63(1–2):121–33.
12. Upjohn MM, Attwood GA, Lerotholi T, et al. Quantitative versus qualitative approaches: A comparison of two research methods applied to identification of key health issues for working horses in Lesotho. Prev Vet Med 2013;108(4):313–20.
13. Wild I, Freeman S, Robles D, et al. Owners' knowledge and approaches to colic in working equids in honduras. Animals 2021;11(7). https://doi.org/10.3390/ani11072087.
14. Proudman CJ. A two year, prospective survey of equine colic in general practice. Equine Vet J 1992;24(2):90–3.
15. Hillyer MH, Taylor FGR, French NP. A cross-sectional study of colic in horses on Thoroughbred training premises in the British Isles in 1997. Equine Vet J 2001; 33(4):380–5.

16. Bowden A, England GCW, Brennan ML, et al. Indicators of 'critical' outcomes in 941 horses seen 'out-of-hours' for colic. Vet Rec 2020;187(12):492.

17. Bowden A, Boynova P, Brennan ML, et al. Retrospective case series to identify the most common conditions seen 'out-of-hours' by first-opinion equine veterinary practitioners. Vet Rec 2020;187(10):404.

18. Dolente BA, Lindborg S, Russell G, et al. Emergency case admissions at a large animal tertiary university referral hospital during a 12-month period. J Vet Emerg Crit Care 2008;18(3):298–305.

19. Cohen ND. Epidemiology of colic. Vet Clin North Am Equine Pract 1997;13(2): 191–201.

20. Archer DC, Proudman CJ. Epidemiological clues to preventing colic. Vet J 2006; 172(1):29–39.

21. Uhlinger C. Effects of three anthelmintic schedules on the incidence of colic in horses. Equine Vet J 1990;22(4):251–4.

22. Banfield pet hospital S of PH. No Title.

23. Surveillance S (Small AV. No Title. https://www.liverpool.ac.uk/savsnet/ Accessed 24 October, 2022.

24. VetCompass. Vet Compass. https://www.vetcompass.org Accessed 24 October, 2022.

25. Dogslife Project. No Title. https://www.ed.ac.uk/roslin/eeragroup/research/dogslife Accessed 24 October, 2022.

26. Paynter AN, Dunbar MD, Creevy KE, et al. Veterinary big data: When data goes to the dogs. Animals 2021;11(7). https://doi.org/10.3390/ani11071872.

27. Welsh CE, Duz M, Parkin TDH, et al. Prevalence, survival analysis and multimorbidity of chronic diseases in the general veterinarian-attended horse population of the UK. Prev Vet Med 2016;131:137–45.

28. Welsh CE, Parkin TDH, Marshall JF. Use of large-scale veterinary data for the investigation of antimicrobial prescribing practices in equine medicine. Equine Vet J 2017;49(4):425–32.

29. EVSNET. Equine Veterinary Surveillance Network. https://www.liverpool.ac.uk/evsnet/. Accessed 24 October, 2022.

30. INCISE. International. Colic Surgery Audit. https://www.internationalcolicaudit.com.

31. Mair TS, White NA II. The creation of an international audit and database of equine colic surgery: Survey of attitudes of surgeons. Equine Vet J 2008; 40(4):400–4.

32. Curtis L, Burford JH, Thomas JSM, et al. Prospective study of the primary evaluation of 1016 horses with clinical signs of abdominal pain by veterinary practitioners, and the differentiation of critical and non-critical cases. Acta Vet Scand 2015;57(1):1–12.

33. Stringer AP. Infectious diseases of working equids. Vet Clin North Am - Equine Pract 2014;30(3):695–718.

34. Stringer AP, Christley RM, Bell CE, et al. Owner reported diseases of working equids in central Ethiopia. Equine Vet J 2017;49(4):501–6.

35. Blikslager AT, Mair TS. Trends in the management of horses referred for evaluation of colic: 2004–2017. Equine Vet Educ 2021;33(4):192–7.

36. Barker I, Freeman SL. Assessment of costs and insurance policies for referral treatment of equine colic. Vet Rec 2019;185(16):508.

37. Archer DC. Colic surgery: Keeping it affordable for horse owners. Vet Rec 2019; 185(16):505–7.

38. Pantaleon L. Why measuring outcomes is important in health care. J Vet Intern Med 2019;33(2):356–62.
39. Erstad BL. Value-Based Medicine: Dollars and Sense. Crit Care Med 2016; 44(2):375–80.
40. Davis E. Donkey and Mule Welfare. Vet Clin North Am - Equine Pract 2019;35(3): 481–91.
41. Scantlebury CE, Perkins E, Pinchbeck GL, et al. Could it be colic? Horse-owner decision making and practices in response to equine colic. BMC Vet Res 2014; 10(Suppl 1):1–14.
42. Bowden A, Burford JH, Brennan ML, et al. Horse owners' knowledge, and opinions on recognising colic in the horse. Equine Vet J 2020;52(2):262–7.
43. The British Horse Society REACT Now to Beat Colic. REACT.
44. Salem SE, Scantlebury CE, Ezzat E, et al. Colic in a working horse population in Egypt: Prevalence and risk factors. Equine Vet J 2017;49(2):201–6.
45. Southwood LL, Dolente BA, Lindborg S, et al. Short-term outcome of equine emergency admissions at a university referral hospital. Equine Vet J 2009; 41(5):459–64.
46. Southwood LL, Gassert T, Lindborg S. Colic in geriatric compared to mature nongeriatric horses. Part 2: Treatment, diagnosis and short-term survival. Equine Vet J 2010;42(7):628–35.
47. Salem SE, Proudman CJ, Archer DC. Prevention of post operative complications following surgical treatment of equine colic: Current evidence. Equine Vet J 2016;48(2):143–51.
48. Curtis L, Burford JH, England GCW, et al. Risk factors for acute abdominal pain (colic) in the adult horse: A scoping review of risk factors, and a systematic review of the effect of management-related changes. PLoS One 2019;14(7). https://doi.org/10.1371/journal.pone.0219307.
49. Scantlebury CE, Archer DC, Proudman CJ, et al. Recurrent colic in the horse: Incidence and risk factors for recurrence in the general practice population. Equine Vet J 2011;43(SUPPL.39):81–8.
50. Cohen ND, Vontur CA, Rakestraw PC. Risk factors for enterolithiasis among horses in Texas. J Am Vet Med Assoc 2000;216(11):1787–94.
51. Hassel DM, Aldridge BM, Drake CM, et al. Evaluation of dietary and management risk factors for enterolithiasis among horses in California. Res Vet Sci 2008;85(3):476–80.
52. Steward SKT, Hassel DM, Martin H, et al. Geographic Disparities in Clinical Characteristics of Duodenitis–Proximal Jejunitis in Horses in the United States. J Equine Vet Sci 2020;93. https://doi.org/10.1016/j.jevs.2020.103192.
53. Archer DC, Costain DA, Sherlock C. Idiopathic Focal Eosinophilic Enteritis (IFEE), An emerging cause of abdominal pain in horses: The effect of age, time and geographical location on risk. PLoS One 2014;9(12):1–19.
54. Archer DC, Pinchbeck GL, Proudman CJ, et al. Is equine colic seasonal? Novel application of a model based approach. BMC Vet Res 2006;2. https://doi.org/10.1186/1746-6148-2-27.
55. Cohen ND, Gibbs PG, Woods AM. Dietary and other management factors associated with colic in horses. J Am Vet Med Assoc 1999;215(1):53–60.
56. Cohen ND, Peloso JG. Risk factors for history of previous colic and for chronic, intermittent colic in a population of horses. J Am Vet Med Assoc 1996;208(5): 697–703.
57. Hudson JM, Cohen ND, Gibbs PG, et al. Feeding practices associated with colic in horses. J Am Vet Med Assoc 2001;219(10):1419–25.

58. Escalona EE, Okell CN, Archer DC. Prevalence of and risk factors for colic in horses that display crib-biting behaviour. BMC Vet Res 2014;10. https://doi.org/10.1186/1746-6148-10-S1-S3.

59. Hillyer MH, Taylor FGR, Proudman CJ, et al. Case control study to identify risk factors for simple colonic obstruction and distension colic in horses. Equine Vet J 2002;34(5):455–63.

60. Reeves MJ, Salman MD, Smith G. Risk factors for equine acute abdominal disease (colic): results from a multi-center case-control study. Prev Vet Med 1996;26(3–4):285–301.

61. Cohen ND, Matejka PL, Honnas CM, et al. Case-control study of the association between various management factors and development of colic in horses. Texas Equine Colic Study Group. J Am Vet Med Assoc 1995;206(5):667–73.

62. Hassel DM, Rakestraw PC, Gardner IA, et al. Dietary risk factors and colonic pH and mineral concentrations in horses with enterolithiasis. J Vet Intern Med 2004;18(3):346–9.

63. Little D, Blikslager AT. Factors associated with development of ileal impaction in horses with surgical colic: 78 Cases (1986-2000). Equine Vet J 2002;34(5):464–8.

64. Suthers JM, Pinchbeck GL, Proudman CJ, et al. Risk factors for large colon volvulus in the UK. Equine Vet J 2013;45(5):558–63.

65. Shirazi-Beechey SP. Molecular insights into dietary induced colic in the horse. Equine Vet J 2008;40(4):414–21.

66. Fan Y, Pedersen O. Gut microbiota in human metabolic health and disease. Nat Rev Microbiol 2021;19(1):55–71.

67. Morais LH, Schreiber HL, Mazmanian SK. The gut microbiota–brain axis in behaviour and brain disorders. Nat Rev Microbiol 2021;19(4):241–55.

68. Sanz MG. Science-in-brief: Equine microbiomics makes its way into equine veterinary medicine. Equine Vet J 2022;54(2):453–4.

69. Costa MC, Arroyo LG, Allen-Vercoe E, et al. Comparison of the fecal microbiota of healthy horses and horses with colitis by high throughput sequencing of the V3-V5 region of the 16s rRNA gene. PLoS One 2012;7(7). https://doi.org/10.1371/journal.pone.0041484.

70. Costa MC, Stämpfli HR, Arroyo LG, et al. Changes in the equine fecal microbiota associated with the use of systemic antimicrobial drugs. BMC Vet Res 2015;11(1):1–12.

71. Peachey LE, Molena RA, Jenkins TP, et al. The relationships between faecal egg counts and gut microbial composition in UK Thoroughbreds infected by cyathostomins. Int J Parasitol 2018;48(6):403–12.

72. Slater R, Frau A, Hodgkinson J, et al. A comparison of the colonic microbiome and volatile organic compound metabolome of Anoplocephala perfoliata infected and non-infected horses: A pilot study. Animals 2021;11(3):1–22.

73. Salem SE, Maddox TW, Berg A, et al. Variation in faecal microbiota in a group of horses managed at pasture over a 12-month period. Sci Rep 2018;8(1):1–10.

74. Salem SE, Hough R, Probert C, et al. A longitudinal study of the faecal microbiome and metabolome of periparturient mares. PeerJ 2019;7:e6687.

75. Weese JS, Holcombe SJ, Embertson RM, et al. Changes in the faecal microbiota of mares precede the development of post partum colic. Equine Vet J 2015;47(6):641–9.

76. Stewart HL, Southwood LL, Indugu N, et al. Differences in the equine faecal microbiota between horses presenting to a tertiary referral hospital for colic compared with an elective surgical procedure. Equine Vet J 2019;51(3):336–42.

77. Stewart HL, Pitta D, Indugu N, et al. Changes in the faecal bacterial microbiota during hospitalisation of horses with colic and the effect of different causes of colic. Equine Vet J 2021;53(6):1119–31.
78. Schoster A. Probiotic Use in Equine Gastrointestinal Disease. Vet Clin N Am Equine Pract 2018;34(1):13–24.
79. Cui L, Morris A, Ghedin E. The human mycobiome in health and disease. Genome Med 2013;5(7). https://doi.org/10.1186/gm467.
80. McGorum BC, Chen Z, Glendinning L, et al. Equine grass sickness (a multiple systems neuropathy) is associated with alterations in the gastrointestinal mycobiome. Anim Microbiome 2021;3(1). https://doi.org/10.1186/s42523-021-00131-2.
81. Kaneene JB, Miller R, Ross WA, et al. Risk factors for colic in the Michigan (USA) equine population. Prev Vet Med 1997;30(1):23–36.
82. Proudman CJ, French NP, Trees AJ. Tapeworm infection is a significant risk factor for spasmodic colic and ileal impaction colic in the horse. Equine Vet J 1998; 30(3):194–9.
83. Peregrine AS, Molento MB, Kaplan RM, et al. Anthelmintic resistance in important parasites of horses: Does it really matter? Vet Parasitol 2014;201(1–2):1–8.
84. Rendle D, Austin C, Bowen M, et al. Equine de-worming: a consensus on current best practice. UK-Vet Equine 2019;3(Sup1):1–14.
85. Sauermann CW, Leathwick DM, Lieffering M, et al. Climate change is likely to increase the development rate of anthelmintic resistance in equine cyathostomins in New Zealand. Int J Parasitol Drugs Drug Resist 2020;14:73–9.
86. Scantlebury CE, Archer DC, Proudman CJ, et al. Management and horse-level risk factors for recurrent colic in the UK general equine practice population. Equine Vet J 2015;47(2):202–6.
87. Cox R, Burden F, Gosden L, et al. Case control study to investigate risk factors for impaction colic in donkeys in the UK. Prev Vet Med 2009;92(3):179–87.
88. Archer DC, Pinchbeck GL, French NP, et al. Risk factors for epiploic foramen entrapment colic in a UK horse population: A prospective case-control study. Equine Vet J 2008;40(4):405–10.
89. Archer DC, Pinchbeck GL, French NP, et al. Risk factors for epiploic foramen entrapment colic: An international study. Equine Vet J 2008;40(3):224–30.
90. Waters AJ, Nicol CJ, French NP. Factors influencing the development of stereotypic and redirected behaviours in young horses: Findings of a four year prospective epidemiological study. Equine Vet J 2002;34(6):572–9.
91. Wickens CL, Heleski CR. Crib-biting behavior in horses: A review. Appl Anim Behav Sci 2010;128(1–4):1–9.
92. Röcken M, Schubert C, Mosel G, et al. Indications, surgical technique, and long-term experience with laparoscopic closure of the nephrosplenic space in standing horses. Vet Surg 2005;34(6):637–41.
93. Nelson BB, Ruple-Czerniak AA, Hendrickson DA, et al. Laparoscopic Closure of the Nephrosplenic Space in Horses with Nephrosplenic Colonic Entrapment: Factors Associated with Survival and Colic Recurrence. Vet Surg 2016;45: O60–9.
94. Munsterman AS, Hanson RR, Cattley RC, et al. Surgical technique and short-term outcome for experimental laparoscopic closure of the epiploic foramen in 6 horses. Vet Surg 2014;43(2):105–13.
95. van Bergen T, Wiemer P, Bosseler L, et al. Development of a new laparoscopic Foramen Epiploicum Mesh Closure (FEMC) technique in 6 horses. Equine Vet J 2016;48(3):331–7.

96. Ragle CA, Yiannikouris S, Tibary AA, et al. Use of a barbed suture for laparoscopic closure of the internal inguinal rings in a horse. J Am Vet Med Assoc 2013;242(2):249–53.

97. Rossignol F, Mespoulhes-Rivière C, Vitte A, et al. Standing laparoscopic inguinal hernioplasty using cyanoacrylate for preventing recurrence of acquired strangulated inguinal herniation in 10 stallions. Vet Surg 2014;43(1):6–11.

98. Wilderjans H, Meulyzer M. Laparoscopic closure of the vaginal rings in the standing horse using a tacked intraperitoneal slitted mesh (TISM) technique. Equine Vet J 2022;54(2):359–67.

99. Pezzanite LM, Hackett ES. Technique-associated outcomes in horses following large colon resection. Vet Surg 2017;46(8):1061–7.

100. Arévalo Rodríguez JM, Grulke S, Salciccia A, et al. Nephrosplenic space closure significantly decreases recurrent colic in horses: A retrospective analysis. Vet Rec 2019;185(21):657.

101. Proudman CJ, Smith JE, Edwards GB, et al. Long-term survival of equine surgical colic cases. Part 2: Modelling postoperative survival. Equine Vet J 2002; 34(5):438–43.

102. Tennent-Brown BS, Wilkins PA, Lindborg S, et al. Sequential plasma lactate concentrations as prognostic indicators in adult equine emergencies. J Vet Intern Med 2010;24(1):198–205.

103. Hackett ES, Embertson RM, Hopper SA, et al. Duration of disease influences survival to discharge of Thoroughbred mares with surgically treated large colon volvulus. Equine Vet J 2015;47(6):650–4.

104. Peloso JG, Cohen ND. Use of serial measurements of peritoneal fluid lactate concentration to identify strangulating intestinal lesions in referred horses with signs of colic. J Am Vet Med Assoc 2012;240(10):1208–17.

105. Henderson ISF. Diagnostic and prognostic use of L-lactate measurement in equine practice. Equine Vet Educ 2013;25(9):468–75.

106. Dondi F, Lukacs RM, Gentilini F, et al. Serum amyloid A, haptoglobin, and ferritin in horses with colic: Association with common clinicopathological variables and short-term outcome. Vet J 2015;205(1):50–5.

107. Kilcoyne I, Nieto JE, Dechant JE. Predictive value of plasma and peritoneal creatine kinase in horses with strangulating intestinal lesions. Vet Surg 2019;48(2): 152–8.

108. Cambiaghi A, Pinto BB, Brunelli L, et al. Characterization of a metabolomic profile associated with responsiveness to therapy in the acute phase of septic shock. Sci Rep 2017;7(1). https://doi.org/10.1038/s41598-017-09619-x.

109. Wang J, Sun Y, Teng S, et al. Prediction of sepsis mortality using metabolite biomarkers in the blood: a meta-analysis of death-related pathways and prospective validation. BMC Med 2020;18(1). https://doi.org/10.1186/s12916-020-01546-5.

110. Bardell D, Milner PI, Goljanek-Whysall K, et al. Differences in plasma and peritoneal fluid proteomes identifies potential biomarkers associated with survival following strangulating small intestinal disease. Equine Vet J 2019;51(6):727–32.

111. Pascoe PJ, Ducharme NG, Ducharme GR, et al. A computer-derived protocol using recursive partitioning to aid in estimating prognosis of horses with abdominal pain in referral hospitals. Can J Vet Res 1990;54(3):373–8.

112. Reeves MJ, Curtis CR, Salman MD, et al. Prognosis in equine colic patients using multivariable analysis. Can J Vet Res 1989;53(1):87–94.

113. Reeves MJ, Curtis CR, Salman MD, et al. Multivariable prediction model for the need for surgery in horses with colic. Am J Vet Res 1991;52(11):1903–7.

114. FURR MO, LESSARD P, II NAW. Development of a Colic Severity Score for Predicting the Outcome of Equine Colic. Vet Surg 1995;24(2):97–101. https://doi.org/10.1111/j.1532-950X.1995.tb01302.x.

115. Farrell A, Kersh K, Liepman R, et al. Development of a Colic Scoring System to Predict Outcome in Horses. Front Vet Sci 2021;8. https://doi.org/10.3389/fvets.2021.697589.

116. Bishop RC, Gutierrez-Nibeyro SD, Stewart MC, et al. Performance of predictive models of survival in horses undergoing emergency exploratory laparotomy for colic. Vet Surg 2022;51(6):891–902.

117. Blikslager AT, Bowman KF, Haven ML, et al. Pedunculated lipomas as a cause of intestinal obstruction in horses: 17 cases (1983-1990). J Am Vet Med Assoc 1992;201(8):1249–52.

118. EDWARDS GB, PROUDMAN CJ. An analysis of 75 cases of intestinal obstruction caused by pedunculated lipomas. Equine Vet J 1994;26(1):18–21.

119. Garcia-Seco E, Wilson DA, Kramer J, et al. Prevalence and risk factors associated with outcome of surgical removal of pedunculated lipomas in horses: 102 Cases (1987-2002). J Am Vet Med Assoc 2005;226(9):1529–37.

120. Cox R, Proudman CJ, Trawford AF, et al. Epidemiology of impaction colic in donkeys in the UK. BMC Vet Res 2007;3. https://doi.org/10.1186/1746-6148-3-1.

Updates on Diagnosis and Management of Colic in the Field and Criteria for Referral

Lauren Bookbinder, DVM, DACVIM[a],*, Amanda Prisk, VMD, DACVS-LA[b]

KEYWORDS

• Colic • Field evaluation • Triage • Palpation per rectum • Analgesia • Referral

KEY POINTS

- A thorough triage colic evaluation aims to define clinical severity and suspected gastrointestinal localization of the colic to inform management recommendations.
- Clinical "red flags" quickly identify critical colic cases, the most important of which are the severity and/or persistence of pain and cardiovascular compromise.
- A definitive etiologic diagnosis of colic is rare in the field and is not required to provide an accurate clinical assessment and guide treatment recommendations.
- Horses with colic that require two or more doses of analgesia over any time period are more likely to require surgery.
- Rapid transportation to a referral center should be prioritized over on-farm stabilization (ie, intravenous fluids) to avoid delay.

INTRODUCTION

Gastrointestinal colic is the most common primary care equine emergency[1] and affects nearly one of four horses per year.[2] Colic is a significant welfare concern for equine patients and a financial and emotional burden for owners.[3,4] However, horse owners may be overconfident and unreliable in defining and identifying colic, which complicates timely and appropriate veterinary intervention.[3,4] Thus, equine primary care practitioners are often tasked with simultaneously educating clients, evaluating patients, and making appropriate management recommendations under emergency circumstances.[5] Despite its importance in primary care practice, most contemporary colic literature is heavily skewed toward referral management. Although field and referral level care are interdependent, they are distinct components of equine practice with unique challenges and decision-making scaffolds.

[a] Large Animal Clinical Sciences, Michigan State University College of Veterinary Medicine, 736 Wilson Road, East Lansing, MI, USA; [b] Department of Clinical Sciences, Cummings School of Veterinary Medicine at Tufts University, 200 Westboro Road, North Grafton, MA, USA
* Corresponding author.
E-mail address: bookbin1@msu.edu

Vet Clin Equine 39 (2023) 175–195
https://doi.org/10.1016/j.cveq.2023.03.001
0749-0739/23/© 2023 Elsevier Inc. All rights reserved.

This article outlines the equine primary care practitioner's role in colic triage and provides decision-making scaffolds for field colic management. Field-appropriate diagnostics, criteria for referral or euthanasia, and options for multimodal pain management are highlighted.

THE EQUINE PRIMARY CARE PRACTITIONER'S ROLE IN COLIC TRIAGE

Up to 80% of horses showing colic signs in the field have no identifable etiologic diagnosis for their colic compared with only 20% of referral colic admissions.[1,2,6–9] Thus, equine primary care practitioners frequently make treatment and management recommendations without a definitive diagnosis of disease. In human medicine, clinical "red flags" inform treatment recommendations in these circumstances,[10] and the same principle can be applied to colic triage.[1] For cases of equine colic, "red flag" parameters are associated with both severity of clinical signs and suspected gastrointestinal localization of the colic. Accurately assigning clinical severity and localizing the general anatomic source of colic can help equine primary care practitioners make timely, appropriate recommendations.

OBJECTIVE AND EFFECTIVE COLIC TRIAGE
Assessing Colic Severity

More than one-third of colic cases evaluated in the field may require repeat veterinary care, hospitalization, or result in natural death or euthanasia.[1] Early recognition and treatment of these critical cases improves outcomes,[9,11] and several studies have defined clinical "red flags" to help practitioners identify critical cases (**Table 1**). These parameters provide an objective guide for treatment and management decisions and can be practically and accurately assessed in the field by obtaining a thorough history and performing a comprehensive colic examination which includes observation, physical examination, transrectal palpation, nasogastric intubation, and ancillary diagnostics such as transcutaneous abdominal ultrasound and percutaneous abdominocentesis.[1,12–20] Specifically, several validated equine pain scoring systems exist and are useful for assessing and monitoring the progression of clinical pain.[19–22] A comprehensive but simple pain scale is outlined in **Table 2**.[21] A triage decision-making tree based on colic severity and gastrointestinal localization is outlined at the end of this article.

Obtaining a Gastrointestinal Localization of Colic

Most sources of colic can be presumably localized to the proximal (stomach, small intestine) or distal (cecum, large colon, small colon) segments of the gastrointestinal tract after a comprehensive diagnostic evaluation (**Table 3**). This localization guides treatment and management decisions[18,23] and is not dependent on a definitive etiologic diagnosis of colic (ie, proximal enteritis vs small intestinal strangulating lesion). During a field colic evaluation, an accurate gastrointestinal localization should be attempted using a combination of diagnostic tools and tests, which include transrectal palpation, nasogastric intubation, transcutaneous abdominal ultrasound, and percutaneous abdominocentesis. Despite their utility, this full complement of diagnostics is rarely performed in a field setting. Transrectal palpation is performed in 75% of primary opinion colic cases,[12] and nasogastric intubation, blood work, and abdominocentesis are performed in less than 40%, 20%, and 10% of colic cases, respectively. Although factors such as patient compliance, facilities, and veterinary safety likely influence these diagnostic omissions in some circumstances, 98% of primary opinion veterinarians believe that diagnostics beyond a physical

Table 1
Clinical "red flags" associated with critical colic cases and used to guide treatment and management decisions after primary evaluation

Pain/pain score	• Moderate or severe pain[7,12] • Persistent or progressive pain despite analgesia[39]
Heart rate	• >48 beats per minute[15] • >60–70 beats per minute is suggestive or severe pain and/or cardiovascular shock[18]
Cardiovascular stability	• Abnormal mucous membrane color[1] • Poor pulse quality[12] • Capillary refill time >2.5 s[12] • Elevated venous lactate[13]
Gastrointestinal sounds	• Reduced or absent in >/ = 1 quadrant[7,12,15]
Diagnostic test results	• Transrectal palpation abnormalities • Transcutaneous abdominal ultrasound abnormalities[13]
Peritoneal fluid characteristics	• Serosanguinous or green/brown[7] ○ ensure blood contamination or enterocentesis does not affect interpretation • Peritoneal lactate >/ = 2x venous[30]
Localization	• Proximal gastrointestinal tract[16] • Cecal dysfunction[16]
Duration of colic	• >1 week[7]

examination and transrectal palpation are "unnecessary for the diagnosis of colic" and are most commonly implemented only *after* severe signs develop.[12] This represents a source of observation bias and intolerable clinical variability in field triage of colic cases. Consistently performing a complete diagnostic evaluation can help

Table 2
Equine acute abdominal pain scale-version 2

Behavior		Occasional/Calm	→	Frequent/Violent	
Depression	1	-	-	-	-
Flank-watching	1	2	-	-	-
Weight-shifting	1	2	-	-	-
Pawing	-	2	3	-	-
Stretching	-	2	3	-	-
Kicking abdomen	-	2	3	-	-
Restlessness	-	2	3	-	-
Sternal recumbency	-	-	3	4	-
Lateral recumbency	-	-	-	4	-
Attempting to lie down	-	-	-	4	-
Rolling	-	-	-	-	5
Collapse	-	-	-	-	5

Adapted from Sutton and colleagues 2019. Pain is graded from mild (1) to severe (5) based on the type of behavior exhibited (rows) and the frequency and character of the behavior when applicable, ranging from occasional and calm (1) to frequent and violent (5). From Wiley publishing and according to STM guidelines.

Table 3
Examination findings that indicate gastrointestinal localization of colic in horses

Examination	Proximal GI Dysfunction (Stomach/Small Intestine)	Distal GI Dysfunction (Cecum, Large, and Small Colon)
Assessment of pain and physical examination	• Moderate-to-severe pain behaviors • Moderate-to-severe cardiovascular compromise	• Absent to severe pain behaviors • Absent to severe cardiovascular compromise
Possible transrectal abdominal palpation findings	• Normal • Distended small intestine	• Normal • Colonic gas • Impacted and/or distended ingesta in the large or small colon • Left dorsal displacement of the large colon into or toward the nephrosplenic space • Horizontal large colon tenia • Taut vertical cecal tenia • Cecal gas or feed accumulation
Possible transcutaneous abdominal ultrasound findings	• Normal • Enlarged stomach (>4 intercostal spaces, or extending caudal to the 13th rib) • Distended small intestine (>4 cm) • Thick-walled small intestine (>4 mm)	• Normal • Large colon obscuring left kidney and spleen • Large colon mesenteric vessels along the body wall • Thick-walled large colon (>5 mm) • Fluid-filled cecum or large colon
Nasogastric intubation	• > 2–3L net accumulation of feed or fluid • Progressive discomfort following enteral fluid therapy	• < 2–3L net accumulation of feed or fluid • Minimal discomfort following enteral fluid therapy

primary care practitioners localize and appropriately manage colic cases in a timely manner.

Transrectal Abdominal Palpation

Transrectal abdominal palpation should be performed during every colic evaluation if patient and veterinarian safety allows. Copious lubrication, adequate restraint, sedation with an alpha-2 agonist, smooth muscle relaxation, and rectal lidocaine infusion (50–60 mL of 2% lidocaine introduced through a flexible red rubber catheter, extension set with clamp and catheter insertion removed, or stallion catheter) facilitate safe palpation.[24] Smooth muscle relaxation via intravenous administration of N-butylscopolammonium bromide is more effective at reducing intra-abdominal pressure and patient straining than rectal lidocaine infusion.[25]

Transrectal tears are the most common complication of palpation and can be fatal.[26] However, this is a rare outcome[26] and concern for this complication should not preclude examination in appropriately sized horses if risks can be mitigated with adequate restraint, sedation, and muscle relaxation. If there is concern for a rectal tear, palpation should immediately stop and the potential tear discussed with the owner and local referral center to determine additional diagnostic and management recommendations.[17,18]

Knowledge of normal and abnormal transrectal palpation findings is requisite for a diagnostic evaluation and thorough palpation is facilitated by a systematic approach.[24] The investigators prefer clockwise palpation beginning at 6 o'clock at the brim of the bony pelvis, moving from caudal to cranial on the left until 12 o'clock, and then from cranial to caudal on the right, returning to the brim of the pelvis to complete the examination. In the normal horse, the following gastrointestinal structures are routinely identified.[17,24] Abnormal structures are included in *italics* where they are typically identified in the abdomen. How these abnormal structures contribute to gastrointestinal localization is categorized in **Table 3**.

BLADDER AND LATERAL LIGAMENTS OF THE BLADDER

- Located at 4 to 8 o'clock, cranial to the bony pelvis (**Fig. 1**).
- The lateral ligaments of the bladder are paired, pencil-width cords that are cranio-caudally oriented and diverge as they travel caudal along the bladder.

Abnormal: Large Colon Gas Distention

- Gas-distended large colon is palpable in the pelvic canal and approximates the feeling of placing your hand through an inflated blood pressure cuff.

Abnormal: Large Colon Displacement

- Horizontally oriented tenia (bands) that do not diverge and cannot be associated with the bladder are the tenia of the large colon.
- These are not normally palpable and their identification signifies a right displacement of the large colon.
- A novice clinician may confuse the lateral ligaments of the bladder with abnormal, horizontally oriented colon tenia or a distended bladder with a gas-distended colon. Careful palpation of the lateral ligaments of the bladder with attention to orientation differentiates these structures.

PELVIC FLEXURE OF THE ASCENDING (LARGE) COLON

- Located at 6 to 9 o'clock, at or cranial to the level of the bladder.

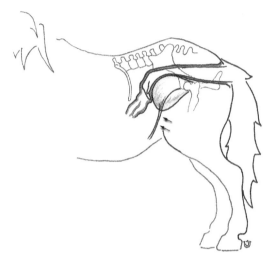

Fig. 1. Schematic representation of transrectal palpation of the bladder and lateral ligaments (*black arrows*). (*From* Southwood, L.L. and Fehr, J. (2012). Abdominal Palpation per
Rectum. In Practical Guide to Equine Colic, L.L. Southwood (Ed.). https://doi.org/10.1002/
9781118704783.ch3.)

- The normal pelvic flexure is soft and margins are relatively indistinct, it is *not
  definitively palpable* in all horses. There are no palpable tenia associated with
  the pelvic flexure.

Abnormal: Pelvic Flexure Impaction

- A readily palpable, rounded ball of feed material in the left caudal abdomen which
  may extend to the right of midline. Size can vary from softball (impacted but not
  distended) to beach ball (impacted and distended).
- The pelvic flexure is both impacted and distended when it is the primary source
  of colic signs. A small, very firm pelvic flexure impaction (that often feels uneven
  and "shrink wrapped") may be secondary to additional sources of colic that
  caused dehydration and desiccation of otherwise normal colon contents, such
  as a small intestinal lesion.

SMALL COLON AND FECAL BALLS

- Located at 6 to 12 o'clock, throughout the left and central caudal abdomen
  (**Fig. 2**).
- Normal fecal balls in the small colon are described as a "string of pearls."
- The broad antimesenteric and fibrous mesenteric tenia of the small colon are
  palpable.

Abnormal: Small Colon Impaction

- Coalescing, tubular-shaped small colon fecal material.
- This can be confused for a small pelvic flexure impaction: the presence of
  palpable small colon tenia differentiates these diagnoses.
- The absence of fecal material in rectum or small colon, or the presence of firm,
  dissected fecal material may indicate a more serious colic.

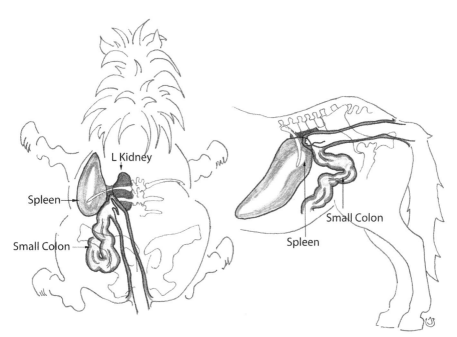

Fig. 2. Schematic representation of transrectal palpation of the small colon, left kidney, and spleen. (*From* Southwood, L.L. and Fehr, J. (2012). Abdominal Palpation per Rectum. In Practical Guide to Equine Colic, L.L. Southwood (Ed.). https://doi.org/10.1002/9781118704783.ch3.)

LEFT KIDNEY AND SPLEEN

- The left kidney is located at 10 to 11 o'clock, cranial to the pelvic flexure and along the dorsal body wall to the left of midline (see **Fig. 2**).
- The caudodorsal border of the spleen is located at 9 to 11 o'clock, abaxial to the kidney.
- Only the caudal pole of the left kidney is palpable and it is differentiated from fecal balls by its proximity to the dorsal body wall and spleen, immovable position, and firm, smooth consistency.
- The nephrosplenic ligament, a horizontal cord of connective tissue between the spleen and kidney, is palpable based on patient and examiner size.

Abnormal: Left Dorsal Displacement of the Colon or Nephrosplenic Entrapment

- Palpation of the large colon between the kidney and the caudodorsal border of the spleen obscuring the nephrosplenic ligament indicates that the horse likely has a nephrosplenic ligament entrapment of the colon. The nephrosplenic space may not be palpable depending on patient and examiner size.
- Large colon in the area of the kidney and spleen displacing the spleen axially and/or ventrally suggests either left dorsal displacement or nephrosplenic ligament entrapment of the colon.

ROOT OF THE MESENTERY AND CENTRAL ABDOMEN

- The root of the mesentery is located at 12 o'clock, at or near the cranial extent of the palpable abdomen; identification depends on the size of the examiner and patient. The caudal abdominal aorta and associated vessels and lymph nodes can be followed from the root of the mesentery caudally along the sublumbar body wall (**Fig. 3**).

- Distended small intestine should be *felt for* within the central abdomen ventral to the root of the mesentery. Specifically, the horizontally oriented duodenum may be identified at root of the mesentery coursing caudal to the cecal base. Normal small intestine is soft and indistinct from other viscera.

Abnormal: Easily Palpable Small Intestine

- Distended small intestine may be encountered anywhere during transrectal palpation but is commonly located ventral to the root of the mesentery in the mid-central abdomen (**Fig. 4**).
- Distended small intestine is not always palpable per rectum, particularly if the proximal portions are affected.

Abnormal: Lymphadenopathy, Vascular Thrombosis

- Vascular anomalies such as verminous arteritis or lymphadenopathy may be identified along the root of the mesentery and sublumbar body wall.

CECAL TENIA

- Located at 2 to 5 o'clock in the right caudal abdomen at approximately the same depth as the pelvic flexure (see **Fig. 3**).

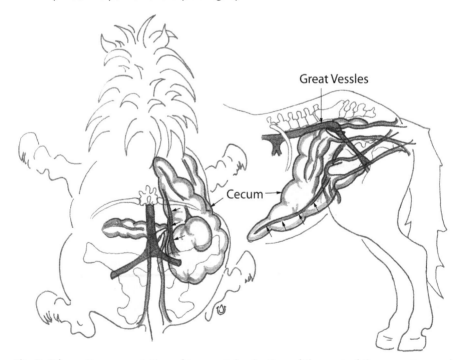

Fig. 3. Schematic representation of transrectal palpation of the root of the mesentery and great sublumbar vessels and medial/ventral cecal band. (*From* Southwood, L.L. and Fehr, J. (2012). Abdominal Palpation per Rectum. In Practical Guide to Equine Colic, L.L. Southwood (Ed.). https://doi.org/10.1002/9781118704783.ch3.)

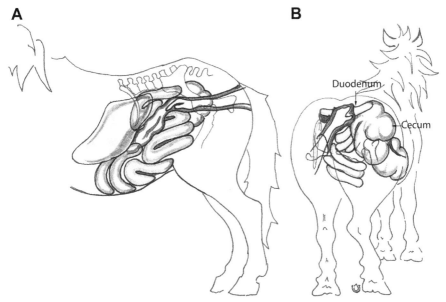

Fig. 4. Schematic representation of transrectal palpation of dilated small intestinal from the lateral (*A*) and caudal (*B*) perspective. (*From* Southwood, L.L. and Fehr, J. (2012). Abdominal Palpation per Rectum. In Practical Guide to Equine Colic, L.L. Southwood (Ed.). https://doi.org/10.1002/9781118704783.ch3.)

- The normal ventral cecal tenia is a pencil width band that is oriented vertically and freely moveable approximately 1 to 2 inches toward the pelvis. The ventral cecal tenia courses from the right caudodorsal abdomen in a cranioventral direction toward midline. Normal cecal haustra are soft and indistinct.

Abnormal: Taut Cecal Tenia or Gas/Feed Distention of the Cecal Haustra

- Fixed position of the cecal tenia on palpation (which may be associated with pain on palpation or manipulation) or persistent gas and/or palpable digesta within the cecum are associated with cecal impaction or atony.
- Unlike other large intestinal impactions, horses with cecal disease show mild pain but are at a high risk of gastrointestinal rupture. Referral should be offered whenever cecal disease is suspected, regardless of clinical pain.

Abdominal masses, such as abscesses or neoplasia, may be palpated based on location and size. Pneumoperitoneum, indicated by loss of negative pressure around the examiners arm, or a large volume of peritoneal effusion may also be appreciated when present.

Nasogastric Intubation

Nasogastric intubation is both a diagnostic and therapeutic procedure that should be performed on all patients evaluated for colic. All horses with moderate-to-severe colic signs should have a nasogastric tube passed urgently during the triage evaluation to relieve gastric distention, if present, and reduce the risk of gastric rupture. A horse showing colic signs with a heart rate $\geq$ 60 beats per minute should have a nasogastric tube passed immediately, and failure to do so may result in litigation if gastric rupture occurs. The presence of greater than 3 L net reflux/ingesta in an adult horse indicates proximal gastrointestinal tract dysfunction. Referral should be discussed when proximal gastrointestinal tract dysfunction is suspected, as these horses often have lesions that require surgery (eg. strangulating small intestinal lesion) or, at a minimum, require frequent nasogastric decompression and continuous intravenous fluid therapy to correct fluid deficits and maintain hydration. The early identification of proximal gastrointestinal dysfunction is imperative for appropriate management.

In the absense of net reflux, enteral fluid therapy through a nasogastric tube can be an effective treatment for several sources of distal gastrointestinal tract colic. Full-size, adult horses with normal proximal gastrointestinal function can tolerate 6 to 10 L of enteral fluids every 2 to 4 hours. Approximately 30 L of enteral fluid therapy over 24 hours resolves most large colon displacements and impactions.[27] Enteral fluid therapy with a balanced electrolyte solution hydrates large colon digesta more effectively than intravenous fluid therapy, despite equivalent effects on systemic hydration.[28] Similarly, enteral fluid therapy with $MgSO_4$ and psyllium (1g/kg daily for 3-7 days) reduces large colon sand accumulation more effectively than in-feed psyllium.[29] Although frequently administered, mineral oil does not soften or lubricate desiccated digesta and largely serves as a marker of gastrointestinal transit. Proximal gastrointestinal tract function must be assessed by checking for net nasogastric reflux before administering enteral fluids; transrectal palpation and transcutaneous abdominal ultrasound can also be used to support proximal gastrointesitnal tract evaluation prior to enteral fluid administration if needed.

Transcutaneous Abdominal Ultrasound

Transcutaneous abdominal ultrasound is accessible to most primary care practitioners and provides useful diagnostic information during colic evaluation with minimal formal training using a transrectal probe.[23] Any abnormal transcutaneous ultrasound findings are associated with more serious gastrointestinal disease. Of note, administering sedatives and/or N-butylscopolammonium bromide will decrease intestinal motility, which particularly affects ultrasonographic interpretation of the small intestine. For this reason, the authors prefer to perform an transcutaneous abdominal ultrasound evaluation following the physical examination, and before transrectal palpation or nasogastric intubation if possible. Easily obtained transcutaneous ultrasound findings that indicate lesion localization are outlined in **Table 2**.

Percutaneous Abdominocentesis

Peritoneal fluid evaluation is a simple diagnostic procedure that is particularly important for determining colic severity, although it does not contribute to lesion localization.[12] In a field setting, peritoneal fluid evaluation is most useful to evaluate for intestinal ischemia/strangulation or gastrointestinal rupture and these can be identified using visual inspection and simple point-of-care analyses. A serosanguinous abdominal fluid is an accurate indicator of intestinal strangulation[30] and the green/brown peritoneal fluid with a fetid odor is associated with gastrointestinal rupture. Because these two peritoneal fluid colors are associated with very severe colic, it is important to ensure an accurate sample is obtained. Subcutaneous bleeding can contaminate and discolor otherwise normal peritoneal fluid. However, when this occurs the sample typically "clears" as fluid drips during collection, and the red blood cells will settle after collection.Careful clinical assessment also differentiates the likelihood of blood contamination versus intestinal strangulation. In addition, the fluid obtained from enterocentesis is grossly identical to free peritoneal fluid following gastrointestinal rupture. Enterocentesis is a fairly benign complication[31] of an abdominocentesis, whereas horses with gastrointestinal rupture should be euthanized and clinical assessment differentiates these two scenarios. Horses with gastrointestinal rupture typically demonstrate that signs of septic shock have a history of severe colic followed by "resolution" after rupture, characteristic loss of negative abdominal pressure on transrectal palpation, and a large volume of free peritoneal fluid on transcutaneous abdominal ultrasound. Abdominocentesis may be performed using ultrasound guidance to prevent enterocentesis or splenocentesis. Ideally, cytology should be used to confirm that the horse indeed has intestinal perforation with the finding of intracellular bacteria and lysis of nucleated cells.

Clinicopathologic evaluation of peritoneal fluid provides additional diagnostic information.[32] In the field, peritoneal lactate concentration can be compared with venous blood concentration as a marker for intestinal ischemia/strangulation.[33] Normal peritoneal fluid lactate is equivalent to systemic lactate concentration and typically less than 2 mmol/L in healthy horses at rest. Peritoneal fluid lactate that is at least twofold higher than systemic lactate indicates intestinal strangulation. Importantly, peritoneal lactate alone is not predictive for intestinal strangulation or ischemia and must be compared with venous concentrations.[30] Additional biochemical and inflammatory markers have been measured in peritoneal fluid in an attempt to identify intestinal strangulation and the need for surgery; however, these markers are not necessarily sensitive or specific for diagnosis of intestinal strangulation or ischemia and are not currently practical.[32–35] Peritoneal serum amyloid A concentrations measured alone or in comparison to blood does not differentiate between inflammatory and strangulating lesions and does not replace lactate measurements for this purpose.[35]

Techniques for percutaneous abdominocentesis in the adult horse are described elsewhere.[36] A teat cannula technique is preferred by the authors and is recommended when small intestinal distention is present. Subcutaneous swelling and enterocentesis are the most common complications of this procedure, but these occur in less than 1% of abdominocentesis attempts, resolve with antimicrobial therapy, and are not associated with user skill level.[31,37] Therefore, abdominocentesis is warranted in any case of adult colic regardless of veterinarian experience, provided they are properly prepared. In cases of marked colon distension or suspected sand impaction, enterocentesis may be more likely and the need for abdominocentesis should be considered in light of this. Of note, milk peritonitis associated with enterocentesis in preweaned foals is very serious; in this population, abdominocentesis should be reserved for cases of severe colic and only performed by experienced practitioners

MANAGEMENT DECISIONS FOLLOWING TRIAGE

Following field evaluation, the equine primary care practitioner must make recommendations for continued on-farm management, referral, or euthanasia. Assessments of colic severity and suspected gastrointestinal localization, as well as frank owner communication inform these recommendations, are described in **Fig. 5**.

Colic pain despite adequate on-farm analgesia is the most important indicator for referral management or euthanasia.[38] As a general principle, colic pain that is refractory to adequate analgesia could be defined as pain that is recurrent, severe, or progressive within a 12-hour period despite full doses of a nonsteroidal anti-inflammatory drug (NSAID) and alpha-2 agonists with or without opioids. Horses with colic that require two or more doses of analgesia over any time period are more likely to require surgery.[39]

In the absence of refractory and/or progressive pain, additional important indications for referral management or euthanasia are outlined in **Fig. 5** and include

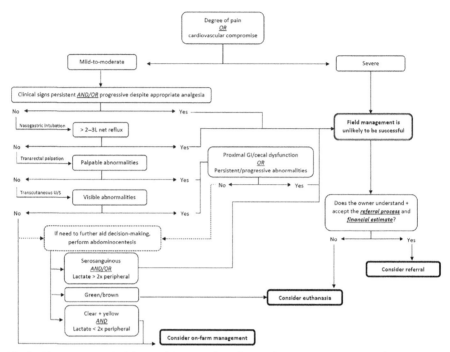

Fig. 5. Management decision-making tree based on colic triage examination findings.

additional indicators of colic severity (see **Tables 1** and **2**) and/or localization to the proximal gastrointestinal tract or cecum (see **Table 3**). Recommendations for stabilizing horses before referral are well-described[18,39] and can be provided for a specific case by the referral center. Typically, rapid transportation to a referral center should be prioritized over on-farm stabilization (ie, intravenous fluids) to avoid delay.

A strong veterinary–client–patient relationship facilitates client decision-making when referral care or euthanasia are considered. Horse owners may have difficulty recognizing quality-of-life concerns[40] and rely heavily on veterinary advice for end-of-life decisions.[41] Although shared decision-making between medical professionals and patients (clients) is a popular and powerful communication tool,[40] it is important to remember that the horse owner is ultimately responsible for taking a veterinarian's management recommendations and making an informed decision that suits their unique situation. Referral care for most common etiologies of care has a good to excellent prognosis for discharge with appropriate medical or surgical treatment, including small intestinal strangulating lesions (>70%), large colon impactions (>90%), and large colon displacements (>90%). Survival rates are comparable for geriatric horses, and age alone should not deter referral or surgical care.[18]

When evaluation supports referral, early referral improves patient outcomes, reduces complications, and frequently decreases the overall cost of care to the owner. Discussing the case with the local hospital before referral ensures the owner has accurate cost and treatment expectations.[18] Referral without providing this information, particularly if a surgical lesion is suspected, can cause owner frustration and prolong patient suffering, and must be avoided. In the authors' experience, some clients will refuse referral until they realize euthanasia is the most likely alternative, which can delay referral of critical cases and negatively affect patient outcomes.[18] Discussing concerns with farm management in light of the horse's clinical examination early and honestly can minimize this frustrating scenario.

If referral is recommended, but declined by the owner, equine primary care practitioners face the additional challenge of advocating for patient welfare within the confines of the client's capabilities. In these instances, euthanasia should be discussed and considered based on the veterinarian's evaluation and the progression and persistence of the horses' clinical abnormalities. Conversely, referral might be elected based on client's needs and preferences when farm management is clinically appropriate. Referral should always be supported if requested by the client or if the client is physically or emotionally unable to closely monitor the horse.

ANALGESIC OPTIONS FOR COLIC CASES

The assessment of comfort is vital to colic triage evaluation, and analgesic and/or sedative medications are frequently required to facilitate a safe examination and treat discomfort. A simple, reliable, descriptive scoring system for equine abdominal pain (equine abdominal pain scale [EAAPS]) is outlined in **Table 2**.[19–21,42] It is important to note the degree of pain before administering any analgesia, and to relay the route, dose, and timing of drug(s) administration to referral veterinarians.

Up to 96% of caretakers report access to at least one type of analgesic medication, and 27% of caretakers acquire these medications outside of a veterinary–client–patient relationship.[43] As such, when evaluating a horse for colic, inquiry as to any prior administration of analgesic medications is paramount to accurately evaluating the patient and guiding drug administration during the evaluation and preventing adverse effects from readministration and overdose. Analgesic medications available and commonly administered in equine patients with colic are discussed below and outlined in **Table 4**.

NONSTEROIDAL ANTI-INFLAMMATORY DRUGS

NSAIDs reduce pain, pyrexia, and inflammation by either nonselectively or selectively inhibiting cyclooxygenase (COX) enzymes. Potential adverse effects of NSAIDs include nephrotoxicity and gastrointestinal disease (right dorsal colitis, gastric ulceration) and are associated with decreased prostaglandin-mediated blood flow, mucous production, and mucosal barrier integrity to the affected organ systems or gastrointestinal dysbiosis.[44] Adverse effects are potentially enhanced in patients with a history of renal disease, NSAID-associated gastrointestinal disease, or concurrent hypovolemia. Combining NSAIDs or administering doses higher than the labeled dose is not supported by current literature and may increase the risk of potential adverse events.[45]

NONSELECTIVE COX INHIBITORS

- Flunixin meglumine and phenylbutazone are nonselective COX-1 and COX-2 inhibitors. Flunixin meglumine provides superior analgesia for visceral pain and is most commonly administered in colic cases with phenylbutazone most commonly prescribed in orthopedic disease.[45,46]
- Oral and injectable forms of flunixin meglumine are available and often administered before evaluation by a veterinarian. In addition to guiding proper dose amount and frequency, caretakers should be cautioned against intramuscular administration of flunixin meglumine due to its association with clostridial myositis.

Table 4
Medications available for sedation and analgesia to facilitate evaluation in an equine patient

Category	Medication	NSAIDs		
		Advantages		Disadvantages

Nonselective COX inhibitor	*Flunixin meglumine*
	0.25 mg/kg PO/IV q8h
	Phenylbutazone
	0.5–1.0 mg/kg PO/IV q12–24 h
	2.2–4.4 mg/kg PO/IV q12–24 h
		• Multiple formulations
		• Dose-dependent effects
		  ○ Anti-endotoxemic
		  ○ Anti-inflammatory
		  ○ Analgesic
		• Rapid onset (IV)
				• Nephrotoxicity
				• GI adverse effects
				  ○ Dysbiosis
				  ○ Right dorsal colitis
				  ○ Gastric ulcers
				• Avoid IM administration

Selective COX-2 inhibitor	*Firocoxib* 0.3 mg/kg PO/IV once (load) 0.1 mg/kg PO/IV q24 h *Meloxicam* 0.6 mg/kg IV/PO	• Multiple formulations • Lesser GI effects • Anti-inflammatory • Analgesic		• Nephrotoxicity • Conflicting data on analgesic potency
Non-traditional	*Acetaminophen* 20 mg/kg PO q12 h *Metamizole* 30 mg/kg IV q12–24 h up to 3 d	• Antipyretic • Analgesic • Coadminister with other NSAIDs • Antipyretic • Analgesic • Antispasmodic		• Limited data in colic • PO administration only • Labeled only for pyrexia • GI adverse effects • Potential coagulopathy
Alpha-2 adrenoreceptor agonists				
Shorter Duration ↓ Longer duration	*Xylazine* 0.2–1.0 mg/kg IV/IM *Romifidine* 0.04–0.12 mg/kg IV/IM *Detomidine* 0.005–0.04 mg/kg IV/IM 0.04 mg/kg sublingually	• Sedation + analgesia • Short duration of action • Oral formulation available (detomidine)		• Sedation may mask discomfort • Reduced GI motility • Hypertension → hypotension

Opioids

Category	Medication	Advantages	Disadvantages
K agonist + μ antagonist	*Butorphanol* 0.01–0.1 mg/kg IV/IM/SQ	• Synergistic with α-2 agonists • Rapid onset of action • Potent analgesia	• Controlled substance • Head twitching (butorphanol) • Reduced GI motility • Excitation • Variable analgesia • Histamine response (morphine)
Partial μ agonist	*Buprenorphine* 0.004–0.006 mg/kg IV/IM/SQ		
μ agonist	*Morphine* 0.05–0.1 mg/kg IV/IIM *Hydromorphone* 0.04 mg/kg IV/IM		

Spasmolytics

Category	Medication	Advantages	Disadvantages
Anticholinergic	*N-butylscopolammonium bromide* 0.3 mg/kg IV/IM	• Facilitates rectal examination • Short duration of action • Spasmolysis → analgesia	• Transient tachycardia • Short duration of action

Abbreviations: GI, gastrointestinal; IM, intramuscular; PO, per os; SQ, sub-cutaneous.

SELECTIVE COX-2 INHIBITORS

- As the results of reduced inhibition of COX-1 enzymes, selective COX-2 inhibitors, such as firocoxib (Equioxx, Boehringer Ingelheim) and meloxicam (Metacam, Boehringer Ingelheim), have reduced mucosal healing time, reduced levels of plasma biomarkers of endotoxemia, and reduced evidence of gastrointestinal insult compared with nonselective COX inhibitors in both experimental and clinical settings.[47–51]
- Despite the evidence of reduced gastrointestinal effects, adverse effects on renal function are equivalent to nonselective medications.
- The analgesic efficacy of COX-2 selective medications is conflicting with both equivalent[47,49,52,53] and inferior[54] analgesia reported.

NONTRADITIONAL NONSTEROIDAL ANTI-INFLAMMATORY DRUGS

- Acetaminophen is one of the most commonly used analgesic and antipyretic medications in human medicine and was historically used in horses as a marker of gastric emptying due to its poor gastric resorption and rapid small intestinal resorption with high oral bioavailability (91%).[55,56] Although its mechanism of action is not entirely understood, its antipyretic and analgesic effects are suspected to be centrally mediated through an inhibitory effect on COX-3.[57]
- With similar pharmacologic profile to selective COX-2 inhibitors, acetaminophen is reported to be an effective analgesic medication for musculoskeletal disease without adverse gastrointestinal, hepatic, or renal effects even when combined with a traditional NSAID.[55,56,58,59] Acetaminophen has not been described as an analgesic for visceral pain in horses but should be considered when traditional NSAIDs are contraindicated.
- Metamizole (dipyrone; Zimeta, Dechra) is a pyrazolone derivative that exerts its effects through a complex mechanism of action involving inhibition of COX-3, activation of the opioidergic system and activation of the cannabinoid system.[60] Metamizole is labeled for treatment of pyrexia but additional effects include mild-to-moderate analgesia and reduced smooth muscle spasms.[60,61]

Alpha-2 Adrenoreceptor Agonists

During a colic evaluation, alpha-2 adrenoreceptor agonists are commonly administered for their sedative and analgesic properties. They are effective at managing patient discomfort and facilitating diagnostic procedures, both critical for safety. Intravenous or intramuscular bolus is the most common route of administration, but an oromucosal detomidine gel (Dormosedan gel, Zoetis) may be administered in patients with aversion to needles or if sedation is required before evaluation and a caretaker is unable to administer an injectable medication.[62]

Xylazine has a short duration of action and is often chosen as the initial alpha-2 agonist during a colic examination; however, several doses may be required. In patients with discomfort refractory to xylazine, administration of a longer-acting alpha-2 agonist (romifidine, detomidine), implementing multimodal analgesia, or coadministration of an opioid should be considered. Discomfort requiring multiple doses of analgesia may be associated with colic that is more serious and should begin raising "red flags" regarding continued on-farm management.

Opioids

Opioids are often coadministered with alpha-2 agonists to enhance sedation and provide neuroleptanalgesia in either noncompliant patients and/or patients with moderate to severe discomfort. Opioids are categorized based on their action on particular opioid receptors. Butorphanol, a schedule IV opioid with mu-receptor antagonism and kappa receptor agonism, can be administered intramuscularly, intravenously, or subcutaneously. It is the most commonly used opioid in equine ambulatory practice, although its analgesic potency for visceral pain has been questioned.[45,63–65] Less common to equine ambulatory practice, mu-opioid agonists (morphine, hydromorphone, buprenorphine) are generally considered to provide superior analgesia. With action on receptors peripherally and centrally, described potential adverse effects of opioids including decreased gastrointestinal motility and hyperactivity are notably dose-dependent and more readily observed in clinically non-painful horses.[66–74] These medications are controlled and cannot be dispensed for non-veterinary administration.

Antispasmodics

N-butylscopolammonium bromide (Buscopan, Boehringer Ingelheim) is an anticholinergic spasmolytic that reduces smooth muscle contraction and is labeled for management of abdominal pain associated with spasmodic colic, flatulent colic, and simple impactions. Although not a labeled indication, it is frequently administered during evaluation of a horse with colic to facilitate more thorough transrectal palpation and decrease risk of rectal trauma by reducing straining against the examiner's arm by up to 68%.[25] Although anecdote follows that reduction of motility is contraindicated for certain causes of colic (impaction), the medication's short duration of action (20–30 minutes) likely provides little detriment to patient outcome and, in fact, reduction of intestinal spasm against impacted digesta may facilitate resolution and improve patient comfort.[75,76]

CLINICS CARE POINTS

- The goals of field colic triage are determining clinical severity of disease and assigning a suspected anatomic localization of the colic signs.
- A thorough history, observation, physical examination, transrectal palpation, and nasogastric intubation are essential components of any colic evaluation. Additional diagnostics include transcutaneous abdominal ultrasound, and percutaneous abdominocentesis can be readily performed in the field and provide useful information for management decisions.
- Clinical "red flags," which are largely related to degree of pain and cardiovascular compromise, alert the clinician to a critical colic, and are the most important considerations for referral or euthanasia.

DISCLOSURE

The authors have no conflicts of interest to disclose.

REFERENCES

1. Bowden A, England GCW, Brennan ML, et al. Indicators of "critical" outcomes in 941 horses seen "out-of-hours" for colic. Vet Rec 2020;187(12):492.
2. Tinker MK, White NA, Lessard P, et al. Prospective study of equine colic incidence and mortality. Equine Vet J 1997;29(6):448–53.

3. Barker I, Freeman SL. Assessment of costs and insurance policies for referral treatment of equine colic. Vet Rec 2019;185(16):508.

4. Bowden A, Burford JH, Brennan ML, et al. Horse owners' knowledge, and opinions on recognising colic in the horse. Equine Vet J 2020;52(2):262–7.

5. Bowden A, Boynova P, Brennan ML, et al. Retrospective case series to identify the most common conditions seen "out-of-hours" by first-opinion equine veterinary practitioners. Vet Rec 2020;187(10):404.

6. Tinker MK, White NA, Lessard P, et al. Prospective study of equine colic risk factors. Equine Vet J 1997;29(6):454–8.

7. van der Linden MA, Laffont CM, Sloet van Oldruitenborgh-Oosterbaan MM. Prognosis in equine medical and surgical colic. J Vet Intern Med 2003;17(3):343–8.

8. Abutarbush SM, Carmalt JL, Shoemaker RW. Causes of gastrointestinal colic in horses in western Canada: 604 cases (1992 to 2002). Can Vet J 2005;46(9): 800–5.

9. Kaufman JM, Nekouei O, Doyle AJ, et al. Clinical findings, diagnoses, and outcomes of horses presented for colic to a referral hospital in Atlantic Canada (2000-2015). Can Vet J 2020;61(3):281–8.

10. Welch E. Red flags in medical practice. Clin Med 2011;11(3):251–3.

11. Hackett ES, Embertson RM, Hopper SA, et al. Duration of disease influences survival to discharge of Thoroughbred mares with surgically treated large colon volvulus. Equine Vet J 2015;47(6):650–4.

12. Curtis L, Burford JH, Thomas JSM, et al. Prospective study of the primary evaluation of 1016 horses with clinical signs of abdominal pain by veterinary practitioners, and the differentiation of critical and non-critical cases. Acta Vet Scand 2015;57:69.

13. Farrell A, Kersh K, Liepman R, et al. Development of a colic scoring system to predict outcome in horses. Front Vet Sci 2021;8:697589.

14. Furr MO, Lessard P, White NA. Development of a colic severity score for predicting the outcome of equine colic. Vet Surg 1995;24(2):97–101.

15. Jennings K, Curtis L, Burford J, et al. Prospective survey of veterinary practitioners' primary assessment of equine colic: clinical features, diagnoses, and treatment of 120 cases of large colon impaction. BMC Vet Res 2014;10(Suppl 1):S2.

16. Mair TS, Smith LJ. Survival and complication rates in 300 horses undergoing surgical treatment of colic. Part 1: Short-term survival following a single laparotomy. Equine Vet J 2005;37(4):296–302.

17. Southwood LJ, Fehr J. Abdominal palpation per rectum. In: Southwood LJ, editor. Practical guide to equine colic. 1st Ed. Hoboken, NJ,: Wiley Blackwell; 2013. p. 23–37.

18. Southwood LJ, Fehr J. Referral of the horse with colic. In: Southwood LJ, editor. Practical guide to equine colic. 1st Ed. Hoboken, NJ: Wiley Blackwell; 2013. p. 71–7.

19. Sutton GA, Dahan R, Turner D, et al. A behaviour-based pain scale for horses with acute colic: Scale construction. Vet J 2013;196:394–401.

20. Sutton GA, Bar L. Refinement and revalidation of the Equine Acute Abdominal Pain Scale (EAAPS) Isr. J Vet Med 2016;71:15–23.

21. Sutton GA, Atamna R, Steinman A, et al. Comparison of three acute colic pain scales: reliability, validity and usability. Vet J 2019;246:71–7.

22. White NA. Prognosticating equine colic. In: Blikslager AT, White NA, Moore JN, et al, editors. The equine acute abdomen. 3rd Ed. Hoboken, NJ: Wiley Blackwell; 2017. p. 289–300.

23. Busoni V, De Busscher V, Lopez D, et al. Evaluation of a protocol for fast localised abdominal sonography of horses (Flash) admitted for colic. Vet J 2011;188(1): 77–82.

24. Mueller POE. Rectal examination. In: Mair T, Divers TJ, Ducharme NG, editors. Manual of equine gastroenterology. Philadelphia, PA: Saunders; 2002. p. 6–8.

25. Luo T, Bertone JJ, Greene HM, et al. A comparison of N-butylscopolammonium and lidocaine for control of rectal pressure in horses. Vet Ther 2006;7(3):243–8.

26. Claes A, Ball BA, Brown JA, et al. Evaluation of risk factors, management, and outcome associated with rectal tears in horses: 99 cases (1985-2006). J Am Vet Med Assoc 2008;233(10):1605–9.

27. Monreal L, Navarro M, Armengou L, et al. Enteral fluid therapy in 108 horses with large colon impactions and dorsal displacements. Vet Rec 2010;166(9):259–63.

28. Lopes MAF, White NA, Donaldson L, et al. Effects of enteral and intravenous fluid therapy, magnesium sulfate, and sodium sulfate on colonic contents and feces in horses. Am J Vet Res 2004;65(5):695–704.

29. Kaikkonen R, Niinistö K, Lindholm T, et al. Comparison of psyllium feeding at home and nasogastric intubation of psyllium and magnesium sulfate in the hospital as a treatment for naturally occurring colonic sand (Geosediment) accumulations in horses: a retrospective study. Acta Vet Scand 2016;58(1):73.

30. Shearer TR, Norby B, Carr EA. Peritoneal fluid lactate evaluation in horses with non-strangulating versus strangulating small intestinal disease. J Equine Vet Sci 2018;61:18–21.

31. Siex MT, Wilson JH. Morbidity associated with abdominocentesis - a prospective study. Equine Vet J 1992;13:22–5.

32. Long A. Clinical insights: Clinicopathological parameters for diagnosing and predicting outcome of horses with colic. Equine Vet J 2022;54(6):1005–10.

33. Kilcoyne I, Nieto JE, Dechant JE. Diagnostic value of plasma and peritoneal fluid procalcitonin concentrations in horses with strangulating intestinal lesions. J Am Vet Med Assoc 2020;256(8):927–33.

34. Pihl TH, Andersen PH, Kjelgaard-Hansen M, et al. Serum amyloid A and haptoglobin concentrations in serum and peritoneal fluid of healthy horses and horses with acute abdominal pain. Vet Clin Pathol 2013;42(2):177–83.

35. Pihl TH, Scheepers E, Sanz M, et al. Influence of disease process and duration on acute phase proteins in serum and peritoneal fluid of horses with colic. J Vet Intern Med 2015;29(2):651–8.

36. Radcliffe RM, Hill JA, Liu SY, et al. Abdominocentesis techniques in horses. J Vet Emerg Crit Care 2022;32(S1):72–80.

37. Duesterdieck-Zellmer KF, Riehl JH, McKenzie EC, et al. Effects of abdominocentesis technique on peritoneal fluid and clinical variables in horses. Equine Vet Edu 2014;26(5):262–8.

38. White NA. Decisions for surgery and referral. In: Blikslager AT, White NA, Moore JN, et al, editors. The equine acute abdomen. 3rd Ed. Hoboken, NJ: Wiley Blackwell; 2017. p. 285–8.

39. White NA, Elward A, Moga KS, et al. Use of web-based data collection to evaluate analgesic administration and the decision for surgery in horses with colic. Equine Vet J 2005;37:347–50.

40. Cameron A, Pollock K, Wilson E, et al. Scoping review of end-of-life decision-making models used in dogs, cats and equids. Vet Rec 2022;191(4):e1730.

41. Clough H, Roshier M, England G, et al. Cross-sectional study of UK horse owner's purchase and euthanasia decision-making for their horse. Vet Rec 2021; 188(6):e56.

42. Maskato Y, Dugdale A, Singer E, et al. Prospective feasibility and revalidation of the equine acute abdominal pain scale (EAAPS) in clinical cases of colic in horses. Animals 2020;10(12):2242.
43. Sellon DC, Sanz M, Kopper JJ. Acquisition and use of analgesic drugs by horse owners in the United States. Equine Vet J 2022;55(1):69–77.
44. Whitfield-Cargile CM, Chamoun-Emanuelli AM, Cohen ND, et al. Differential effects of selective and non-selective cyclooxygenase inhibitors on fecal microbiota in adult horses. PLoS One 2018;13(8):e0202527.
45. Bowen IM, Redpath A, Dugdale A, et al. BEVA primary care clinical guidelines:analgesia. Equine Vet J 2020;52(1):13–27.
46. Duz M, Marshall JF, Parkin TD. Proportion of nonsteroidal anti-inflammatory drug prescription in equine practice. Equine Vet J 2019;51(2):147–53.
47. Cook VL, Meyer CT, Campbell NB, et al. Effect of firocoxib or flunixin meglumine on recovery of ischemic-injured equine jejunum. Am J Vet Res 2009;70(8):992–1000.
48. Raidal SL, Hughes KJ, Charman AL, et al. Effects of meloxicam and phenylbutazone on renal responses to furosemide, dobutamine, and exercise in horses. Am J Vet Res 2014;75(7):668–79.
49. Urayama S, Tanaka A, Kusano K, et al. Oral administration of meloxicam suppresses low-dose endotoxin challenge-induced pain in thoroughbred horses. J Equine Vet Sci 2019;77:139–43.
50. Ziegler AL, Blikslager AT. Sparing the gut: COX -2 inhibitors herald a new era for treatment of horses with surgical colic. Equine Vet Educ 2020;32(11):611–6.
51. Ziegler AL, Freeman CK, Fogle CA, et al. Multicentre, blinded, randomised clinical trial comparing the use of flunixin meglumine with firocoxib in horses with small intestinal strangulating obstruction. Equine Vet J 2019;51(3):329–35.
52. Gobbi FP, Di Filippo PA, de Macêdo Mello L, et al. Effects of flunixin meglumine, firocoxib, and meloxicam in equines after castration. J Equine Vet Sci 2020;94:103229.
53. Lemonnier LC, Thorin C, Meurice A, et al. Comparison of flunixin meglumine, meloxicam and ketoprofen on mild visceral post-operative pain in horses. Animals (Basel) 2022;12(4):526.
54. Naylor RJ, Taylor AH, Knowles EJ, et al. Comparison of flunixin meglumine and meloxicam for post operative management of horses with strangulating small intestinal lesions: does meloxicam improve survival in horses following small intestinal strangulation? Equine Vet J 2014;46:427–34.
55. Mercer MA, McKenzie HC, Davis JL, et al. Pharmacokinetics and safety of repeated oral dosing of acetaminophen in adult horses. Equine Vet J 2020;52(1):120–5.
56. Mercer MA, McKenzie HC, Byron CR, et al. Pharmacokinetics and clinical efficacy of acetaminophen (Paracetamol) in adult horses with mechanically induced lameness. Equine Vet J 2022;55(3):524–33.
57. Chandrasekharan NV, Dai H, Roos KL, et al. COX-3, a cyclooxygenase-1 variant inhibited by acetaminophen and other analgesic/antipyretic drugs: cloning, structure, and expression. Proc Natl Acad Sci U S A 2002;99:13926–31.
58. Pesko B, Habershon-Butcher J, Muir T, et al. Pharmacokinetics of paracetamol in the Thoroughbred horse following an oral multi-dose administration. J Vet Pharmacol Ther 2022;45(1):54–62.
59. West E, Bardell D, Morgan R, et al. Use of acetaminophen (Paracetamol) as a short-term adjunctive analgesic in a laminitic pony. Vet Anaesth Analg 2011;38(5):521–2.

60. Jasiecka A, Maslanka T, Jaroszewski JJ. Pharmacological characteristics of metamizole. Pol J Vet Sci 2014;17(1):207–14.
61. Roelvink M, Goossens L, Kalsbeek H, et al. Analgesic and spasmolytic effects of dipyrone, hyoscine-N-butylbromide and a combination of the two in ponies. Vet Rec 1991;129(17):378–80.
62. Dai F, Rausk J, Aspegren J, et al. Use of detomidine oromucosal gel for alleviation of acute anxiety and fear in horses: a pilot study. Front Vet Sci 2020;7:573309.
63. Taylor PM, Hoare HR, de Vries A, et al. A multicentre, prospective, randomised, blinded clinical trial to compare some perioperative effects of buprenorphine or butorphanol premedication before equine elective general anaesthesia and surgery. Equine Vet J 2016;48:442e450.
64. Love EJ, Taylor PM, Clark C, et al. Analgesic effect of butorphanol in ponies following castration. Equine Vet J 2009;41(6):552–6.
65. Chiavaccini L, Claude AK, Lee JH, et al. Pharmacokinetics and pharmacodynamics comparison between subcutaneous and intravenous butorphanol administration in horses. J Vet Pharmacol Ther 2015;38(4):365–74.
66. Boscan P, Van Hoogmoed LM, Farver TB, et al. Evaluation of the effects of the opioid agonist morphine on gastrointestinal tract function in horses. Am J Vet Res 2006;67:992–7.
67. Figueiredo JP, Muir WW, Sams R. Cardiorespiratory, gastrointestinal, and analgesic effects of morphine sulfate in conscious healthy horses. Am J Vet Res 2012;73:799–808.
68. Flynn H, Cenani A, Brosnan RJ, et al. Pharmacokinetics and pharmacodynamics of a high concentration of buprenorphine (Simbadol) in conscious horses after subcutaneous administration. Vet Anaesth Analg 2021;48(4):585–95.
69. Martins FC, Keating SC, Clark-Price SC, et al. Pharmacokinetics and pharmacodynamics of hydromorphone hydrochloride in healthy horses. Vet Anaesth Analg 2020;47:509–17.
70. Reed R, Barletta M, Mitchell K, et al. The pharmacokinetics and pharmacodynamics of intravenous hydromorphone in horses. Vet Anaesth Analg 2019;46: 395–404.
71. Reed RA, Knych HK, Barletta M, et al. Pharmacokinetics and pharmacodynamics of hydromorphone after intravenous and intramuscular administration in horses. Vet Anaesth Analg 2020;47:210–8.
72. Reed R, Trenholme N, Skrzypczak H, et al. Comparison of hydromorphone and butorphanol for management of pain in equine patients undergoing elective arthroscopy: a randomized clinical trial. Vet Anaesth Analg 2022;49(5):490–8.
73. Skrzypczak H, Reed R, Barletta M, et al. A retrospective evaluation of the effect of perianesthetic hydromorphone administration on the incidence of postanesthetic signs of colic in horses. Vet Anaesth Analg 2020;47:757–62.
74. Tessier C, Pitaud JP, Thorin C, et al. Systemic morphine administration causes gastric distention and hyperphagia in healthy horses. Equine Vet J 2019;51(5): 653–7.
75. Hart KA, Sherlock CE, Davern AJ, et al. Effect of N -butylscopolammonium bromide on equine ileal smooth muscle activity in an ex vivo model: Effects of N-butylscopolammonium bromide on equine ileum. Equine Vet J 2015;47(4):450–5.
76. Boatwright CE, Fubini SL, Grohn YT, et al. A comparison of N-butylscopolammonium bromide and butorphanol tartrate for analgesia using a balloon model of abdominal pain in ponies. Can J Vet Res 1996;60(1):65–8.

Abdominal Sonographic Evaluation
In the Field, at the Hospital, and After Surgery

Cristobal Navas de Solis, LV, PhD[a],*, Michelle Coleman, DVM, PhD[b]

KEYWORDS

• Ultrasound • Sonography • Colic • Gastrointestinal • Abdominal

KEY POINTS

- The use of abdominal sonography provides useful diagnostic and monitoring information in the evaluation of horses with colic in the field, hospital, and postoperative setting.
- During the last 4 decades, veterinarians have created a large body of literature informative to clinicians using sonography to diagnose horses with colic.
- It is likely that this technique will continue to advance in the near future as sonography becomes more available and affordable and newer generations of veterinarians receive more and earlier training.

INTRODUCTION

Abdominal sonography is currently a routine procedure in the evaluation of horses with colic. This imaging technique is used to assess horses presenting in the emergency setting with acute colic and the horse presenting for chronic or recurrent colic in the nonemergency setting. Sonography for colic evaluation is used by specialists in different disciplines and by general practitioners in the ambulatory and hospital setting. It is likely that the most common use of sonography for the assessment of colic is as a point-of-care ultrasound (POCUS) modality to answer pointed questions using specific anatomic windows while complete abdominal sonograms are reserved for other clinical scenarios.

Because the description of protocols for the evaluation of the horse with acute colic[1] and later of the popular fast abdominal sonogram of horses (FLASH) protocol,[2] there has been an interest in defining information obtained by limited, point-of-care sonograms compared with information obtained by complete transcutaneous sonographic evaluation.

---

[a] Clinical Studies New Bolton Center, University of Pennsylvania; [b] Department of Large Animal Medicine, University of Georgia
* Corresponding author.
E-mail address: navasdes@vet.upenn.edu

Vet Clin Equine 39 (2023) 197–210
https://doi.org/10.1016/j.cveq.2023.03.006
0749-0739/23/© 2023 Elsevier Inc. All rights reserved.

Financial and technological factors are important considerations. Financially, it is advantageous for practitioners to have the ability to transcutaneously image horses with probes traditionally available in equine practice, such as the rectal probes. The use of the rectal probe for the transcutaneous evaluation of colic in the horse has been partially explored.[3,4] In normal horses, viscera in the right side of the abdomen can be identified with similar frequency using rectal and curvilinear probes transcutaneously. On the left side, the stomach, liver, and kidney were less likely to be detected with rectal probes. This information may be useful when deciding which equipment a practitioner invests in or if available equipment can be used for a particular examination. It should be considered that the clinician is interested in not only to identify an organ but also in the ability to identify relevant lesions and describe their sonographic characteristics. With the rapid development of more affordable POCUS equipment, capable of obtaining images equine practitioners seek to obtain in the point of care setting,[5] questions regarding which organs can be imaged will be less relevant. Rather, diagnostic accuracy, indications, and the training and skills needed for different protocols will become more important.[6] In this review, we will focus on indications, clinical interpretation of imaging findings, and recent literature on transcutaneous sonographic evaluation of the colic patient. Equipment, animal preparation, imaging technique, and didactic description of lesions have been thoroughly described recently.[7,8]

Another important aspect of the comparison of limited, localized sonograms and complete sonograms is which pathologic conditions are visible using each protocol. This question has been partially investigated in a study,[4] in which authors compared a focused examination (different than FLASH) to complete sonograms in normal horses. Focused sonograms identified most key structures, yet had some limitations compared with a detailed, complete examination. Specifically, the cecum, sacculated large colon, spleen, liver, and right kidney were consistently identified with a focal examination, yet the left kidney was inconsistently identified. Further, more imaging sites or repeated examinations were required to identify normal small intestine with the limited, focused protocol. The authors proposed that less frequent identification of the kidney could have been due to poor images due to limited preparation and not clipping with the focused technique or the limited windows. The role of sonography in the evaluation of the horse with acute colic has been studied by comparing abdominal palpation per rectum and transcutaneous sonographic findings.[9] The authors of the latter study reported that small intestinal obstruction and large colon volvulus (LCV) was more frequently identified with transcutaneous sonography. Displacements of the colon (except for left dorsal displacements), impactions, and diseases of the cecum were more frequently identified on palpation per rectum.[9] It was concluded that in the hospital setting, it is highly advisable to include ultrasonography in the routine examination of the equine acute abdomen; however, this technique does not replace examination per rectum.[9]

When deciding on the type of examination, multiple variables including the probability of each type of lesion (pretest probability), diagnostic accuracy to determine the presence or absence of these lesions (specificity and sensitivity of the test or likelihood ratios), the clinical consequence of a positive or negative result, and consequence of an incorrect diagnosis should be considered. A recent review of the use of transcutaneous abdominal sonography includes tables showing its diagnostic accuracy for different diseases.[10] The use of Fagan's nomograms is an interesting approach to the use of this information in specific clinical situations. The use of Fagan's nomograms allows using the estimated pretest probability and known specificity and sensitivity of a diagnostic test to calculate a posttest probability. The posttest probability becomes a relevant piece of information for the clinical management.[11]

The current limitation of using this approach for decision-making is that pretest probabilities are described in some situations yet hard to define in every setting, region, or practice. Therefore, the clinical acumen of the veterinarian is key in the diagnostic process. Furthermore, sonography is an operator-dependent technique and the diagnostic accuracy described in the literature may not apply to all operators. Finally, a posttest probability is used differently for decision-making depending on the clinical situation and therapies available.

SMALL INTESTINAL STRANGULATED VERSUS NONSTRANGULATED OBSTRUCTION

Traditional sonographic criteria to identify strangulated obstructions include the presence of distended, turgid, nonmotile, thickened loops of small intestine. Small intestinal ileus and nonstrangulated obstructions typically result in small intestine that is hypomotile and dilated (more open or filled than usual) but not thickened or turgid (circular and completely filled).[7] The diagnostic accuracy of finding distended or thickened small intestine for small intestinal obstruction or strangulation has been evaluated.[1,2,12] Sonographic identification of distended small intestine had a specificity and sensitivity of 73% to 76% for small intestinal strangulation.[12] Amotile, distended, "edematous" small intestine was 100% specific and sensitive for a diagnosis of small

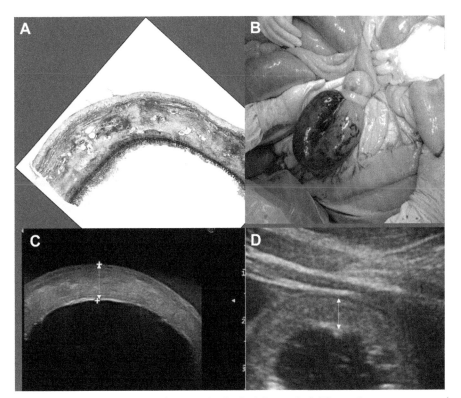

Fig. 1. Small intestinal strangulation. Histologic (*A*), surgical (*B*), ex-vivo sonogram and sonogram of the small intestine of a horse with a strangulated small intestinal lesion. Note the distended nonmotile thickened intestine (*D*) and diffusely echoic wall corresponding histopathologically to transmural hemorrhage (*C*). The *yellow double headed arrow* (*C* and *D*) mark the small intestinal wall.

intestinal strangulation.[1] The ability of a FLASH seems similar to a more detailed sonogram to detect small intestinal strangulation[13] (**Fig. 1**).

The presence of increased peritoneal fluid, sedimented digesta within small intestine or "two populations of intestine" with different appearance are often used as supportive findings of strangulated lesions but the diagnostic accuracy of these findings and overlap with other diseases such as nonstrangulated obstructions, functional obstructions, or an inflammatory processes is problematic. Overlap exists between the sonographic findings in horses with strangulating lesions, nonstrangulating lesions, and proximal enteritis. For example, early strangulated lesions may have intestine with normal wall thickness.[7] An elegant study investigated the association between oxygen saturation in intestinal capillaries of horses with strangulated lesions and the thickness of the wall measured sonographically.[14] There was no association between oxygen saturation and small intestinal wall thickness at the ischemic site. There was, however, a negative correlation (thicker wall with decreasing oxygen saturation) in the adjacent aboral segment. The authors suggested that venous occlusion leads to decreasing oxygen saturation being associated with increasing wall thickness (perhaps enhanced by surgical manipulation), and with arteriovenous occlusion, the association is lost. Consequently, making conclusions about oxygen saturation based on intestinal wall thickness is not possible. Intestinal wall thinning may be a late stage of ischemia preceding rupture; however, it is rarely identified in the horse. Other recent studies[15,16] have investigated the association between sonographic and pathologic findings in normal intestine and pathologic conditions (**Fig. 2**). Bevevino and collaborators showed that intestinal wall layering and thickness of the different layers were associated with the histologic appearance of the intestine and speculated that beyond the intestinal wall thickness other sonographic characteristics may be useful to diagnose equine intestinal disease (**Fig. 3**). Characterization of the intestinal wall layering, echogenicity, and blood flow may help, in the future, define further the presence and stage of progression of strangulated or nonstrangulated lesions similar to the described conditions such as necrotizing enterocolitis in humans.[17,18] Pneumatosis intestinalis (gas within the intestinal wall) is more commonly described in neonates with necrotizing gastrointestinal disease[19] and rarely in horses with strangulating lesions. Pneumatosis intestinalis is seen with other conditions causing necrosis such as clostridial diseases, *Lawsonia intracellularis* infection (proliferative enteropathy),[20] vascular compromise, or infarcts.

The sonographic appearance of the intestinal wall blood flow[21] has not been thoroughly studied in the horse. In a preliminary study,[21] the intestine blood flow could not be detected in neonates using Doppler interrogation raising concerns about the feasibility of this procedure. Since this study was performed, technology has improved and equipment with more sensitive color-flow Doppler and motion correction algorithms are currently available. Color-flow Doppler could be a useful technique in the adult horse with colic similarly to its use in humans where Doppler signal with different types of intestinal lesions is associated with histopathological findings and can be used to guide therapeutic interventions.[22–24] This concept would need to be tested prospectively.

VISUALIZATION OF COLONIC MESENTERIC VESSELS

A high-yield finding in the evaluation of a horse with acute colic is the identification of malpositioned mesenteric vessels. This finding has been reported in several studies.[25–27] Colonic blood vessels are normally located in the mesentery along the medial aspect of the large colon and, therefore, obscured by digesta or gas. Colonic

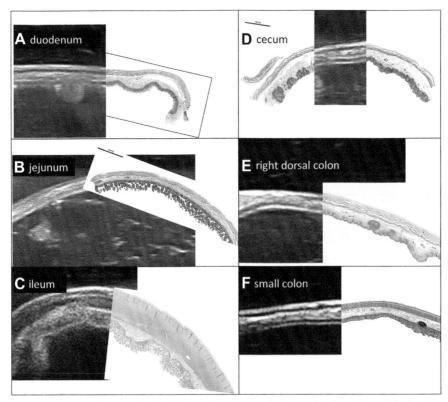

Fig. 2. Composite depicts the histology of segments of the equine intestine with the basic layers (mucosa, submucosa, muscularis, serosa) and corresponding in vitro sonographic appearance of the basic sonographic layers. Inner hyperechoic layer = interface of contents and mucosa, inner hypoechoic layer = mucosa, intermediate echoic layer = submucosa, inner hypoechoic layer = muscularis, outer echoic layer = serosa. In the ileum, the muscularis propria is thicker and the inner and outer muscularis layers separated by an echoic band are more obvious than in the jejunum and duodenum. (A) Dudenum, (B) Jejunum, (C) Ileum, (D) Cecum, (E) Right dorsal colon, (F) Small colon.

displacement or 180° volvulus leads to the medially located vessels becoming sonographically visible laterally adjacent to the body wall. Medial colonic vessels occasionally are visible in their normal location if the large intestine is fluid-filled. It is important to recognize that 2 lateral cecal vessels (lateral cecal vessels and vessels of the cecal arch) can be visible in the normal horse adjacent to the body wall from the middle portion of the right flank caudal to costal arch and coursing cranioventrally. Therefore, 2 or more hypoechoic circular structures situated directly adjacent to the colon wall is the sonographic criteria used to define this abnormality. These vessels are more frequently identified in the middle aspect of the flank but the cranial to caudal, dorsal to ventral location, and the number of intercostal spaces varies considerably[27] (**Fig. 4**). The changes in the diameter of the normal mesenteric vasculature or flow patterns with different diagnoses have not been described.

Manso-Diaz and colleagues[27] reported 34 horses presenting with acute colic associated with large intestinal disease and sonographically visible dilated large colon mesenteric vasculature. The visible vasculature on the right side of the abdomen was associated with a diagnosis of right dorsal displacement of the large colon,

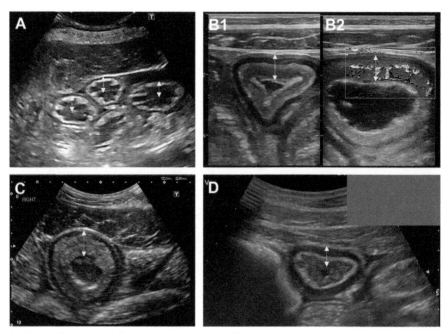

Fig. 3. Small intestinal thickening. Sonogram of a thickened loop of small intestine with a prominent hypoechoic mucosa in a horse with anterior enteritis (*A*). Thickened (*B1*) and hypervascular (*B2*) small intestinal wall with echoic loss of layering of the mucosa and submucosa in a weanling with *Lawsonia intracellularis* infection (*C*). Thickened small intestine with the loss of layering and echoic wall in a horse with a strangulating small intestinal lesion (*D*). Thickened wall with prominent mucosa and muscularis in a horse with lymphoplasmacytic inflammatory bowel disease. *Double headed arrows* mark small intestinal walls (*A-D*).

180° LCV, 540° LCV, or large colon impaction. A 540° LCV is uncommon, and clinical findings of severe pain and shock often preclude transabdominal sonographic evaluation and emergency surgery or euthanasia is indicated. When the vessels were imaged on the left side of the abdomen, left dorsal displacement of the left colon, 180° LCV, or right dorsal displacement of the left colon were the described diagnoses. If the malpositioned vessel was at the dorsal aspect of the left abdomen, left colon displacement was the only diagnosis in this case series. Colonic vessels were imaged bilaterally in one horse with a 180° LCV. Earlier studies had reported that sonographic visualization of colonic mesenteric vessels provided a sensitivity of 67.7%, specificity of 97.9%, positive predictive value of 95.8%, and negative predictive value of 81% for right dorsal displacement or 180° LCV, or both.[26] It is important to recognize that the sonographic identification of colonic vessels adjacent to the body wall does not always necessitate exploratory laparotomy. This sonographic finding may, however, be clinically useful to narrow the differential diagnosis list and to guide therapy in conjunction with other clinical information.

SEVERELY THICKENED LARGE INTESTINE

The sonographic finding of severely thickened large intestine during the evaluation of a horse with acute colic is interesting. The sonographic thickness of the intestine in clinically normal horses and ponies is mean ± SD 1.8 ± 0.03 mm to 4.2 ± 0.3 mm.[28,29] Severe large intestinal thickening (defined as wall thickness ≥9 mm) in the ventral

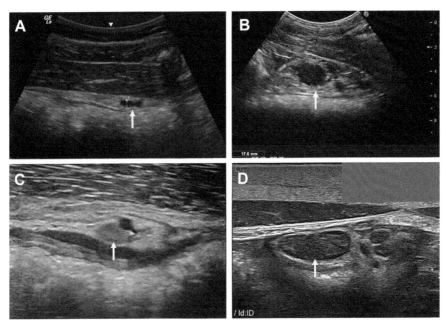

Fig. 4. Mesenteric vasculature and lymph nodes. Normal sonographic appearance of the lateral cecal band (*yellow arrow, A*). Displaced and distended mesenteric vasculature in a horse with colon volvulus (*yellow arrow, B*). Sonographically mild mesenteric lymphadenopathy in a horse with colitis (*white arrow, C*). Sonographically severe mesenteric lymphadenopathy in a horse with peritonitis (*white arrow, D*).

abdomen has been reported as a specific finding for the diagnosis of horses with LCV[30] in a population of horse with acute colic. It is important to recognize that other causes of severe large intestinal thickening have been described including infectious colitis, nonsteroidal anti-inflammatory drugs (NSAID) enteropathy/right dorsal colitis, inflammatory bowel disease, colonic displacement, intestinal neoplasia, or intestinal histoplasmosis. Although these diseases should be distinguishable from an LCV based on clinical presentation, occasionally horses with these diseases can present with acute and moderate-to-severe colic.[31] For this reason, the 100% specificity described by Pease and colleagues[30] for their population, although informative, may not be applicable to all clinical scenarios and the finding of a severely thickened colon cannot always be attributed to LCV (**Fig. 5**).

A controversial finding is the presence of nonsacculated large colon in the left ventral portion of the abdomen as an indication of LCV (180° or 540°). This finding is anatomically logical because these degrees of rotation position the nonsacculated dorsal colon ventrally and the sacculated ventral colon dorsally away from the ventral abdomen.[32] However, the diagnostic accuracy of this finding is uncertain,[33] and it is likely that other clinical scenarios that cause slight rotations, colonic distension, or heavy contents can cause the loss of ventral sacculations (eg, impactions or sand enteropathy among others).

SAND IMPACTIONS AND ENTEROPATHY

Sand impactions are often seen sonographically as a flattened colon in the ventral abdomen with hyperechoic contents that cast an acoustic shadow and reduced or

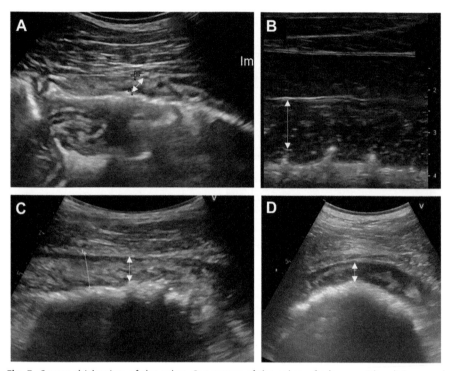

Fig. 5. Severe thickening of the colon. Sonogram of the colon of a horse with colitis caused by salmonellosis (*A*). Sonogram of the colon of a horse with left dorsal displacement that resolved without surgery (*B*). Sonogram of the colon in the cranial abdomen of a horse with a LCV (*C*). Sonogram of the colon present in the caudal abdomen of horse (same horse as in *C*) with a colon volvulus (*D*). Note the severely thickened colon in all images (*yellow arrows*) that is echoic in (*A*) and (*C*), hypoechoic and striated in (*B*), and hypoechoic with echoic submucosal patches in (*D*).

absent motility.[7] The specificity of sonography in detecting sand accumulations has been reported as 87.5% and the sensitivity as 87.5%.[34] Quantifying the amount of sand, however, is best performed radiographically.[34] For this reason, sonography can help increase the index of suspicion about the presence of sand yet cannot replace radiography as a quantitative tool. In the author's experience, a large area of visible sand and a flattened appearance of the colon are useful sonographic characteristics to describe sand accumulation and monitor resolution when radiography is not available. Imaging the colon with high-frequency probes can provide information about the colonic wall thickness and layering pattern. These sonographic characteristics with color flow Doppler interrogation can help determine if enteropathy accompanies the presence of sand. The diagnostic accuracy of this approach is unknown (**Fig. 6**).

LEFT DORSAL DISPLACEMENT OF THE LARGE COLON WITH OR WITHOUT NEPHROSPLENIC LIGAMENT ENTRAPMENT

The inability to see the left kidney sonographically from the left flank has been classically used to diagnose nephrosplenic ligament entrapment of the large colon.[35] Nephrosplenic entrapment and displacement of the large colon lateral to the spleen are

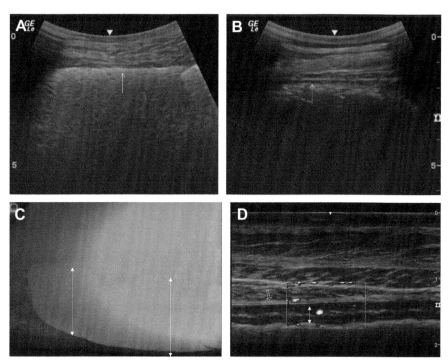

Fig. 6. Sonogram of a horse with sand impaction and enteropathy showing hyperechoic contents (sand) in the colon (A), white single-headed arrow and echoic (normal digesta) in another area of the colon (B), yellow single-headed arrow. The sonographic appearance of the contents suggests sand and the radiograph confirms and quantifies the area of sand (C). The high-frequency sonogram (D) shows the layered wall with mildly prominent submucosa and subjectively mildly increased color flow signal suggesting enteropathy associated with the presence of sand. The white double headed arrow (C) marks the sand dorsoventral height.

collectively referred to as left dorsal displacement of the large colon. Lateral displacements can resolve spontaneously whereas nephrosplenic ligament entrapments more commonly require specific interventions.[36] It has been suggested that if the sonographic appearance of the dorsal aspect of the spleen is obliterated by a gas echo, a diagnosis of nephrosplenic ligament entrapment can be made, whereas if the entire image of the spleen was obscured by gas, lateral displacement of the colon without nephrosplenic entrapment is more likely.[36] A colonic mesenteric vessel is often seen laterally in cases of nephrosplenic ligament entrapment (adjacent to the medial aspect of the spleen or abdominal wall)[27] due to this entrapment being often accompanied by a 180° rotation of the colon. False-positive and false-negative findings exist, and diagnostic accuracy testing is complicated by the lack of a reliable reference method in horses where the displacement resolves without laparotomy. Some horses with other displacements of the large colon, and even LCV can have colon dorsal to the spleen and a nonvisible left kidney chronically and without signs of coli[8] (Fig. 7).

POSTOPERATIVE MONITORING

Sonography may have some applications in monitoring horses postoperatively. The use of sonography to assess intestinal motility, the response to prokinetics, and

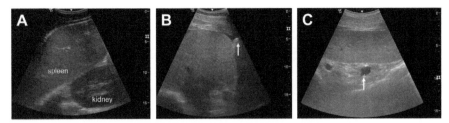

Fig. 7. Sonogram of the normal nephrosplenic area (*A*) with the spleen adjacent to the left kidney. A horse with a nephrosplenic ligament entrapment of the large colon. The colon is dorsal and lateral to the spleen and the dorsal edge of the spleen is not visible (*B, yellow arrow*). A horse with a nephrosplenic entrapment where the malpositioned colonic vessel is adjacent to the medial aspect of the spleen (*C, white arrow*).

the amount of fluid in the stomach seem reliable.[37–39] The number of intercostal spaces in which fluid is observed sonographically is correlated with the volume of obtained reflux (r = 0.77, *P* < .001) in horses with gastrointestinal disease, and the sonographically estimated height of the stomach wall at the 12th intercostal space is

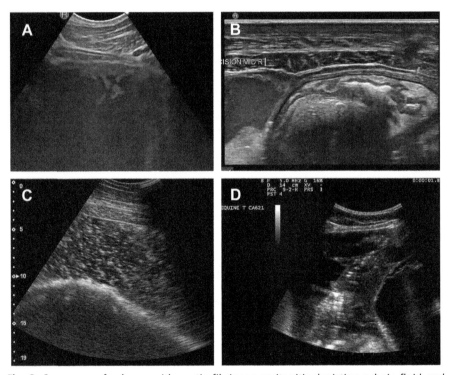

Fig. 8. Sonogram of a horse with septic fibrinous peritonitis depicting echoic fluid and echoic material (fibrin) adhered to the peritoneal lining (*A*). Sonogram of a horse with septic peritonitis depicting echoic fluid and an adhesion between and small intestinal loop and the peritoneal lining (*B*). Sonogram of a horse with peritonitis and ruptured viscus showing a large amount of echoic fluid with large particles (*C*). Sonogram of a horse with septic fibrinous peritonitis due to gastrointestinal rupture showing hypoechoic fluid, echoic materials (fibrin) and hyperechoic echoes of gas adhered to the fibrin (*D*).

correlated with the volume of fluid administered via nasogastric tube in normal hors-es.[38,39] In recent studies, an average of 5.7 to 7.4 L of reflux was obtained in horses with gastric distension secondary to intestinal problems when the fluid-filled stomach was imaged in 5 to 6 intercostal spaces.[38] After administration of 6 L of fluid via naso-gastric tube, the fluid-filled stomach was seen in 2 to 7 intercostal spaces.[40] These findings led the authors to conclude that sonography may be useful clinically to iden-tify horses likely to have gastric reflux although the variability between horses needs to be considered.

The intestinal wall thickness has been monitored in horses after surgical correction of an LCV.[41] In this interesting study, horses that recovered from LCV surgery without signs of multiorgan dysfunction syndrome (MODS) had a significantly shorter period to colon wall involution ($\leq$5 mm) compared with horses diagnosed with MODS (mean $\pm$ standard error 19.6 h $\pm$ 2.5 and 39.7 h $\pm$ 6.7, respectively; $P =$ .006). This is a physiologically interesting finding, informative to the understanding of clinical pro-gression of horses in the postoperative period. However, despite differences in mean thicknesses between groups, the overlap of individual measurements and the lack of association with survival limit its use as a sole criterion in monitoring. Cuevas Ramos and colleagues[42] showed that horses with large or small intestinal disease that did not need resection and anastomosis had small intestinal wall thickness and loop diameter that normalized during the 3 days postoperatively, whereas horses with small intesti-nal pathologic condition needing resection and anastomosis remained abnormal dur-ing these 3 days.

Sonography may be used for an early diagnosis of incisional infections. A high sensi-tivity (100%) and specificity (88%)[43–45] have been described for this application when discharge of the wound is used as diagnostic criteria for clinical incisional infection.

The sonographic signs in horses with septic peritonitis include corrugation of the small and/or large intestinal walls, increased or echoic peritoneal fluid, heteroechoic flocculent peritoneal fluid with dorsal accumulations of free gas in the case of gastro-intestinal rupture, mesenteric lymphadenopathy and, masses or abscesses.[7] It is interesting to recognize that increased free peritoneal fluid was only found in 17 out of 25 cases of confirmed peritonitis in a recent case series[46] (**Fig. 8**).

SUMMARY

The use of abdominal ultrasonography provides useful diagnostic and monitoring in-formation in the evaluation of horses with colic in the field, hospital, and postoperative setting. Sonographic findings should be interpreted in light of clinical signs and other diagnostic tests. During the last 4 decades, veterinarians have created a large body of literature informative to clinicians using sonography in horses with colic. It is likely that this technique will continue to advance in the near future as sonography becomes more available and affordable and newer generations of veterinarians receive more and earlier training in sonography.

DISCLOSURE

The authors have no finical disclosures related to this article.

ACKNOWLEDGMENTS

The authors want to acknowledge Kari Bevevino for contributing to figures in this article.

REFERENCES

1. Klohnen A, Vachon AM, Fischer AT. Use of diagnostic ultrasonography in horses with signs of acute abdominal pain. J Am Vet Med Assoc 1996;209:1597–601.
2. Busoni V, De Busscher V, Lopez D, et al. Evaluation of a protocol for fast localised abdominal sonography of horses (FLASH) admitted for colic. Vet J 2011;188: 77–82.
3. Haardt H, Romero AE, Boysen SR, et al. Incidence of superficial abdominal organ identification is similar using high-frequency linear (transrectal) and low-frequency curvilinear (abdominal) transducers in clinically healthy horses: A pilot study. Vet Radiol Ultrasound 2022;345–52.
4. Williams S, Cooper J, Freeman S. Evaluation of normal findings using a detailed and focused technique for transcutaneous abdominal ultrasonography in the horse. BMC Vet Res 2014;10(1):S5.
5. Deacon LJ, Reef VB, Leduc L, et al. Pocket-sized ultrasound versus traditional ultrasound images in equine imaging: a pictorial essay. J Equine Vet Sci 2021; 104:103672.
6. Eberhardt C, Schwarzwald CC. Focused cardiac ultrasound examination in the emergency and critical care horse: Training for non-specialist veterinarians and evaluation of proficiency. J Vet Intern Med 2022;36:1471–80.
7. Slack, J. (2012). Abdominal sonographic evaluation. In Practical guide to equine colic, L.L. Southwood (Ed.). Available at: https://doi.org/10.1002/9781118704783.ch12.
8. le Jeune S, Whitcomb MB. Ultrasound of the equine acute abdomen. Vet Clin North Am Equine Pract 2014;30(2):353–viii.
9. Scharner D, Bankert J, Brehm W. Vergleich rektaler und sonographischer Untersuchungsbefunde bei der Kolik des Pferdes [Comparison of the findings of rectal examination and ultrasonographic findings in horses with colic]. Tierarztl Prax Ausg G Grosstiere Nutztiere 2015;43:278–86.
10. Cribb NC, Arroyo LG. Techniques and Accuracy of Abdominal Ultrasound in Gastrointestinal Diseases of Horses and Foals. Vet Clin North Am Equine Pract 2018;34(1):25–38.
11. Safari S, Baratloo A, Elfil M, et al. Evidence Based Emergency Medicine; Part 4: Pre-test and Post-test Probabilities and Fagan's nomogram. Emerg (Tehran) 2016;4:48–51.
12. Beccati F, Pepe M, Gialletti R, et al. Is there a statistical correlation betweenultrasonographicfindings and definitive diagnosis in horses withacute abdominal pain? Equine Vet J 2011;43:98–105.
13. Fairburn A. Fast vs. detailed ultrasound scan for decision making in colic. Equine Vet Educ 2017;29:466–7.
14. Mirle E, Wogatzki A, Kunzmann R, et al. Correlation between capillary oxygen saturation and small intestinal wall thickness in the equine colic patient. Vet Rec Open 2017;4:e000197.
15. Bevevino KE, Edwards JF, Cohen ND, et al. Ex vivo comparison of ultrasonographic intestinal wall layering with histology in horses: A feasibilty study. Vet Radiol Ultrasound 2021;62:316–30.
16. Diana A, Freccero F, Giancola F, et al. Ex vivo ultrasonographic and histological morphometry of small intestinal wall layers in horses. Vet Radiol Ultrasound 2022; 63:353–63.

17. Epelman M, Daneman A, Navarro OM, et al. Necrotizing enterocolitis: Review of state-of the- art imaging findings with pathologic correlation. Radiographics 2007;27:285–305.
18. Faingold R, Daneman A, Tomlinson G, et al. Necrotizing enterocolitis: Assessment of bowel viability with color doppler US. Radiology 2005;235:587–94.
19. de Solis CN, Palmer JE, Boston RC, et al. The importance of ultrasonographic pneumatosis intestinalis in equine neonatal gastrointestinal disease. Equine Vet J Suppl 2012;(41):64–8.
20. Page AE, Fallon LH, Bryant UK, et al. Acute deterioration and death with necrotizing enteritis associated with Lawsonia intracellularis in 4 weanling horses. J Vet Intern Med 2012;26:1476–80.
21. Abraham M, Reef VB, Sweeney RW, et al. Gastrointestinal ultrasonography of normal Standardbred neonates and frequency of asymptomatic intussusceptions. J Vet Intern Med 2014;28(5):1580–6.
22. Reginelli A, Genovese E, Cappabianca S, et al. Intestinal Ischemia: US-CT findings correlations. Crit Ultrasound J 2013;5(Suppl 1):S7.
23. Danse EM, Kartheuser A, Paterson HM, et al. Color Doppler sonography of small bowel wall changes in 21 consecutive cases of acute mesenteric ischemia. JBR-BTR 2009;92:202–6.
24. Sasaki T, Kunisaki R, Kinoshita H, et al. Doppler ultrasound findings correlate with tissue vascularity and inflammation in surgical pathology specimens from patients with small intestinal Crohn's disease. BMC Res Notes 2014;7:363.
25. Grenager NS, Durham MG. Ultrasonographic evidence of colonic mesenteric vessels as an indicator of right dorsal displacement of the large colon in 13 horses. Equine Vet J Suppl 2011;(39):153–5.
26. Ness SL, Bain FT, Zantingh AJ, et al. Ultrasonographic visualization of colonic mesenteric vasculature as an indicator of large colon right dorsal displacement or 180° volvulus (or both) in horses. Can Vet J 2012;53:378–82.
27. Manso-Díaz G, Bolt DM, López-Sanromán J. Ultrasonographic visualisation of the mesenteric vasculature in horses with large colon colic. Vet Rec 2020;186:491.
28. Epstein K, Short D, Parente E, et al. Gastrointestinal ultrasonography in normal adult ponies. Vet Radiol Ultrasound 2008;49:282–6.
29. Bithell S, Habershon-Butcher JL, Bowen M, et al. Repeatability and reproducibility of transabdominal ultrasonographic intestinal wall thickness measurements in Thoroughbred horses. Vet Radiol Ultrasound 2010;51:647–51.
30. Pease AP, Scrivani PV, Erb HN, et al. Accuracy of increased large-intestine wall thickness during ultrasonography for diagnosing large-colon torsion in 42 horses. Vet Radiol Ultrasound 2004;45:220–4.
31. Biscoe EW, Whitcomb MB, Vaughan B, et al. Clinical features and outcome in horses with severe large intestinal thickening diagnosed with transabdominal ultrasonography: 25 cases (2003-2010). J Am Vet Med Assoc 2018;253:108–16.
32. Abutarbush SM. Use of ultrasonography to diagnose large colon volvulus in horses. J Am Vet Med Assoc 2006;228:409–13.
33. Pease A, Cook V, Jones S, et al. Views conclusions in ultrasound study as unsupported. J Am Vet Med Assoc 2006;228:1011–2.
34. Korolainen R, Ruohoniemi M. Reliability of ultrasonography compared to radiography in revealing intestinal sand accumulations in horses. Equine Vet J 2002;34:499–504.
35. Hardy J, Minton M, Robertson JT, et al. Nephrosplenic entrapment in the horse: a retrospective study of 174 cases. Equine Vet J Suppl 2000;95–7.

36. Santschi EM, Slone DE Jr, Frank WM 2nd. Use of ultrasound in horses for diagnosis of left dorsal displacement of the large colon and monitoring its nonsurgical correction. Vet Surg 1993;22:281–4.

37. Beder NA, Mourad AA, Aly MA. Ultrasonographic evaluation of the effects of the administration of neostigmine and metoclopramide on duodenal, cecal, and colonic contractility in Arabian horses: A comparative study. Vet World 2020;13: 2447–51.

38. Bankert J, Winter K, Scharner D. Vergleich zwischen sonografischen Untersuchungsbefunden am Magen und gewonnener Refluxmenge beim Warmblutpferd [Comparison between gastric ultrasonography findings and the obtained reflux amounts in warmblood horses - First results]. Tierarztl Prax Ausg G Grosstiere Nutztiere 2019;47:366–71.

39. Lores M, Stryhn H, McDuffee L, et al. Transcutaneous ultrasonographic evaluation of gastric distension with fluid in horses. Am J Vet Res 2007;68:153–7.

40. Epstein KL, Hall MD. Effect of Nasogastric Tube Placement, Manipulation, and Fluid Administration on Transcutaneous Ultrasound Visualization and Assessment of Stomach Position in Healthy Unfed and Fed Horses. Animals 2022;12:3433.

41. Sheats MK, Cook VL, Jones SL, et al. Use of ultrasound to evaluate outcome following colic surgery for equine large colon volvulus. Equine Vet J 2010;42: 47–52.

42. Cuevas-Ramos G, Domenech L, Prades M. Small Intestine Ultrasound Findings on Horses Following Exploratory Laparotomy, Can We Predict Postoperative Reflux? Animals (Basel) 2019;9:1106.

43. Wilson DA, Badertscher RR, Boero MJ, et al. Ultrasonographic evaluation of the healing of ventral midline abdominal incisions in the horse. Equine Vet J 1989; 21(S7):107–10.

44. Shearer TR, Holcombe SJ, Valberg SJ. Incisional infections associated with ventral midline celiotomy in horses. J Vet Emerg Crit Care 2020;30:136–48.

45. Protopapas A, Marr CM, Archer FJ, et al. Ultrasonographic assessment and factors associated with incisional infection and dehiscence following celiotomy in horses. Vet Surg 2000;29:289.

46. Arndt S, Kilcoyne I, Vaughan B, et al. Clinical and diagnostic findings, treatment, and short- and long-term survival in horses with peritonitis: 72 cases (2007-2017). Vet Surg 2021;50:323–35.

Early Identification of Intestinal Strangulation

Why It Is Important and How to Make an Early Diagnosis

Louise L. Southwood, BVSc, PhD

KEYWORDS

- Colic • Laparotomy • Celiotomy • Equine • Strangulation • Ischemia • Reperfusion
- Survival

KEY POINTS

- Early diagnosis and surgical treatment improves survival, decreases complications, and decreases expense associated with treatment.
- A strangulating obstruction should be ruled out based on diagnostic tests in any older horse presenting for colic.
- Avoid enteral fluids in horses with a suspected small intestinal strangulating obstruction.
- Horses with small intestinal strangulating obstructions often have desiccated contents of the left ventral colon often mistaken for a pelvic flexure impaction.
- Prognosis is best determined at surgery in horses presenting with acute and persistent colic signs.

Importance of early diagnosis

The most important contributing factor to a successful outcome for horses with intestinal strangulation is early identification and prompt surgical correction of the lesion. Irreversible intestinal injury occurs within hours of strangulation. Death can occur within 3 to 4 hours of a large colon volvulus (LCV) developing. In one study of horses presenting to a surgical facility with an LCV, longer colic duration was associated with higher odds of death.[1] Compared to horses with a colic duration of 2 or fewer hours, horses with a colic duration of 2 to 4 hours had increased odds of death of 3.0 (95% confidence interval [CI] 1.3–7.1) and with a colic duration over 4 hours odds of death of 11.6 (95% CI 5.1–26.5).[1] These data highlight the importance of early referral and the critical need for efficiency following hospital admission to surgical resolution of the LCV.

Clinical Studies New Bolton Center, University of Pennsylvania, 382 West Street Road, Kennett Square, PA 19348, USA
E-mail address: southwoo@vet.upenn.edu

Vet Clin Equine 39 (2023) 211–227
https://doi.org/10.1016/j.cveq.2023.03.007
0749-0739/23/© 2023 Elsevier Inc. All rights reserved.

Although it is arguable that, distinct from the situation with LCV, the segment of the strangulated small intestine or small colon can be resected making early diagnosis less critical, in fact, early referral and surgical correction of horses with these lesions is just as vital to a successful outcome. Often small colon strangulations, most commonly a strangulating pedunculated lipoma, affects the aboral small colon and cranial rectum with a delay in surgical treatment leading to an inoperable section of bowel affected. Similarly, ileal ischemia (**Fig. 1**) and subsequent necrosis can complicate a jejunocecostomy procedure. In one study, horses with a small intestinal strangulating obstruction undergoing surgery sufficiently early that the bowel was viable and resection and anastomosis unnecessary, had a better outcome compared to horses undergoing intestinal resection.[2,3] That being said, horses requiring intestinal resection and anastomosis can still do very well. Recently reported survival rates have exceeded 80%.[2–4] In one study, survival to hospital discharge for jejunojejunostomy, jejunoileostomy, and jejunocecostomy was 89%, 88%, and 87%, respectively, excluding horses euthanized due to salmonellosis. For horses surviving to hospital discharge, subsequent survival to 1 year was 97% for jejunojejunostomy, 100% for jejunoileostomy, and 83% for jejunocecostomy. Only five horses were euthanized due to colic in the first year. Four of the five horses had a jejunocecostomy one of which had the jejunocecostomy performed during a repeat celiotomy. The fifth horse also had a repeat celiotomy following a jejunojejunostomy. Therefore, all horses euthanized due to colic in the first year had either a repeat celiotomy or jejunocecostomy.[4] Therefore, althougha it is optimal to operate sufficiently early not to require a resection, if circumstances are such that a resection of affected bowel is necessary, the horse can do well post-resection.

An important yet often overlooked feature is the function of the intestinal segment orad to the strangulating obstruction and subsequent resection and anastomosis site (**Fig. 2**). In a series of experimental studies using jejunal distention and decompression as well as ischemia-reperfusion models, Dabareiner and colleagues[5–9] demonstrated that intraluminal distention caused low-flow ischemia as well as mesothelial cell loss, moderate serosal edema, lymphatic dilation, and erythrocyte infiltration with a further increase in these histological changes following decompression. An increase in vascular permeability was observed in addition to neutrophil infiltration adjacent to the serosal basement membrane, with degranulating neutrophils observed migrating through damaged serosal capillaries into the serosa and longitudinal muscle. A fibrinous exudate covered the damaged serosal basement membrane associated with swelling, vacuolation, and mitochondrial damage of capillary endothelial cells. The jejunal seromuscular layer showed more extensive evidence of serosal injury

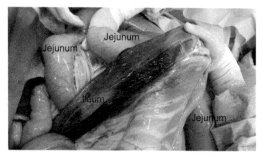

Fig. 1. A geriatric Quarter Horse gelding with an acute onset of colic. The horse had a pedunculated lipoma strangulating the ileum. The affected bowel extended to the ileocecal orifice; the most affected segment of ileum could not be exteriorized. Although there are several surgical options, the owner requested an uncomplicated recovery and the horse was euthanized.

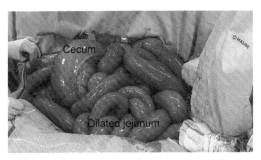

Fig. 2. Multiple dilated loops of jejunum. The distention can lead to ischemia and intestinal injury. Decompression of the bowel requires manipulation causing further injury. Intestinal edema, hemorrhage, and inflammation potentially lead to ileus and adhesions. Although horses do often recover successfully following decompression, early referral and surgical treatment and avoiding enteral fluids in horses with a suspected small intestinal obstruction can prevent extensive decompression and improve recovery.

compared to the ascending (large) colon after experiencing the same periods of ischemia and reperfusion. Similarly, Gerard and colleagues reported that the oral resection margins had serosal hemorrhage, edema, and an increase in neutrophils in horses with a small intestinal strangulating obstruction.[10] More recently, and at a molecular level, an elevation of ubiquitin in the enterocytes' nucleus, HSP70, in the smooth muscle cells' nucleus and c-jun in enteric neurons was observed at the oral border of jejunal resection margins.[11] The activation of these protective and degenerative pathways provide evidence of cellular stress potentially triggering protein damage in the apparently healthy non-resected tissue in case of strangulation obstruction.[11] In a related study, the smooth muscle layer from the oral resection margin showed degradation specifically vacuolar degeneration, and at a molecular level, a decrease in myosin protein and an increase in desmin and heat shock protein 20.[12] Intestinal injury in these bowel segments as evidenced by edema, hemorrhage, and inflammation likely cause ileus, anastomosis complications, and adhesion formation prolonging hospitalization, increasing expense of treatment, leading to problems with recurrent colic, and ultimately euthanasia. Findings from these clinical and research studies reinforce the critical need for early surgical management of horses with strangulating obstruction, particularly small intestinal strangulating obstruction, prior to injury occurring from distention orad to the obstruction.

Of note is that administration of enteral fluids to horses with a small intestinal strangulating obstruction markedly exacerbates distention-induced ischemia, requires more bowel manipulation during surgery to achieve decompression, and worsens the aforementioned histological and molecular changes in the oral bowel segment. Enteral fluid administration in these horses should be avoided. Furthermore, surgeons should resect sufficient bowel such that the anastomosis is performed in both grossly viable and functional bowel. Achieving this may require resecting an additional 1 to 1.5 m of bowel; however, it decreases complications and potentially improves survival. Yet this may not be feasible in horses administered enteral fluids or with a prolonged colic duration.

HOW TO MAKE AN EARLY DIAGNOSIS

Early recognition of a horse with intestinal strangulation is essential to enhance recovery of these critical patients with much information being attainable with thorough history taking and meticulous physical examination. Diagnostic procedures such as transabdominal ultrasonography and peritoneal fluid analysis are used to solidify the diagnosis in some instances where the intestinal strangulations is not obvious or when surgery is not an option to support a decision for humane euthanasia. Although it is easy to make the aforementioned statements, the information provided below will hopefully aid with clinical application.

Signalment, History, and Physical Examination

Signalment is import when considering a particular equid's propensity for a strangulating obstruction. In one study, using light breeds as a reference, ponies/miniature horses had decreased odds of colon displacements and, importantly, ponies had higher odds of having small intestinal strangulation by a pedunculated lipoma with an odds ratio of 2.3 (95% CI 1.3–4.1). Miniature horses had decreased odds of strangulating small intestinal lesions and draft breeds increased odds of cecal disease.[13] In the latter study, the odds of having a strangulating small intestinal lesion, increased with aging (odds ratio 1.1 [95% CI 1.1–1.2]); meaning that for every 10 years increase in age, the odds of having a small intestinal strangulation, primarily strangulation by a pedunculated lipoma, increased by 100%.[13] Age and breed are typically confounded, with a higher percentage of Arabian and pony breeds in geriatric age ranges.[14] Two studies reported that geriatric horses (15 years and older) had an odds ratio of 2.05 (95% CI 1.25–3.38) for strangulating obstruction[15] and 2.57 (95% CI 1.19–5.54) for small intestinal strangulating obstruction.[14] A strangulating obstruction, therefore, should be suspected, and the diagnosis thoroughly excluded, in any horse in their teens or older showing signs of colic. It is important to communicate with clients that geriatric horses with intestinal strangulation do not have a poor prognosis[15] and if the horse is otherwise healthy, they can live and perform successfully post-colic surgery.

Broodmares with an acute onset of moderate to severe colic signs and abdominal distention are highly likely to have an LCV. This is particularly so for 8- to 10-year-olds thoroughbred mares and for mares during the first 1 to 3 months post-partum.[16–19] In fact, this is one emergency where referral without first being evaluated by a primary care veterinarian is indicated assuming the owner or caregiver is able to safely transport the mare to a surgical facility. It is important to recognize that non-broodmares and geldings as well as stallions can also develop an LCV with almost half of the horses in one study population being geldings or stallions.[20] As mentioned, moderate to severe signs of pain, pain unresponsive to analgesia, and abdominal distention, particularly in a broodmare are indications for immediate referral.

Colic duration should always be taken into account when evaluating horses with colic particularly when interpreting clinical findings. In a recent study using a statistical model to predict intestinal strangulation, colic duration (OR 95 [95% CI 0.90–0.99]) was included in the final multivariable model with age, reflux, pain at admission, abdominal palpation per rectum findings, and the difference between peritoneal and blood lactate concentrations.[21] Interpretation of these findings is that for every 1 hour *decrease* in colic duration, the odds of having a strangulating obstruction increases by 5% for horses with a given age, reflux volume, pain category, palpation per rectum finding, and peritoneal fluid analysis (more details below).[21] Specific signs being shown by the horse and any change in signs over time should be part of the history for any horse described by an owner as having colic.

Any previous colic episodes and the diagnosis should be considered including previous colic surgery. It is not uncommon for horses with a particular cause of colic, such as a colonic displacement or impaction, to have recurrence of that problem. Multiple colic episodes in the preceding 12 months were identified as a risk factor for having an

LCV in one UK study (OR 8.73 [95% CI 1.78–42.74]).[17] Anecdotally, geriatric horses presenting with acute colic and diagnosed with a strangulating pedunculated lipoma have no prior history of colic. This observation is supported by the finding that horses which *did not* have a small intestinal strangulation had higher odds of a previous history of colic (OR 12 [95% CI 1.5–95]).[22]

Although there is much overlap in specific physical examination finding between horses with a non-strangulating and strangulating obstruction, there are several key findings that should prompt pursuing diagnostic tests to rule-in or rule-out a strangulating obstruction. Horses with intestinal strangulation are moderately to severely painful at least at some point in time following lesion development. Horses with an LCV are usually severely painful, unresponsive to analgesia, and have marked abdominal distention. Although the horse may not be demonstrating colic signs at the time of veterinary examination, observation of abrasions on head, tuber coxae, or limbs particularly over bony prominences can be a key finding for recognition of the potential for a strangulating lesion (**Fig. 3**). Older horses often display more subtle signs of pain such as occasional flank watching and pawing. Strained or dilated nostrils and tachypnea are often seen. Grimace, a vacant expression, or lack of concern for surroundings (**Figs. 4** and **5**) is often observed. The horse grimace scale and other pain scales have been described[23,24] and may be helpful in assessing older horses in particular, and prompting further diagnostic evaluation with transabdominal ultrasonography and peritoneal fluid analysis. Evaluation of pain should always be made taking into consideration any analgesic medication given and preferably before administration of analgesia including sedation. Some horses may not show pain during an examination; however, when moved to a bedded stall signs become apparent. Moving a horse to a bedded stall earlier during an examination and before administering analgesia can help with pain assessment (**Fig. 6**).

Horses may have only mild tachycardia (48–56 beats/minutes) or even a heart rate within normal limits. As mentioned above, tachypnea is often observed. Rectal temperature is typically within normal limits and mucous membrane moistness and color are also often normal in horses with a small intestinal strangulating obstruction. Mucous membranes, however, may become tacky, injected with a more prolonged capillary refill time with longer colic duration. Borborygmi are often decreased to absent; however, normal borborygmi do not mean that the horse does not have a strangulating obstruction. In one survey, horses with colic having decreased or absent borborygmi had higher odds of needing surgery compared to horses with normal borborygmi (OR 7.55 [95% CI 1.07–331.35])[25]

Medications administered should always be considered when evaluating vital signs. Furthermore, it is best to evaluate any horse presenting for colic prior to sedation whenever possible because a lot of important clinical information is lost once the horse is sedated. In the aforementioned survey,[25] constant pain (OR 96.48 [95% CI 14.38-∞]) and the need for a second analgesic (OR 14.89 [95% CI 4.7–56.4]) were the two other significant risk factors for the horse having a surgical lesion.

Often it is not safe or necessary to perform abdominal palpation on horses with an LCV because of the severity of the horse's colic signs necessitating surgery (or euthanasia). On palpation per rectum, horses with small intestinal strangulating obstructions often have desiccated contents of the left ventral colon which is often mistaken for a pelvic flexure impaction. Sequestration of enteral secretions in the oral portion of the gastrointestinal tract leads to dehydration of the colonic contents creating somewhat of a pseudo-impaction. Identification of dilated small intestine should raise suspicion of a strangulating obstruction. In the multivariable model mentioned above,[21] horses having small intestinal distention on palpation per rectum had odds of 29.54 (95%

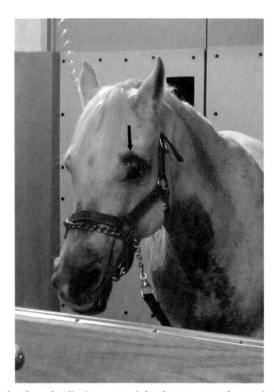

Fig. 3. The horse developed colic signs overnight that were unobserved. At presentation to the hospital the following morning, the horse was not demonstrating classic colic signs. However, there were multiple abrasions to the head (*arrow*), obvious nostril flare or strained nostrils, and the horse was sweating and had muscle fasciculations. At surgery, a diagnosis of strangulating obstruction affecting at least 80% of the small intestine was identified. Humane euthanasia was recommended.

CI 6.33–137) of having a strangulating obstruction. Of note is that the latter study was performed in a hospital with a very low prevalence of ileal impaction (see Peritoneal Fluid Analysis). Strangulating obstruction of the small colon is uncommon; however, approximately 10% of strangulating pedunculated lipomas involve the small colon. These older horses often have abdominal distention. On palpation per rectum, dilated small colon distinguishable by its broad antimesenteric and prominent mesenteric bands is often identified. Frequently the lipoma pedicle can be felt encircling the aboral small colon-cranial rectum.

Reflux on nasogastric intubation is associated with either functional or mechanical obstruction, the latter of which may be strangulating or non-strangulating. Functional obstructions are most commonly ileus or enteritis, most often proximal enteritis. The volume of reflux is greater for horses with a more orad obstruction, particularly in horses with a short colic duration. Horses with proximal enteritis (or primary ileus) often have large volumes of reflux, by definition.[26,27] Strangulating small intestinal obstructions more commonly affect the aboral jejunum and ileum and it takes time for fluid to accumulate and lead to reflux on nasogastric intubation. In fact, in the aforementioned multivariable model,[21] for every 1 L *decrease* in reflux volume, the odds of intestinal strangulation increased by 15% (OR 0.85 [95% CI 0.77–0.94]) for a given age, colic duration, pain score, and palpation per rectum finding.

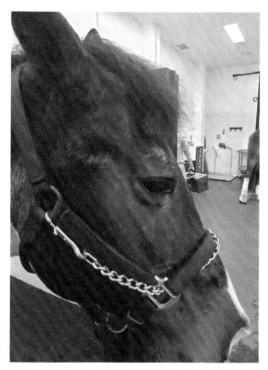

Fig. 4. A geriatric gelding presenting for colic. Similar to the horse in **Fig. 3**, he was not demonstrating classic colic signs; however, he had a small abrasion on his head, strained and dilated nostrils, a vacant expression, and lack of interest in surroundings.

Importantly, all historical and clinical findings must be taken into consideration when deciding if a horse may or may not have an intestinal strangulating obstruction. Geography should also be considered when interpreting these findings. If there is any indication that the horse may have an intestinal strangulating obstruction based on signalment, history, pain, physical examination, palpation per rectum, or reflux, a more detailed evaluation should be pursued to rule out a strangulating lesion unless the horse is persistently painful in which instance emergency surgery is indicated.

Transabdominal Sonography

With the development and clinical evaluation of techniques such as Fast Localized Abdominal Sonography of Horses (FLASH), rapid identification of dilated small intestine (**Figs. 7** and **8**) which, in conjunction with regional differences in lesion occurrence and other clinical signs, is used to increase the likelihood of identifying a horse with intestinal strangulation early. FLASH is similar in concept to the Focused Assessment with Sonography in Trauma (FAST) protocol used in human patients. The FLASH protocol focuses on seven topographical areas (1) ventral abdomen; (2) gastric area (left cranioventral); (3) renosplenic area (left flank); (4) left middle third of the abdomen; (5) duodenal area (right); (6) right middle third of the abdomen; and (7) cranioventral thorax.[28] The FLASH protocol was useful for identifying an increased volume of peritoneal fluid and dilated small intestinal loops.[28] Identification of dilated small intestinal loops had positive and negative predictive values of 89% and 81%, respectively, for detecting a surgical lesion.[28] It is important to keep in mind that such findings are dependent

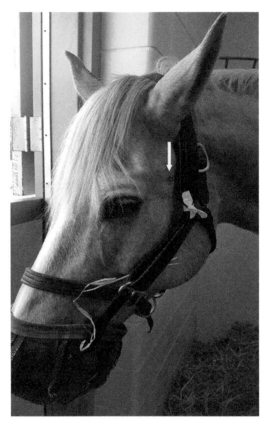

Fig. 5. This horse had an unremarkable physical examination on presentation for colic. He was noted, however, to have a small abrasion on his head (*arrow*), and when placed in a stall, stood at the window with his ears back, his head below the window, and did not respond to his surroundings. The abrasion and his demeanor raised concern for a strangulating obstruction.

on the study population. The inguinal region can also be useful for identifying dilated and thickened small intestine. Similarly, in another study, distended, amotile small intestinal loops were associated with a strangulating small intestinal obstruction.[29] An increase in peritoneal fluid volume, dilated small intestine with abnormal motility, and thickened small intestine were associated with a small intestinal lesion.[29] In the latter study,[29] a thick large colon was associated with an LCV similar to the study by Pease and colleagues.[30] Most horses with LCV, however, are markedly painful and distended and sonography is unnecessary. Furthermore, occasionally horses with severe colitis can present similarly to an LCV and these horses have a thick large colon on sonographic evaluation making this procedure less useful for distinguishing LCV from colitis. See Chapter 3: Abdominal sonographic evaluation: in the field, at the hospital, and after surgery.

As with any test, the value of the results are dependent on the skill of the operator, quality of image obtained, and the experience of the clinician interpreting the findings. Importantly, a negative finding or the sonographic findings deemed within normal limits, does not completely rule-out an intestinal strangulation.

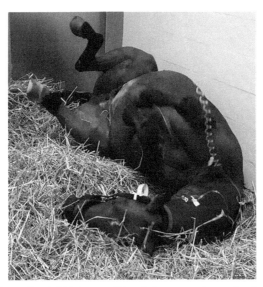

Fig. 6. The horse from **Fig. 1**. This horse did not show any signs of colic and had a normal physical examination at hospital admission. The horse was moved to a stall and began to show obvious signs consistent with a strangulating obstruction (persistent rolling).

Point-of-Care Laboratory Data

Although there have been several studies evaluating various plasma or blood and peritoneal laboratory values to diagnose surgical or strangulation lesions in horses presenting with colic,[31–39] values that can be obtained at the point-of-care tend to

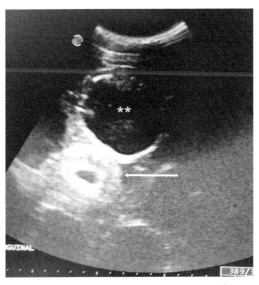

Fig. 7. Point-of-care transabdominal ultrasonographic image of horse in **Fig. 4** showing dilated (*asterisks*) and thickened (*arrow*) small intestine. A large volume of serosanguineous peritoneal fluid was obtained on abdominocentesis. Surgery was not an option for this horse and humane euthanasia was recommended.

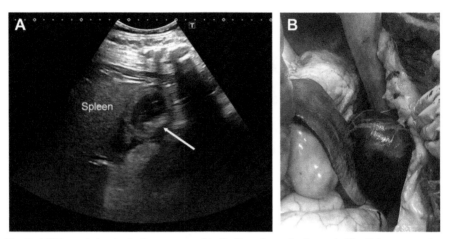

Fig. 8. (*A*) Transabdominal ultrasonographic findings from the horse in **Fig. 5** demonstrating one loop of dilated and thickened small intestine in the left cranioventral abdomen (*arrow*). Surgery was not an option for this horse. He eventually began to show colic signs and was diagnosed with a gastrosplenic ligament entrapment on necropsy (*B*).

be most economical, convenient, and efficient. Point-of-care analyzers should be meticulously maintained and validated to avoid spurious results. When reviewing the literature, it is critical to differentiate between a statistical association and the predictive value of a test. This means that while there may be a significant association between a particular variable and the diagnosis of a strangulating obstruction if there is a lot of variability or overlap between horses with strangulating and non-strangulation obstructions, it is unlikely to be predictive of an intestinal strangulation. Furthermore, most information provided in the literature on variables associated with or used to predict intestinal strangulation is obtained from tertiary referral hospitals and care must be taken with extrapolating to a primary care setting or even other hospital populations.

Packed cell volume (PCV) and total solids (TS) are measured point-of-care as long as a centrifuge and refractometer are available. PCV and TS are useful for providing some prognostic information at the extreme values (eg, it is difficult to give an owner a good prognosis for an uncomplicated recovery for a horse presenting with acute and persistent colic with a PCV of 67% and a TS of 5.8 g/dL). Notwithstanding, it is not necessarily useful for early identification of intestinal strangulation. Prognosis is best determined at surgery for most horses presenting with acute colic.

Horses with a small intestinal obstruction can develop hypochloremic metabolic alkalosis. Point-of-care chemistry analyzers allow clinicians access to easy and inexpensive measurement of electrolyte concentrations and acid–base status. Although the association between a hypochloremic metabolic alkalosis is not diagnostic for an intestinal strangulation per se, observation of this abnormality should prompt further diagnostic tests such as transabdominal sonography and peritoneal fluid analysis.

Blood glucose is tightly regulated between 80 and 120 mg/dL (4.4–7.2 mmol/L) by insulin and glucagon. A decrease in insulin production and an increase in insulin resistance can lead to hyperglycemia in adult horses. Stress, sepsis, systemic inflammatory response syndrome (SIRS)/endotoxemia, and pain can all lead to failure to maintain blood glucose within an acceptable range. Although alpha-2 agonists such as xylazine HCl and detomidine HCl can increase blood glucose concentration, the increase was modest for xylazine (<150 mg/dL, dose rate 1.1 mg/kg) and detomidine (<170 mg/dL, dose rate 30 μg/kg) in normal horses and horses with insulin dysregulation.[40] Admission hyperglycemia is common in horses with colic.[41–43] A mean blood glucose of 155 mg/dL was observed in one study of horses presenting for colic.[42] Blood glucose concentration is associated inversely with survival.[41,42] Hyperglycemia also has a strong association with strangulating obstruction.[41,44] Blood glucose concentration was associated with surgical, small intestinal, and strangulating lesions in one study[41]; however, the predictive value was not calculated. Although a blood glucose concentration within reference range does not rule out an intestinal strangulation, diagnostic tests such as peritoneal fluid analysis should be performed in horses presenting with hyperglycemia, particularly moderate to marked hyperglycemia (>150 mg/dL).

Blood L-lactate (lactate) concentration is not as precisely controlled as blood glucose concentration. Normal blood lactate concentration is < 1 mmol/L (albeit some reports utilize <2 mmol/L as a reference value). Signalment should be considered when interpreting blood lactate concentration.[45,46] Blood lactate concentrations in ponies with large intestinal disease, non-strangulating lesions, undergoing medical treatment, and surviving were significantly higher than in horses in the same categories.[45] In the latter study, the median (range) blood lactate concentrations on admission were higher in ponies (2.8 [0.7–18.0] mmol/L) than in horses (1.6 [0.4–8.1] mmol/L) and, unlike horses, for ponies, there were no differences in blood lactate concentrations between ponies with medical versus surgical lesions, strangulating versus non-strangulating lesions, and survivors versus nonsurvivors. A marked increase in blood lactate concentration (>10 mmol/L) is associated with a grave prognosis for survival in horses and, in one study, no horses with an LCV and blood lactate concentration >10.6 mmol/dL survived.[47] Blood lactate concentration can be highly variable and while an association with strangulating obstruction in horses has been identified (median [range]: non-strangulating 1.2 [0.4–7.4] mmol/L vs strangulating 3.0 [0.8–8.1] mmol/L),[45] it is not necessarily predictive because of the wide variation and overlap between horses with and without intestinal strangulation. Peritoneal fluid L-lactate (lactate) concentration is a better indication of intestinal strangulation than blood lactate concentration.[48]

Peritoneal Fluid Analysis

Abdominocentesis is performed aseptically in a location to the right of the ventral midline using an 18-gauge needle or a teat cannula.[49] Peritoneal fluid is evaluated based on its color, clarity, and volume as well as the nucleated cell count (NCC), total protein (TP), and lactate concentration. Note that TP and lactate concentration can be measured using a point-of-care refractometer or lactate meter.[48,50] Normal peritoneal fluid is yellow, clear, and a small volume (<10 mL) is usually obtained. The normal NCC is < 10 × 10^6 cells/μL (and in most horses <5 × 10^6 cells/uL) and TP < 2.5 g/dL. Serosanguineous peritoneal fluid, particularly if it is a large volume, is strongly associated with the need for surgical treatment.[51,52] In one study,[51] 98% (47/48) of serosanguineous peritoneal samples were from surgical cases; sensitivity, specificity, positive and negative predictive values of serosanguineous peritoneal fluid for determining the need for surgery were 48%, 99%, 98%, and 64%, respectively. The latter findings suggest if a horse has serosanguineous peritoneal fluid, it has a strangulating or surgical lesion; however, if the peritoneal fluid is not serosanguineous, it does not rule-out an intestinal strangulation or surgical lesion. Similarly, in the same study,[51] a high peritoneal fluid TS concentration (>2.0 g/dL) had a sensitivity, specificity, positive and negative predictive value of 86%, 75%, 77%, and 85%, respectively, for identifying the need for surgery. Importantly, these variables can be measured point-of-care.

The usefulness of peritoneal fluid lactate concentration for determining the need for surgery and identifying horses with intestinal strangulation has been evaluated in several studies. Normal peritoneal fluid lactate concentration is < 1 mmol/L and should be less than blood lactate concentration. Peritoneal fluid:plasma lactate concentration ratio >2 is highly suggestive of a strangulating obstruction. In one study, horses with a strangulating obstruction had a peritoneal fluid lactate of 8.45 mmol/L and non-strangulating obstruction of 2.09 mmol/L.[53] However, gross appearance of the peritoneal fluid was also useful for distinguishing a strangulating from a non-strangulating obstruction.[53] Serial peritoneal fluid lactate concentration was a good predictor for differentiating horses with a strangulating from a non-strangulating lesion.[54] Samples were taken at admission and 1 to 6 hours post admission.[54] An increase in peritoneal fluid lactate concentration over time had high odds of being associated with a strangulating obstruction (odds ratio 62 [95% CI 8–519]) with a sensitivity of 92% and specificity of 77%.[54] Although this approach may be useful for hospital populations with a high proportion of non-strangulating small intestinal obstructions (eg, ileal impactions), waiting 1 to 6 hours delays surgery in horses with a strangulating obstruction. It is important to recognize that in many of these studies, there are no horses with enteritis, colitis, or peritonitis, and the interpretation of peritoneal fluid lactate concentration in horses with these diseases has not been investigated.

Multivariable models are likely to prove more valuable than individual variables for predicting which horses presenting for colic have an intestinal strangulation. Age, colic duration, admission pain and reflux volume, abdominal palpation per rectum and/or transabdominal sonographic findings, blood glucose and lactate concentrations, and peritoneal fluid color and lactate concentration relative to blood lactate concentration appear to be the most useful variables for model building.[21]

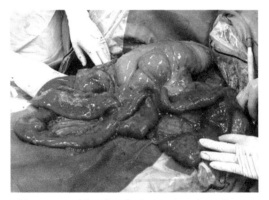

Fig. 9. A geriatric Arabian mare with colic of 4 hours duration. The mare was recumbent on the trailer with muscle fasciculations, tachycardia, dilated small intestinal loops on palpation per rectum, and no reflux on nasogastric intubation. She had a PCV of 39%, TS of 7.4 g/dL, blood lactate concentration of 4.9 mmol/L, and blood glucose concentration of 236 mg/dL. No additional diagnostic tests were needed. On exploratory laparotomy, the mare was diagnosed with a strangulating pedunculated lipoma affecting approximately 10 m of distal jejunum and ileum. Fortunately, because of early referral and surgical treatment, no resection was necessary and the mare recovered without complication.

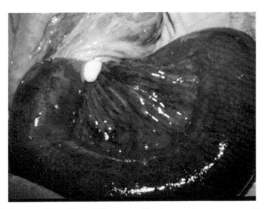

Fig. 10. A strangulating pedunculated lipoma affecting a short segment of jejunum. With a short segment of jejunum needing resection and the orad segments of bowel not being markedly distended for a prolonged period, these horses can have a good prognosis for an uncomplicated recovery.

SUMMARY

Early identification of horses with a strangulating obstruction is vital for an uncomplicated recovery from surgery. In fact, the goal should be to identify horses sufficiently early such that resection is unnecessary (**Fig. 9**).[2,3] Even if a resection and anastomosis are necessary, horses can have an uncomplicated recovery particularly horses with a short segment of jejunum affected (**Fig. 10**). Attention to detail during the initial examination, considering all clinical findings, pursuing diagnostic tests early when indicated based on the initial examination, and effective client communication are critical for a successful outcome. Client communication should be effective so that misinformation about diagnosis, procedure, cost, and prognosis does not delay referral and surgery.[55] Most importantly, a team approach involving owners, caregivers, primary care veterinarians, hospital nursing staff, emergency clinicians, and surgeons is necessary to continue to improve the prognosis for horses with intestinal strangulation.

CLINICS CARE POINTS

- Horses with intestinal strangulating obstruction can have a good prognosis for survival and athletic performance.
- Horses undergoing surgical correction of the lesion early have a better long-term prognosis, fewer complications, and less expense associated with treatment than horses with delayed referral and surgery.
- Careful consideration of signalment, history, and physical examination in conjunction with point-of-care blood work and targeted diagnostic tests can help with early diagnosis of intestinal strangulating in cases where it is not obvious based on pain and unresponsiveness to analgesia.

DISCLOSURE

The author has no financial disclosures related to this article

REFERENCES

1. Hackett ES, Embertson RM, Hopper SA, et al. Duration of disease influences survival to discharge of Thoroughbred mares with surgically treated large colon volvulus. Equine Vet J 2015;47(6):650–4.
2. Rudnick MJ, Denagamage TN, Freeman DE. Effects of age, disease and anastomosis on short- and long-term survival after surgical correction of small intestinal strangulating diseases in 89 horses. Equine Vet J 2022;54(6):1031–8.
3. Freeman DE, Schaeffer DJ, Cleary OB. Long-term survival in horses with strangulating obstruction of the small intestine managed without resection. Equine Vet J 2014;46(6):711–7.
4. Stewart S, Southwood LL, Aceto HW. Comparison of short- and long-term complications and survival following jejunojejunostomy, jejunoileostomy and jejunocaecostomy in 112 horses: 2005-2010. Equine Vet J 2014;46(3):333–8.
5. Dabareiner RM, Sullins KE, White NA, et al. Serosal injury in the equine jejunum and ascending colon after ischemia-reperfusion or intraluminal distention and decompression. Vet Surg 2001;30(2):114–25.
6. Dabareiner RM, White NA, Donaldson LL. Effects of intraluminal distention and decompression on microvascular permeability and hemodynamics of the equine jejunum. Am J Vet Res 2001;62(2):225–36.
7. Dabareiner RM, Snyder JR, White NA, et al. Microvascular permeability and endothelial cell morphology associated with low-flow ischemia/reperfusion injury in the equine jejunum. Am J Vet Res 1995;56(5):639–48.
8. Dabareiner RM, Sullins KE, Snyder JR, et al. Evaluation of the microcirculation of the equine small intestine after intraluminal distention and subsequent decompression. Am J Vet Res 1993;54(10):1673–82.
9. Dabareiner RM, Snyder JR, Sullins KE, et al. Evaluation of the microcirculation of the equine jejunum and ascending colon after ischemia and reperfusion. Am J Vet Res 1993;54(10):1683–92.
10. Gerard MP, Blikslager AT, Roberts MC, et al. The characteristics of intestinal injury peripheral to strangulating obstruction lesions in the equine small intestine. Equine Vet J 1999;31(4):331–5.
11. De Ceulaer K, Delesalle C, Van Elzen R, et al. Morphological data indicate a stress response at the oral border of strangulated small intestine in horses. Res Vet Sci 2011;91(2):294–300.
12. De Ceulaer K, Delesalle C, Van Elzen R, et al. Morphological changes in the small intestinal smooth muscle layers of horses suffering from small intestinal strangulation. Is there a basis for predisposition for reduced contractility? Equine Vet J 2011;43(4):439–45.
13. Dunkel B, Buonpane A, Chang YM. Differences in gastrointestinal lesions in different horse types. Vet Rec 2017;181(11):291.
14. Silva AG, Furr MO. Diagnoses, clinical pathology findings, and treatment outcome of geriatric horses: 345 cases (2006-2010). J Am Vet Med Assoc 2013;243(12):1762–1768.2.
15. Southwood LL, Gassert T, Lindborg S. Colic in geriatric compared to mature non-geriatric horses. Part 2: Treatment, diagnosis and short-term survival. Equine Vet J 2010;42(7):628–35.
16. Petersen JL, Lewis RM, Embertson R, et al. Preliminary heritability of complete rotation large colon volvulus in Thoroughbred broodmares. Vet Rec 2019; 185(9):269.

17. Suthers JM, Pinchbeck GL, Proudman CJ, et al. Risk factors for large colon volvulus in the UK. Equine Vet J 2013;45(5):558–63.

18. Moore JN, Dreesen DW, Boudinot DF. Colonic distention, displacement and torsion in Thoroughbred broodmares: results of a two-year study. In: Moore JM, editor. Proceedings of the 4th equine colic research symposium. 1991. p. 23–5.

19. Weese JS, Holcombe SJ, Embertson RM, et al. Changes in the faecal microbiota of mares precede the development of post partum colic. Equine Vet J 2015;47(6): 641–9.

20. Southwood LL, Bergslien K, Jacobi A, et al. Trumble TN 2002 Large colon displacement and volvulus in horses: 495 cases (1987-1999). Proceedings of the 7th Equine Colic Research Symposium 2002;32–3.

21. Southwood LL, Lindborg S. Early identification of horses with strangulating lesions: can we do better with point-of-care evaluation? Equine Vet Educ 2021; 33(S12):21.

22. Southwood LL, Lindborg S. Variables associated with a prior history of colic in horses admitted to a tertiary referral hospital for colic. Equine Vet Educ 2021; 33(S12):10–1.

23. Dalla Costa E, Minero M, Lebelt D, et al. Development of the horse grimace scale (HGS) as a pain assessment tool in horses undergoing routine castration. PLoS One 2014;9:e29981.

24. De Grauw JC, van Loon JPAM. Systematic pain assessment in horses. Vet J 2016;209:14–22.

25. White NA, Elward A, Moga KS, et al. Use of web-based data collection to evaluate analgesic administration and the decision for surgery in horses with colic. Equine Vet J 2005;37(4):347–50.

26. Seahorn TL, Cornick JL, Cohen ND. Prognostic indicators for horses with duodenitis-proximal jejunitis. 75 horses (1985-1989). J Vet Intern Med 1992; 6(6):307–11.

27. Underwood C, Southwood LL, McKeown LP, et al. Complications and survival associated with surgical compared with medical management of horses with duodenitis-proximal jejunitis. Equine Vet J 2008;40(4):373–8.

28. Busoni V, De Busscher V, Lopez D, et al. Evaluation of a protocol for fast localized abdominal sonography of horses (FLASH) admitted for colic. Vet J 2011;188(1): 77–82.

29. Beccati F, Pepe M, Gialletti R, et al. Is there a statistical correlation between ultrasonographic findings and definitive diagnosis in horses with acute abdominal pain? Equine Vet J Suppl 2011;39:98–105.

30. Pease AP, Scrivani PV, Erb HN, et al. Accuracy of increased large-intestine wall thickness during ultrasonography for diagnosing large-colon torsion in 42 horses. Vet Radiol Ultrasound 2004;45(3):220–4.

31. Long A. Clinical insights: Clinicopathological parameters for diagnosing and predicting outcome of horses with colic. Equine Vet J 2022;54(6):1005–10.

32. Krueger CR, Ruple-Czerniak A, Hackett ES. Evaluation of plasma muscle enzyme activity as an indicator of lesion characteristics and prognosis in horses undergoing celiotomy for acute gastrointestinal pain. BMC Vet Res 2014;10 Suppl 1(Suppl 1):S7.

33. Kilcoyne I, Nieto JE, Dechant JE. Diagnostic value of plasma and peritoneal fluid procalcitonin concentrations in horses with strangulating intestinal lesions. J Am Vet Med Assoc 2020;256(8):927–33.

34. Kilcoyne I, Nieto JE, Dechant JE. Predictive value of plasma and peritoneal creatine kinase in horses with strangulating intestinal lesions. Vet Surg 2019;48(2): 152–8.

35. Delesalle C, van de Walle GR, Nolten C, et al. Determination of the source of increased serotonin (5-HT) concentrations in blood and peritoneal fluid of colic horses with compromised bowel. Equine Vet J 2008;40(4):326–31.

36. Grulke S, Franck T, Gangl M, et al. Myeloperoxidase assay in plasma and peritoneal fluid of horses with gastrointestinal disease. Can J Vet Res 2008;72(1): 37–42.

37. Barton MH, Collatos C. Tumor necrosis factor and interleukin-6 activity and endotoxin concentration in peritoneal fluid and blood of horses with acute abdominal disease. J Vet Intern Med 1999;13(5):457–64.

38. Saulez MN, Cebra CK, Tornquist SJ. The diagnostic and prognostic value of alkaline phosphatase activity in serum and peritoneal fluid from horses with acute colic. J Vet Intern Med 2004;18(4):564–7.

39. Weiss DJ, Evanson OA. Evaluation of activated neutrophils in the blood of horses with colic. Am J Vet Res 2003;64(11):1364–8.

40. Kritchevsky JE, Muir GS, Leschke DHZ, et al. Blood glucose and insulin concentrations after alpha-2-agonists administration in horses with and without insulin dysregulation. J Vet Intern Med 2020;34(2):902–8.

41. Hollis AR, Boston RC, Corley KT. Blood glucose in horses with acute abdominal disease. J Vet Intern Med 2007;21(5):1099–103.

42. Hassel DM, Hill AE, Rorabeck RA, et al. Association between hyperglycemia and survival in 228 horses with acute gastrointestinal disease. J Vet Intern Med 2009; 23(6):1261–5.

43. Underwood C, Southwood LL, Walton RM, Johnson AL. Hepatic and metabolic changes in surgical colic patients: a pilot study. J Vet Emerg Crit Care 2010; 20(6):578–86.

44. Roessner H, Jacobs C, Stefanovski D, et al. Blood glucose in horses with colic. Seattle, WA: Proceedings of the American College of Veterinary Surgeons; 2016.

45. Dunkel B, Kapff JE, Naylor RJ, et al. Blood lactate concentrations in ponies and miniature horses with gastrointestinal disease. Equine Vet J 2013;45(6):666–70.

46. Dunkel B, Mason CJ, Chang YM. Retrospective evaluation of the association between admission blood glucose and l-lactate concentrations in ponies and horses with gastrointestinal disease (2008-2016): 545 cases. J Vet Emerg Crit Care 2019;29(4):418–23.

47. Johnston K, Holcombe SJ, Hauptman JG. Plasma lactate as a predictor of colonic viability and survival after 360 degrees volvulus of the ascending colon in horses. Vet Surg 2007;36(6):563.

48. Delesalle C, Dewulf J, Lefebvre RA, et al. Determination of lactate concentrations in blood plasma and peritoneal fluid in horses with colic by an Accusport analyzer. J Vet Intern Med 2007;21(2):293–301.

49. Walton RM, Southwood LL. Abdominocentesis and peritoneal fluid analysis. In: Southwood LL, editor. Practical guide to equine colic. Ames IA: Wiley-Blackwell; 2012. p. 87–98.

50. Nieto JE, Dechant JE, le Jeune SS, et al. Evaluation of 3 handheld portable analyzers for measurement of L-lactate concentrations in blood and peritoneal fluid of horses with colic. Vet Surg 2015;44(3):366–72.

51. Matthews S, Dart AJ, Reid SWJ, et al. Predictive values, sensitivity and specificity of abdominal fluid variables in determining the need for surgery in horses with an acute abdominal crisis. Aust Vet J 2002;80(3):132–6.

52. Freden GO, Provost PJ, Rand WM. Reliability of using results of abdominal fluid analysis to determine treatment and predict lesion type and outcome for horses with colic: 218 cases (1991-1994). J Am Vet Med Assoc 1998;213(7):1012–5.
53. Latson KM, Nieto JE, Beldomenico PM, et al. Evaluation of peritoneal fluid lactate as a marker of intestinal ischaemia in equine colic. Equine Vet J 2005;37(4):342–6.
54. Peloso JG, Cohen ND. Use of serial measurements of peritoneal fluid lactate concentration to identify strangulating intestinal lesions in referred horses with signs of colic. J Am Vet Med Assoc 2012;240(10):1208–17.
55. Freeman DE, Southwood LL, Epstein K, et al. Referral of horses with colic: a time to review. Proceedings of the 68th Annual Convention of the American Association of Equine Practitioners 2022;470–5.

Current Topics in Medical Colic

Michelle Henry Barton, DVM, PhD[a],*, Gayle D. Hallowell, MA, VetMB, PhD, CertVA, FRCVS[b]

KEYWORDS

- Gastric • Stomach • Impaction • Ulceration • Colon • Displacement • Trocarization
- Inflammatory bowel disease

KEY POINTS

- Gastric impaction is a relatively uncommon cause of colic in horses that can lead to gastric rupture and death if not identified. Clinical signs are often vague with definitive ante-mortem diagnosis achievable via gastroscopy. A successful treatment option in recent years is gastric intubation and/or lavage with carbonated beverages.
- Diagnosis of gastric glandular disease is on the increase. Clinical signs include none to poor performance, cutaneous hypersensitivity, and signs of colic. Gastroscopy is used to diagnose this condition. The epidemiology is not well understood. A variety of treatment options have been used with some success.
- Displacement of the colon is a common cause of either acute, chronic, or recurrent colic in the horse. Diagnosis is often achievable via transrectal examination and transabdominal ultrasonography. Successful treatment may be achieved medically with prudent use of analgesics, enteral and parenteral fluid therapy, enteral laxatives, and transabdominal trocarization.
- Inflammatory bowel disease is a common cause of weight loss, diarrhea, and recurrent colic in horses. Diagnosis is obtained by using transabdominal ultrasonography, oral glucose absorption tests, and intestinal biopsies (partial-thickness rectal mucosal or transendoscopic duodenal or full thickness obtained via laparoscopy or laparotomy). This is a chronic condition and needs management using corticosteroids and other immunosuppressive agents, anthelmintics, and dietary changes.

GASTRIC IMPACTION
Introduction

Gastric impactions are relatively rare, comprising less than 5% of causes of colic in horses.[1] Prompt diagnosis can be hindered by the often vague and mild clinical signs. Medical management is preferred with enteral treatment, particularly with carbonated beverages. Although many horses with a primary gastric impaction respond favorably

The authors have no conflicts of interest with the material contained in this article.
[a] College of Veterinary Medicine, University of Georgia, 2200 College Station Road, Room 1903, Athens, GA 30602, USA; [b] IVC Evidensia, Valley View, Main Road, Upper Broughton, Nottinghamshire, UK LE14 3BG
* Corresponding author.
E-mail address: bartonmh@uga.edu

to treatment, a subset of horses with gastric impactions will experience recurrence or gastric rupture as a terminal complication.

History and Clinical Signs

Any breed or age equidae can be affected, although gastric impaction is unusual in equidae under 1 year of age.[1,2] In the largest retrospective study to date, the Friesian breed was significantly overrepresented compared with the study center's overall hospital population.[3] Horses with gastric impactions may have an acute (less than 24 hours to several days), chronic, or recurrent history of illness. Clinical signs reported by owners are typically mild and nonspecific. The most commonly reported historical complaint is anorexia that may be accompanied by nonspecific signs of mild abdominal discomfort. When signs of abdominal pain are apparent or severe, concurrent distal intestinal disease is more commonly present.[1,2] Less frequently reported clinical findings include dysphagia, reduced fecal output, low-grade fever, salivation, and diarrhea.[1,2]

Cause and Pathophysiology

Gastric impactions may be categorized as primary or secondary, although the distinction may be difficult to prove without a celiotomy or postmortem examination to exclude secondary contributors. Gastric impactions may also be categorized by whether the material retained in the stomach is regarded as an acceptable equine feedstuff or represents the ingestion of poorly or indigestible material, such as persimmon seeds (phytobezoar) or a mixture of hair and plant-based material (tricho phytobezoar). Primary gastric impaction implies that it arose spontaneously with no other underlying cause or prior disease.[1] In one retrospective study, approximately two-thirds of the cases were presumptively primary, as no additional intestinal disorder was identified.[2] Bird and colleagues[1] reported that 6 of 7 horses with primary gastric impaction that died or were euthanized had gross evidence of thickening of the muscle layers of the wall of the saccus caecus at postmortem, measuring up to 10 times the thickness of unaffected control horses. It was unclear if the thickened stomach wall was the cause or the result of the gastric impaction. Histopathology revealed focal fibrosis or myositis of the stomach wall. Two horses also had gross thickening of the distal esophagus or pylorus.[1] Despite the postmortem signs of chronicity, some of those cases presented with clinical signs of less than 24 hours' duration, two of which had gastric ruptures. In contrast, in a more recent report of 113 cases of gastric impaction diagnosed by gastroscopy or celiotomy, only approximately one-third were classified as primary disease. The remaining two-thirds of cases had concurrent intestinal disease,[4] which included both simple and strangulating obstructive disorders of the distal intestinal tract.[1]

A recent report of concurrent gastric impaction identified during celiotomy for colonic volvulus was particularly intriguing and demonstrates the difficulty in distinguishing primary from secondary disease.[5] Given the severity of the gastric impactions in the latter case series, it seems improbable that the volvulus caused the gastric impaction, although chronic partial colonic displacement before to the development of the volvulus could not be ruled out as a potential inciting contribution to gastric outflow obstruction leading to gastric impaction. It was proposed that chronic primary gastric impaction contributed to the development of colonic volvulus through changes in normal anatomic alignment of the colon and alternations in microbiota, intraabdominal pressure, or motility. Additional reported conditions associated with gastric impaction are water deprivation, overindulgence of pelleted feed, poor dentition, hepatic disease, and suspicion of gastric dysmotility.[1]

Diagnosis

Given the vague and often mild signs of primary gastric impaction or the presence of more pronounced signs of distal intestinal disease that may occur with secondary gastric impaction, the prompt diagnosis of gastric impaction in horses can be challenging. Physical examination and laboratory findings are often within normal limits or include nonspecific findings. Hyperfibrinogenemia is a sign of chronicity and may indicate the presence of mural inflammation or peritonitis.[1,2] Although typically there is no gastric reflux, it may be difficult to pass the nasogastric tube into the stomach lumen or the patient may appear anxious or uncomfortable when attempting to obtain gastric reflux. Caudal extension of the stomach as evidence of gastric distension may be present on transabdominal ultrasonography if the wall of the greater curvature can be visualized at or beyond the left 14th intercostal space.[1,2] If a horse has been anorexic for at least 24 hours or nasogastric intubation fails to correct ultrasonographically identified caudal extension of the stomach wall, gastroscopy is recommended as the preferred method for obtaining a definitive diagnosis. Gastric impactions can vary in appearance from a well-formed concretion of ingesta that obscures ability to see the margo plicatus (**Fig. 1**) to the inability to enter the stomach lumen if the impacted material extends to the esophageal sphincter (**Fig. 2**).[2] Impacted material may be covered with mucus. If not detected via gastroscopy, a gastric impaction can be diagnosed during exploratory laparotomy.

Treatment

Initially food should be withheld until progress is made in reducing the size of the gastric impaction. In one retrospective study with 20 cases, enteral fluid therapy with or without laxatives was reported to lead to resolution in 5 days in 90% of horses with primary gastric impaction.[2] Recently, Giusto and colleagues[6] reported development of colonic volvulus in 4 horses following treatment with a single large volume ($\geq$8 L) of enteral fluid given to patients with concurrent gastric impaction that were not identified until celiotomy. It could not be definitively determined if the gastric impaction and enteral fluid treatment led to the volvulus. In all 4 cases, intense signs of abdominal pain and the need for a celiotomy occurred shortly after receiving the enteral fluids, leading to the conclusion that the additional gastric distension precipitated the volvulus. Thus, frequent enteral administration of smaller volumes of water or crystalloids (4 to 10 mL/kg) through gravity flow was recommended.

The use of an enteral carbonated cola beverage for the treatment of gastric phytobezoars in people was introduced approximately 2 decades ago, with the first report of its use in a horse in 2007.[7] Subsequently, a case series highlighted its use for treatment of equine gastric phytobezoars with doses ranging from less than one-half liter to 2 L twice daily to 1 L every hour for 1 to 3 days.[8] One horse was given the cola beverage with an equine complete feed pellet consumed voluntarily as a mash.

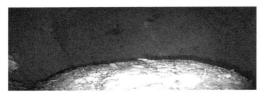

Fig. 1. Endoscopic appearance of a discrete concretion of ingesta covered with mucus in a horse with vague signs of anorexia and reduced performance under saddle. The greater curvature of the stomach is in the background.

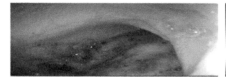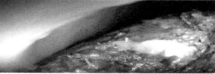

Fig. 2. Endoscopic appearance of a gastric impaction extending to the cardia in a donkey (*left*) and a horse (*right*).

Caffeinated and high-sugar preparations should be used with caution.[9] Subsequently, 2 recent large case studies on gastric impactions in horses revealed a significantly improved likelihood of survival to discharge for horses treated with enteral carbonated cola.[3,4] The mechanism of cola-mediated phytobezoar or ingesta dissolution remains unknown, but it may be associated with the mucolytic effect of sodium bicarbonate, the acidifying effect of carbonic and phosphoric acid, or penetration and breakdown by carbon dioxide bubbles.[9] There is suggestion that any carbonated beverage would be beneficial for treatment.[10] Soft drink beverages, such as colas, are likely most affordable for use in horses. Additional enteral treatments that have been used successfully for gastric impactions are magnesium sulfate, dioctyl sodium sulfosuccinate, and sorbitol.[2,6] Medical treatment is preferred, although there are recent successful reports of gastrotomy in the adult horse.[11,12]

Follow-up gastroscopy is highly recommended at the end of therapy to ensure definitive resolution of the impaction and to fully assess the gastric mucosa, as both nonglandular and glandular gastric ulcerations are reported.[2] Impaction recurs in some cases, particularly when it is diagnosed as primary disease; thus, additional follow-up gastroscopy after discharge is advised.[1,2]

Outcome

Treatment success for gastric impaction is variable with survival to discharge ranging from 0% in horses with concurrent colonic volvulus[5] to 90% for horses with primary gastric impaction.[2] The overall survival rate on data comprising 238 cases from 2 recent reports was approximately 60%.[3,4] There was no difference in survival to discharge for horses with primary (23/40; 58%) and secondary (45/73; 62%) disease.[4] The complication rate with primary disease may be higher with reports of recurrence[1,2] and a greater likelihood to progress to gastric rupture.[4]

EQUINE GASTRIC GLANDULAR DISEASE
Introduction

It is now widely accepted that equine gastric glandular disease (EGGD) is a separate entity to equine squamous gastric disease (ESGD),[13] and this section provides an update. Recent studies have demonstrated that the risk factors[14] and response to treatment[15,16] of EGGD differ from ESGD. This is likely due to differences in the anatomy and physiology of the 2 regions of the stomach. Over the last 10 to 15 years, there have been increased identification and reported prevalence of EGGD, and most think that this is a true change in disease prevalence. However, despite many recent publications, there is still knowledge lacking on this condition.

History and Clinical Signs

Clinical signs likely associated with EGGD include changes in temperament, including nervousness and aggression, changes in rideability, including reduced willingness to work and reluctance to move forward; unexplained weight loss, likely concurrently associated with reduced appetite or altered eating patterns; cutaneous sensitivity manifested as flank-biting, resentment to girthing, leg aids, or rugging; mild and/or recurrent abdominal pain.[13] Changes in coat condition, stereotypical behavior, bruxism, and diarrhea are unlikely to be associated with EGGD.[13]

Cutaneous sensitivity seems an implausible clinical sign of gastric disease. However, data from other species suggest that afferent pathways from abdominal viscera and the sixth to ninth thoracic spinal nerves are pooled, such that afferent signals from the skin may be affected by input from the stomach and misinterpreted within the brain. In addition, viscerosomatic reflexes can result in pain and sensitivity in segmentally related structures, such as the skin.[17]

Cause and Pathophysiology

The prevalence of EGGD in clinical and abattoir studies of various horse types worldwide is between 47% and 65%.[18–23] Anecdotally, the prevalence of this condition is thought to have increased over the last 15 years or so.

Risk factors for EGGD are limited and occasionally contradictory but are very different from those for ESGD. Warmbloods are at increased risk of developing EGGD compared with other horse types.[20,24] In thoroughbred racehorses, the trainer was identified as a risk independent of other management factors.[14] Exercising for more than 4 or 5 days per week has been shown to be a risk factor in racehorses[14] and sports horses,[25] whereas intensity of exercise was not. The more experienced a horse is at its discipline, the lower the prevalence of EGGD,[25,26] which may suggest work adaptation or management differences of elite horses.[13] A study in endurance horses demonstrated a higher prevalence of EGGD in the competition season,[23] which may relate to reduced gastric blood flow during prolonged exercise.

Horses with severe EGGD have increased cortisol in response to novel stimuli[27] and in response to exogenous ACTH,[28] suggesting more sensitivity to stress. The association between EGGD and stereotypies is conflicting; no association was found in one study,[14] whereas an association with crib-biting was found in another.[29] These differences may be explained by high prevalence of EGGD and stereotypic behavior in these populations predominantly of racehorses,[14,29] particularly as stereotypies are deemed a coping strategy in horses.[29] It would be more interesting to evaluate disease prevalence in horses prevented from exhibiting stereotypical behavior, as removal of coping strategies, in humans at least, is deemed stressful. The lower prevalence of EGGD in more experienced polo ponies and show jumpers[25,30] may relate to adaptation to physiologic stress. More experienced show and show jumping horses have lower plasma cortisol concentrations than less experienced horses.[31,32] It is challenging to know what is "stressful" to an individual horse, and as such, changes to minimize stress should be tailored to an individual and ideally kept consistent.

Thus far, no association has been documented for involvement of infectious agents,[19,21] nonsteroidal anti-inflammatory drug use in clinical cases,[14,24] diet, or lameness with EGGD.[13,14]

Lesions of the glandular mucosa are usually not ulcerative. These lesions are erosive and inflammatory in nature, consisting of a mixed inflammatory population (lymphocytes, plasmacytes, and neutrophils), and as such, the lesions are best described as glandular gastritis.[19,21,33] The glandular mucosa differs from the squamous mucosa in that it is adapted to the highly acidic (pH 1 to 3) environment in which it is usually bathed.[34] It is thus likely that EGGD may result from a breakdown of the normal defense mechanisms that protect the mucosa (bicarbonate and gastric mucus consisting of glycoproteins, water, electrolytes, lipids, and antibodies).[35]

The proposed pathophysiology of these lesions includes changes in blood flow with or without perpetuation of these lesions owing to exposure to acid or as an extension of inflammatory bowel disease (IBD).[13] Reductions in blood flow may be secondary to "stress," which influences gastrin production or relates to exercise and feeding.[13] A recent study found horses with EGGD had upregulated salivary proteins relating to immune activation compared with normal horses, which may support the proposal that EGGD is a manifestation of IBD, as this suggested further evidence that EGGD is an inflammatory disease.[36]

Diagnosis

Gastroscopy remains the only reliable method for diagnosis with most lesions located around the pylorus and in the antrum (**Fig. 3**).[14–16] It is now widely accepted that the grading system for EGGD does not reflect the severity of disease. Until a better system is developed, describing lesions based on the ECEIM-ACVIM consensus statement is recommended.[37] These descriptors include the following: focal, multifocal, and diffuse; mild, moderate, and severe; nodular, raised, flat, or depressed; erythematous, hemorrhagic, or fibrinosuppurative. A more recent consensus statement focusing on EGGD suggested that flat, erythematous lesions were likely to heal more rapidly than lesions with a nodular, raised, fibrinosuppurative or hemorrhagic appearance.[38] The agreement regarding these descriptors varies from fair to moderate[39] and moderate to good[40] and was better between ACVIM/ECEIM Diplomates than other equine clinicians.[39] Lack of consensus and lack of reliable methods for grading severity of lesions make it challenging to perform clinical and experimental studies on this disease.

Differences in the gastric microbiota between healthy horses and those with EGGD have been documented,[41,42] but what is currently uncertain is if these are cause or effect and how they can be used clinically.

Treatment

It is now widely accepted that treatment and management options for ESGD and EGGD are different. Three or 4 combinations of treatments have been proposed in a recent consensus statement: oral omeprazole (4 mg/kg every 24 hours) combined with sucralfate (12 mg/kg every 12 hours), oral misoprostol (5 µg/kg every 12 hours) with or without sucralfate (12 mg/kg every 12 hours); long-acting intramuscular omeprazole (4 mg/kg every 5–7 days), which is available in some locales or therapeutic combinations for IBD (see inflammatory bowel disease section in later discussion).

Sucralfate provides a physical barrier preventing acid diffusion, stimulates mucus secretion, which blocks acid diffusion, inhibits pepsin and bile acid secretion,

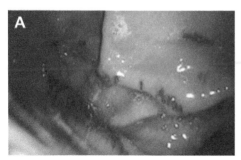
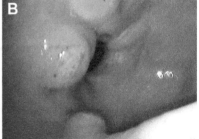

Fig. 3. Two common, but very different appearances of glandular gastric lesions. (*A*) Some multifocal, flat, hemorrhagic lesions. (*B*) A unifocal, raised, fibrinosuppurative lesion.

promotes epithelialization by preventing fibroblast degradation, stimulates epidermal and insulin-like growth factors, and increases mucosal blood flow through increased production of prostaglandin E_2 (PGE). Response to oral omeprazole and sucralfate therapy varies with healing reported in 22% to 63% of horses[35,43]; this difference likely relates to differing definitions of healing. When used, omeprazole should be administered on an empty stomach and fasted for an additional 30 to 60 minutes after administration.[13]

Misoprostol is a PGE analogue that likely improves mucosal blood flow. It also suppresses acid production in the horse[44] and inhibits neutrophilic inflammation.[45] One study[43] demonstrated EGGD healing in 73% of horses. Side effects are rare and include mild, transient diarrhea, mild abdominal pain, and urticaria. Care must be taken in administration to pregnant mares, as this drug could induce abortion, although there are some safety data to suggest it can be administered between 100 and 130 days of gestation.[46] Because of abortigenic potential, misoprostol should not be dispensed to women who may be pregnant or planning to become pregnant. There is no rationale for combining this drug with oral omeprazole.[13]

Long-acting intramuscular omeprazole is more effective than oral formulations at acid suppression when pH is measured in the ventral portion of the stomach.[47] Acid suppression is maintained for 4 to 7 days and as such should be administered at 5- to 7-day intervals. Healing reportedly occurred in 64% to 75% of horses.[47,48] Transient swelling at the injection site has been reported in less than 10% of cases, and it is thus recommended that it be administered after warming. The author (G.H.) has had one injection site reaction many weeks after the last injection; no others have been reported in the literature.

There may be some rationale for administration of glucocorticoids, which have anecdotally been reported to be efficacious. Initial administration of 1 mg/kg prednisolone orally every 24 hours or 0.05 to 0.1 mg/kg dexamethasone orally every 24 hours, which is then gradually tapered over 4 to 5 weeks, has been proposed.[13] Other recommendations include dietary simplification, whereby cereal proteins or alfalfa may play a role in initiation or perpetuation of IBD. A small proportion of cases develop very large hyperplastic nodules (**Fig. 4**) that are at risk of obstructing pyloric outflow. These cases may require transendoscopic removal using thermocautery.[13]

There is no evidence for administration of antibiotics, ranitidine, aloe vera, pectin-lecithin complexes, polysaccharides, kaolin, bismuth subsalicylate, sea buckthorn, acupuncture, or homeopathy for the treatment of EGGD.[13] For concurrent ESGD and EGGD lesions, treatment should be aimed at the EGGD.

Outcome and Prevention of Recurrence

Rates of EGGD healing are slow compared with ESGD and unpredictable. Raised, nodular, and fibrinosuppurative lesions may take longer to heal than flat, hemorrhagic lesions. Although mucosal restitution can occur within 3 to 5 weeks, EGGD may take several months to completely resolve, especially where raised areas or nodules are visible.

Ideally, evaluation should be performed every 6 to 8 weeks using gastroscopy until resolution has occurred, and only then should treatment be discontinued. There is no rationale for reducing the dose of the drugs except for glucocorticoids. The author (G.H.) usually starts at 1 mg/kg prednisolone or 0.1 mg/kg dexamethasone (preferred) orally once daily for a week and then reduces the dose by 25% weekly.

If there is no improvement or deterioration in lesion appearance at the reexamination, it is recommended to change to an alternative treatment. If there is improvement,

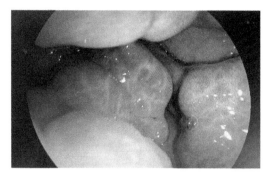

Fig. 4. Some multifocal, raised lesions surrounding the pylorus in a 12-year-old Irish-draught cross horse that presented with recurrent colic and intermittent gastric impactions. These lesions failed to respond to commonly used treatment combinations for EGGD (injectable omeprazole; oral misoprostol and sucralfate; oral dexamethasone) and so were removed using a transendoscopic cautery technique. Since removal, the horse's clinical signs have resolved.

treatment should be continued for a maximum of 3 months, and at this point, consider alternative treatments if not healed.

Prevention of EGGD is problematic. Based on known risk factors, horses should have 2 rest days per week; stress should be minimized (calm environments, minimal number of caregivers, and the same equine field companions), and turn out should be maximized. Avoid any irritating supplements, such as magnesium sulphate. Corn oil (150 to 250 mL/d/500 kg) may be beneficial as a preventative, as it decreases gastric acid output and increases PGE,[49] as may the use of pectin-lecithin as a mucosal protectant at 150 g every 12 hours (or feeding sugar beet pulp) despite its lack of efficacy as a treatment.[50]

INFLAMMATORY BOWEL DISEASE
Introduction

IBD is associated with clinical signs of weight loss, diarrhea, and/or recurrent colic.[51] Clinical signs are likely due to changes in absorption of nutrients and water and effects on gastrointestinal motility.[51] IBD is likely driven by an inappropriate immune response to bacteria, viruses, parasites, and dietary allergens.[51] Diagnosis of IBD is achieved using a variety of techniques, including abnormal oral glucose or xylose absorption tests, increased intestinal wall thickness on transabdominal ultrasonographic evaluation, partial-thickness rectal and transendoscopic duodenal biopsies, or full-thickness intestinal biopsies.[52] The sentinel publication in the early 2000s made for grim reading.[51] This poor prognosis was recently challenged in another, larger prospective publication, whereby initial response to therapy was 75% with 3-year survival reported to be 65%.[52]

History and Clinical Signs

The most common presenting signs are weight loss, combined weight loss and recurrent colic, and recurrent colic alone,[52] and in certain subtypes of IBD, diarrhea and inappetence.[52] Ventral edema is seen secondary to hypoalbuminemia.[52,53]

Epidemiology and Pathophysiology

Little is known about the epidemiology of IBD in horses. However, extrapolating knowledge from others species, particularly humans and dogs, it can be surmised that there is a complex relationship between genetics, the environment, bacteria, viruses and parasites, and cereal and meat proteins.[54] The relative roles of these factors are somewhat controversial; however, it is accepted that the enteric microbiota in humans play a central role in the pathogenesis of IBD.[55,56] There is one study suggesting that gluten may play a role in IBD in the horse, but further studies are required to ascertain if this is the case.[57]

Five types of IBD are described in the horse that can affect the small and large intestine: lymphocytic-plasmocytic enterocolitis, granulomatous enteritis (GE), diffuse eosinophilic enterocolitis, idiopathic focal eosinophilic enterocolitis, and multisystemic eosinophilic epitheliotropic disease (MEED).[51] A sixth subtype affecting only the large intestine has been proposed with identification at postmortem and resembles ulcerative colitis in humans both grossly and histopathologically; the clinical relevance is yet to be elucidated (Kerbyson and Knottenbelt, personal communication, 2014). MEED and GE are the only subtypes of IBD with disease in tissues beyond the intestinal tract. In MEED, changes in the skin and other organs are commonly reported, and in GE, changes in the skin and lymph nodes can be seen.[53] GE and MEED have most commonly been reported in horses less than 4 years of age with an increased prevalence in standardbreds[51]; the breed predilection may suggest that there is a genetic component.[58] The other 3 subtypes have been identified in any age of horse and in a variety of breeds.[51–53]

It has been proposed that lymphocytic-plasmocytic enterocolitis may be a precursor to intestinal lymphoma as in other species.[51,53,59,60] GE has histopathologic similarities to Crohn disease in humans and can be associated with anemia, likely secondary to reduced absorption of nutrients or associated with chronic disease.[51]

Diagnosis

Initial evaluation for clinical presentations of weight loss, diarrhea, and recurrent colic should include ruling out dental, parasitic, and other infectious disease, sand accumulation, renal or hepatic failure, intestinal motility disorders, and gastric disease.[52] Specific tests for evaluation of suspected IBD include fecal worm egg count, serum biochemistry, oral glucose or xylose absorption test, transabdominal (**Fig. 5**) and transrectal ultrasonography, partial-thickness transendoscopic duodenal and rectal mucosal biopsies, and full-thickness intestinal biopsies obtained by laparoscopy or laparotomy.[52,53,58] Increased fecal worm egg counts have been reported to be negative or have a low prevalence in horses diagnosed with IBD.[52,53]

Clinicopathologic signs most commonly identified are hypoproteinemia, hypoalbuminemia, and abnormal absorption of glucose or xylose.[51–53,58] Anemia was reported in one study.[51] Increased serum activity of gamma-glutamyl transferase was reported in cases of MEED.[51]

Thickening of the intestinal wall using transabdominal ultrasonography was seen in 40% to 50% of cases.[52,53] Abnormalities on partial-thickness transendoscopic duodenal and rectal mucosal biopsies are variable and likely to relate to the type of IBD and extent of disease. Abnormalities on rectal mucosal biopsies are found in approximately 40% to 50% of cases (range, 0% to 82%).[51–53,58] Transendoscopic duodenal biopsies did not yield a diagnosis in one study.[58]

Treatment

There is little evidence regarding the effective management of IBD in horses. Recommendations for treatment in horses include parasiticides, corticosteroids, and azathioprine (3–5 mg/kg once daily).[52] Horses that did not respond to corticosteroids and required the addition of azathioprine had a poorer outcome.[52] Anecdotally, cetirizine

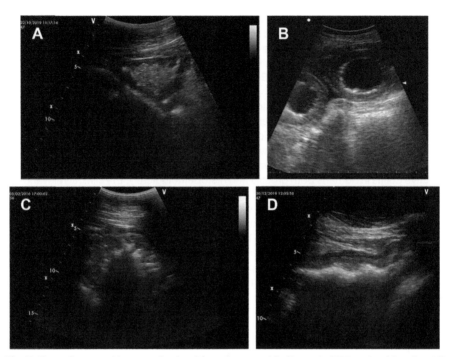

Fig. 5. Four ultrasound images obtained from horses with diagnosed IBD, using biopsies. All displayed marked thickening of the intestinal wall with changes in layer demarcation. (*A-D*) (*top left*) Thickened duodenal wall obtained from the right 11th intercostal space with a diagnosis of lymphocytic-plasmocytic enteritis from a transendoscopic duodenal biopsy. (*top right*) Thickened small intestine obtained from the right caudoventral abdomen; increased eosinophils were identified from a transendoscopic duodenal biopsy. (*bottom left*) Thickened right ventral colon obtained from the right ventral abdomen with a diagnosis of eosinophilic colitis from a full-thickness biopsy obtained at exploratory laparotomy. (*bottom right*) Thickened left ventral colon obtained from the left ventral abdomen with a diagnosis of lymphocytic-plasmocytic colitis from a rectal mucosal biopsy.

and oclacitinib, synthetic cyclohexylamino pyrrolopyrimidine janus kinase inhibitors, have been successfully used for the management of eosinophilic colitis and disease associated with MEED and warrant further investigation (M.H. Barton, personal communication, 2014).

Because of the multifactorial nature of IBD, cases do not always respond to the same management; however, anti-inflammatories and antibiotics are used for treatment in humans and dogs, and both species usually require further intervention to manage "flare-ups."[61] In addition to traditional corticosteroids (prednisolone and dexamethasone), other agents that modulate the inflammatory response are used and include sulfasalazine, budesonide, and cyclosporine. Sulfasalazine (canine dose of 12.5 mg/kg every 6 hours orally reducing in frequency and dose over time) has immunosuppressive, antibacterial, and anti-inflammatory properties; as it is metabolized to its active component in the large intestine, it is probably most useful for large intestinal disease.[62] Budesonide is regarded as a very potent glucocorticoid that may be associated with fewer side effects and is used in dogs at doses of 1 or 5 mg orally once daily for animals 3 to 30 kg and greater than 30 kg, respectively.[63] Cyclosporine is an immunosuppressive agent and is used in dogs at doses of 5 mg/kg orally once daily.[62] Antibiotics that are commonly implemented for IBD in dogs that have concurrent anti-inflammatory effects include metronidazole and tylosin. These antibiotics not only remove pathogenic organisms but also change the microbiota and reduce the commensal bacterial load that are not tolerated by dogs with IBD because of their dysfunctional gastrointestinal immune system.[61] Other newer agents being used include chlorambucil, cyclophosphamide, which are immunosuppressants and immunomodulators, and second-generation 2-aminocyclates (mesalazine and olsalazine)[62]; these drugs can be used in conjunction with corticosteroids or as an alternative.[64] There is currently limited evidence in the literature for consistent benefits of prebiotics and probiotics.[61] Fecal transplantation may allow manipulation of the microbiota, in the short and medium term. Surgery to undertake resection and anastomosis may be curative for focal idiopathic eosinophilic enterocolitis.[51,65]

Outcome

Assuming the pathophysiology of IBD in the horse is like other species, simplifying treatment and treating IBD like it is a short-term condition that will resolve with corticosteroids are likely to be ineffective. In fact, one needs to appreciate the multifactorial nature and attempt to address the inciting cause and attempt to simplify the dietary management: change the fiber source, reduce the carbohydrate content, and simplify to 1 or 2 cereal sources and supplement with corn oil and vitamin D. Surgical management to resect focal lesions may be beneficial when medical management is unsuccessful. Client expectations need to be managed so that it is understood that this is a chronic condition and may need ongoing treatment for recurrence.

Assuming similarities with human disease, use of anthelmintics and antibiotics early in life, exposure to gastrointestinal infections, and rearing in very clean conditions may increase the risk of IBD in adulthood. Ultimately, large, multicenter studies with definitive diagnoses, thorough case histories, and ultimately an understanding of the natural history of IBD in the horse are lacking.

COLON DISPLACEMENT
Introduction

Displacement of the large colon is second to colon impaction as the most common reason for colic in horses and the second most common reason for colic referral.[66–68] The 2 most commonly described types of colon displacement are dorsal displacement of the left ascending colon over the nephrosplenic ligament (renosplenic entrapment, nephrosplenic ligament entrapment, or left dorsal displacement of large colon, LDDLC) and right dorsal displacement of large colon (RDDLC). Although colon displacement is often cited as the most common cause for colic surgery, medical treatment for colon displacement can often be successfully achieved with enteral fluids, laxatives, feed restriction, and analgesics. Under some conditions, transabdominal or transrectal trocarization of the cecum or ascending colon may relieve gas distension that is contributing to pain and sustaining the displacement. In general, the long-term survival rate for colon displacement is excellent.

History and Clinical Signs

There are no historical facts that are unique to horses with an RDDLC or LDDLC, although RDDLC is reported in broodmares, and LDDLC is reported more commonly in large breed horses.[69,70] Clinical signs of pain are variable and depend on the degree of extramural luminal compression of the colon, retention of ingesta, and gas distension of the proximal segments of the ascending colon and cecum. Clinical signs of colic are most commonly acute, although, in some cases, signs of recurrent colic are apparent in cases with chronic displacement. Clinical findings are consistent with a nonstrangulating obstruction and may include signs of mild to moderate dehydration in an otherwise cardiovascularly stable patient.[69,71]

Cause and Pathophysiology

Left dorsal displacement of the large colon describes the clinical scenario whereby the left colon is displaced between the left kidney and the spleen and left body wall, dorsal to the nephrosplenic ligament (**Fig. 6**). The RDDLC is easiest to describe as the clinical scenario whereby the ascending colon moves lateral to the base of the cecum such that a section of it lies between the cecum and the right body wall.[72] In the most common situation of an RDDLC, the pelvic flexure retroflexes toward the cranioventral abdomen, and gas-distended sternal and diaphragmatic flexures end up at the pelvic inlet (**Fig. 7**).[72] Less commonly, the pelvic flexure crosses the pelvic inlet directly and migrates lateral to the cecum and the right body wall.[72] In either scenario, a portion of the sternal and diaphragmatic flexures crosses the pelvic inlet and can be palpated traversing the caudal abdomen during transrectal examination.

The exact cause of colon displacement is not known and is likely multifactorial. Displacement is facilitated by the fact that the pelvic flexure is not fixed in its location, enabling freer movement of the ascending colon. Diet (particularly those higher in fermentable carbohydrates), changes in diet and exercise, changes in fecal microbiota, and colon impaction are listed as potential predisposing causes.[70,72]

Diagnosis

A presumptive diagnosis of colon displacement can be achieved by transrectal palpation. In horses with an LDDLC, the spleen is often ventrally and/or medially displaced

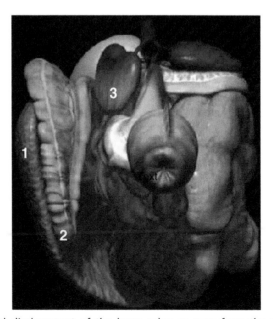

Fig. 6. Left dorsal displacement of the large colon as seen from the caudal abdomen. 1 = spleen; 2 = pelvic flexure; 3 = left kidney. (*From* the Glass Horse, University of Georgia, with permission of Science In 3D, Inc.)

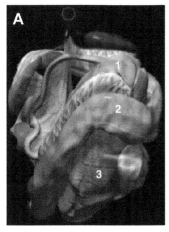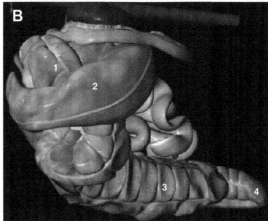

Fig. 7. Right dorsal displacement of the large colon as seen from the caudal abdomen (*A-D*) (*left*: 1 = ventral colon; 2 = dorsal colon; 3 = cecum) and from the right abdomen (*right*: 1 = ventral colon; 2 = dorsal colon; 3 = cecum; 4 = pelvic flexure). (*From* the Glass Horse, University of Georgia, with permission of Science In 3D, Inc.)

from the left body wall, and the large colon is palpable in the nephrosplenic space. The latter finding may be difficult to appreciate if there is minimal gas distension of the left colon. In the situation of an RDDLC, gas-distended large colon, most often the sternal and diaphragmatic flexures, and their associated tenia coli are palpable horizontally crossing the abdomen cranial to the pelvic inlet. The displaced colon makes it difficult to identify the cecum. Similar to an LDDLC, the latter finding may be difficult to appreciate if there is no gas distension of the displaced colon.

The following ultrasonographic findings have been attributed to horses with LDDLC: the dorsal aspect of the spleen or the left kidney is obliterated by gas shadowing from the displaced left colon or fluid-filled colon is visualized in the nephrosplenic space. The inability to visualize the left kidney is not always diagnostically accurate with both false positive and negative diagnoses reported.[73] The left kidney may be visualized ultrasonographically in cases in which there is minimal gas distension of the entrapped colon. More common than a false negative, a false positive diagnosis is encountered when gas is in the rectum after recent examination per rectum or gas distension of non-entrapped left colon is obscuring visualization of the left kidney.[74]

In horses with RDDLC, the colon often rotates 180° on its long axis, and normal medially located colonic vessels are displaced to the right lateral body wall (**Fig. 8**). Thus, careful dorsal to ventral transabdominal ultrasonographic interrogation of each right-sided intercostal space should be performed in horses suspected with RDDLC. Identification of colonic mesenteric vessels adjacent to the right body wall in at least 2 intercostal spaces dorsal to the costochondral junction that are distinct from lateral cecal vessels can be identified in approximately half of horses with surgically confirmed RDDLC.[75] Although the ultrasonographic presence of the displaced colon's vasculature is highly associated with RDDLC or 180° large colon volvulus, absence does not rule out displacement. Ness and colleagues found that visualization of the colonic mesenteric vessels was 89% specific for RDDLC and 68% sensitive, whereas Scharner and colleagues found a higher specificity of 100% but much lower sensitivity of 9%.[73] In this latter study, examination per rectum had an impressively higher sensitivity (96%) ultrasonography.

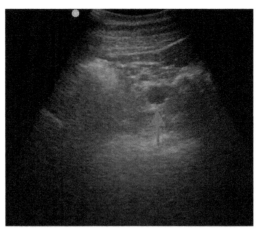

Fig. 8. Transabdominal ultrasonography at the right 12th intercostal space of a horse with an RDDLC. Dorsal is to the left of the image. The arrow points at the medial colonic vessels that were displaced laterally to the right body wall.

With the exception of clinicopathologic signs of mild to moderate dehydration, a complete blood count, serum chemistry profile, and peritoneal fluid analysis should be within normal limits.[71] In some cases of RDDLC, serum gamma-glutamyl transferase activity may be increased, presumptively from occlusion of the common bile duct by the displaced colon.[76]

Treatment

The prognosis for survival to discharge and long-term survival for horses with colon displacement is excellent.[69,77] The progress on successful medical management for LDDLC and RDDLC has been positive in the last decade.[71,78] In the largest study to date that included both types of displacements, medical management had a good success rate for treatment of suspected RDDLC (49/77; 64%) and even better success rate for horses with suspected LDDLC (38/50; 76%).[71] Although all cases were examined by a surgery specialist, the cases treated medically did not have an exploratory celiotomy to confirm a definitive diagnosis, so it is possible that other causes of simple obstruction of the large colon were miscategorized, and the success of medical therapy was slightly overestimated.

For both types of displacements, the treatment themes that are in common included use of enteral and intravenous fluids, enteral laxatives, analgesics (alpha-two agonists, opioids, nonsteroidal anti-inflammatory drugs, antispasmotic agents such as N-butylscopolammonium bromide, and continuous rate infusion of lidocaine), feed restriction, and cecal or colonic trocarization.[69,71,77,79] Administration of tap water rectally at a maintenance rate has been shown to be effective in providing hydration and is well tolerated, affordable, and safe.[80] Rectal fluids could be considered adjunct medical treatment for horses with colon displacement that are experiencing gastric reflux and financial limitations preclude the use of intravenous fluids. Furthermore, compared with healthy horses that received isotonic fluids enterally or intravenously, horses that received rectal tap water had improved intestinal sounds and greater fecal output.[80]

Transabdominal or transrectal trocarization of the cecum or large colon has gained favor as adjunct medical therapy for nonstrangulating simple obstructions of the large colon accompanied with moderate to severe gas distension, with recent detailed reviews on how to perform the transabdominal procedure in the paralumbar fossa with a 14-gauge catheter (**Fig. 9**).[81,82] Trocarization reduces luminal distension that contributes to pain and hinders perfusion. Trocarization can be a low-cost method to help manage pain from gas distension, although it should not replace surgical intervention when affordable for an owner and deemed necessary for the patient. Complications are purportedly rare and include fever, peritonitis, cellulitis or abscess formation, and hemorrhage, but no fatal complications associated with trocarization were reported by the authors of 2 recent reviews.[82,83] Multiple trocarizations were associated with nonsurvival, but this was attributed to severity of the disease and not the process of trocarization, as the complication rate was not associated with the number of trocarizations performed on a single patient.[83]

Two additional medical treatment options specifically used for LDDLC are jogging or strategically rolling under anesthesia, with or without concurrent treatment with phenylephrine, and treatment only with phenylephrine (3 μg/kg/min given in 1 L 0.9% saline over 15 minutes) without jogging or rolling.[71,78,79] Use of phenylephrine should be carefully considered in older horses. In one report, the risk of developing phenylephrine-associated hemorrhage, mostly fatal, was significantly higher in horses greater than or equal to 15 years old.[84] Risk of hemorrhage was not associated with the dose of phenylephrine.

Interestingly, in a recent 2020 meta-analysis on LDDLC in which 19 studies met inclusion criteria, treatment strategy, including medical versus surgical therapy, did not affect the likelihood of resolution of LDDLC.[79] Patients treated via the rolling technique were no more likely to resolve with medical management than those treated via jogging, and patients treated with phenylephrine were no more likely to exhibit medical resolution than patients that did not receive phenylephrine, either when all medical treatment methods were considered or when rolling under general anesthesia was used.[79] In a single report published after the meta-analysis, inclusion search reported 90% of LDDLC cases were resolved by rolling the horse under general anesthesia.[78]

Outcome

The short- and long-term survival is good to excellent for both RDDLC and LDDLC. Recurrence is reported with both types of colon displacement, although the actual rate of true recurrence is unknown. For horses with LDDLC, recurrence rate is reported

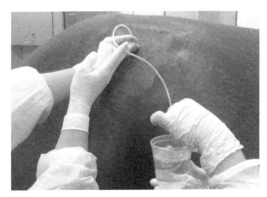

Fig. 9. Trocarization of a gas-distended cecum. A 14-gauge catheter was used and attached to an extension set with the end placed in a cup of water. Note the gas bubbles in the cup of water.

to be significantly lower in horses that have laparoscopic-assisted surgical closure of the nephrosplenic space.[85] When making decisions on treatment, it might be of interest to note that 2 retrospective studies found that compared with horses with other causes of nonstrangulating obstruction of the large colon requiring surgery, horses with RDDLC were more likely to have postoperative colic, complications that adversely affected short-term survival, and an increased likelihood of a relaparotomy.[86,87] It was not possible to determine if medical treatment could have reduced the complication rate and/or improved short-term outcome. There was no reported difference in long-term survival for RDDLC treated medically versus surgically.

REFERENCES

1. Bird AR, Knowles EJ, Sherlock CE, et al. The clinical and pathological features of gastric impaction in twelve horses. Equine Vet J 2012;44(S43):105–10.
2. Vainio K, Sykes BW, Blikslager AT. Primary gastric impaction in horses: a retrospective study of 20 cases (2005-2008). Equine Vet Educ 2011;23:186–90.
3. Hagedoorn S, Witt P, Kranenburg LC, et al. The use of cola for the treatment of gastric impactions in horses. Equine Vet Ed 2021;33:38.
4. Tallon R, Hayes C, Dunkel K. Comparison of outcomes for lone and concurrent gastric impactions in 113 hospitalized horses. Equine Vet J 2020;52:5.
5. McGovern KF, Suthers JM, James FM, et al. Gastric impaction associated with displacement and volvulus of the large colon in seven mature horses. Equine Vet Educ 2015;27:453–9.
6. Giusto G, Cerullo A, Gandini M. Gastric and Large Colon Impactions Combined With Aggressive Enteral Fluid Therapy May Predispose to Large Colon Volvulus: 4 Cases. J Equine Vet Sci 2021;102:103617.
7. Hurtado IR, Stewart A, Pellegrini-Masini A. Successful treatment for a gastric persimmon bezoar in a pony using nasogastric lavage with a carbonated cola soft drink. Equine Vet Educ 2007;19:571–4.
8. Banse HE, Gilliam LL, House AM, et al. Gastric and enteric phytobezoars caused by ingestion of persimmon in equids. J Am Vet Med Assoc 2011;239:1110–6.
9. Banse HE. Management of phytobezoars. Equine Vet Educ 2020;32:515–7.
10. Iwamuro M, Yamauchi K, Shiraha H, et al. All carbonated beverages effectively dissolve phytobezoars. Clin Res Hepatol Gastroenterol 2018;42:e66–7.
11. Parker RA, Barr ED, Dixon PM. Treatment of equine gastric impaction by gastrotomy. Equine Vet Educ 2011;23:169–73.
12. Bauck AG, Nelson E, McLain A, et al. J-incision to approach the cranial abdomen in the adult horse. Vet Surg 2021;50:600–6.
13. Rendle D, Bowen M, Brazil T, et al. Recommendations for the management of equine glandular gastric disease. UK-Vet Equine. 2018;2:2–11.
14. Sykes B, Bowen M, Habershon-Butcher J, et al. Management factors and clinical implications of glandular and squamous gastric disease in horses. J Vet Intern Med 2019;33:233–40.
15. Sykes BW, Sykes KM, Hallowell GD. A comparison of two doses of omeprazole in the treatment of equine gastric ulcer syndrome: A blinded, randomised, clinical trial. Equine Vet J 2014;46:416–21.
16. Sykes BW, Sykes KM, Hallowell GD. A comparison of three doses of omeprazole in the treatment of equine gastric ulcer syndrome: A blinded, randomised, dose-response clinical trial. Equine Vet J 2015;47:285.
17. deLaHunta A, Glass E, Kent M. Veterinary neuroanatomy and clinical neurology. 4th edition. St. Louis, MO: Elsevier; 2014.

18. Begg LM, O'Sullivan CB. The prevalence and distribution of gastric ulceration in 345 racehorses. Aust Vet J 2003;81:199–201.

19. Husted L, Jensen TK, Olsen SN, et al. Examination of equine glandular stomach lesions for bacteria, including Helicobacter spp by fluorescence in situ hybridisation. BMC Microbiol 2010;10. Article number 84.

20. Luthersson N, Nielsen KH, Harris P, et al. The prevalence and anatomical distribution of equine gastric ulceration syndrome (EGUS) in 201 horses in Denmark. Equine Vet J 2009;41:619–24.

21. Martineau H, Thompson H, Taylor D. Pathology of gastritis and gastric ulceration in the horse. Part 1: Range of lesions present in 21 mature individuals. Equine Vet J 2009;41:638–44.

22. Nieto JE, Snyder JR, Beldomenico P, et al. Prevalence of gastric ulcers in endurance horses - a preliminary report. Vet J 2004;167:33–7.

23. Tamzali Y, Marguet C, Priymenko N, et al. Prevalence of gastric ulcer syndrome in high-level endurance horses. Equine Vet J 2011;43:141–4.

24. Mönki J, Hewetson M, Virtala AMK. Risk factors for equine gastric glandular disease: a case-control study in a Finnish referral hospital population. J Vet Intern Med 2016;30:1270–5.

25. Pedersen SK, Cribb AE, Windeyer MC, et al. Risk factors for equine glandular and squamous gastric disease in show jumping Warmbloods. Equine Vet J 2018;50:747.

26. Banse HE, MacLeod H, Crosby C, et al. Prevalence of and risk factors for equine glandular and squamous gastric disease in polo horses. Can Vet J 2018;59:880–4.

27. Malmkvist J, Poulsen JM, Luthersson N, et al. Behaviour and stress responses in horses with gastric ulceration. Appl Anim Behav Sci 2012;142:160–7.

28. Scheidegger MD, Gerber V, Bruckmaier RM, et al. Increased adrenocortical response to adrenocorticotropic hormone (ACTH) in sport horses with equine glandular gastric disease (EGGD). Vet J 2017;228:7–12.

29. Scott L, de Lavis I, Daniels S. Crib Biting and Equine Gastric Ulcer Syndrome, is there an Anatomical link? Equine Vet Educ 2017;S8:11.

30. MacLeod H, Windeeyer C, Crosby C, et al. Prevalence and risk factors for gastric ulceration in polo horses. J Vet Intern Med 2015;27:1244.

31. Cayado P, Muñoz-Escassi B, Domínguez C, et al. Hormone response to training and competition in athletic horses. Equine Vet J 2006;274–8.

32. Covalesky ME, Russoniello CR, Malinowski K. Effects of show-jumping performance stress on plasma cortisol and lactate concentrations and heart rate and behavior in horses. J Equine Vet Sci 1992;12:244–51.

33. Crumpton SM, Baiker K, Hallowell GD, et al. Diagnostic Value of Gastric Mucosal Biopsies in Horses with Glandular Disease. Equine Vet J 2015;47:9.

34. Merritt AM, Sanchez LC, Burrow JA, et al. Effect of GastroGard and three compounded oral omeprazole preparations on 24 h intragastric pH in gastrically cannulated mature horses. Equine Vet J 2003;35:691–5.

35. Hepburn R. Equine Glandular Ulceration: Epidemiology and Pathophysiology. Proceedings of the Annual Veterinary Medical Forum - American College of Veterinary Internal Medicine, New Orleans. 2012;289-289.

36. Muñoz-Prieto A, Contreras-Aguilar MD, Cerón JJ, et al. Changes in Proteins in Saliva and Serum in Equine Gastric Ulcer Syndrome Using a Proteomic Approach. Animals 2022;12:1169–83.

37. Sykes BW, Hewetson M, Hepburn RJ, et al. European College of Equine Internal Medicine Consensus Statement–Equine Gastric Ulcer Syndrome in Adult Horses. J Vet Intern Med 2015;29:1288–99.

38. Gough S, Hallowell GD, Rendle D. A study investigating the treatment of equine squamous gastric disease with long-acting injectable or oral omeprazole. Vet Med Sci 2020;6:235–41.

39. Tallon R, Hewetson M. Inter-observer variability of two grading systems for equine glandular gastric disease. Equine Vet J 2021;495-502.

40. Pratt S, Bowen I, Hallowell G, et al. Assessment of agreement using the equine glandular gastric disease grading system in 84 cases. Vet Med Sci 2022;8:1472–7.

41. Paul C, Ericsson C, Andrews F, et al. Gastric microbiome in horses with and without equine glandular gastric disease. J Vet Intern Med 2021;35:2458–64.

42. Voss SJ, McGuinness DH, Weir W, et al. A study comparing the healthy and diseased equine glandular gastric microbiota sampled with sheathed transendo-scopic cytology brushes. J Equine Vet Sci 2022;116:104002.

43. Varley G, Bowen IM, Habershon-Butcher JL, et al. Misoprostol is superior to combined omeprazole-sucralfate for the treatment of equine gastric glandular disease. Equine Vet J 2019;51:575–80.

44. Sangiah S, MacAllister C, Amouzadeh H. Effects of misoprostol and omeprazol on basal gastric pH and free acid content in horses. Res Vet Sci 1989;47:350–4.

45. Martin EM, Schirmer JM, Jones SL, et al. Pharmacokinetics and ex vivo anti-inflammatory effects of oral misoprostol in horses. Equine Vet J 2019;51:415–21.

46. Jacobson CC, Sertich PL, McDonnell SM. Mid-gestation pregnancy is not disrupted by a 5-day gastrointestinal mucosal cytoprotectant oral regimen of misoprostol. Equine Vet J 2013;45:91–3.

47. Sykes BW, Kathawala K, Song Y, et al. Preliminary investigations into a novel, long-acting, injectable, intramuscular formulation of omeprazole in the horse. Equine Vet J 2017;49:795–801.

48. Gough S, Hallowell G, Rendle D. Evaluation of the treatment of equine glandular gastric disease with either long-acting-injectable or oral omeprazole. Vet Med Sci 2022;561-567.

49. Cargile JL, Burrow JA, Kim I, et al. Effect of dietary corn oil supplementation on equine gastric fluid acid, sodium, and prostaglandin E2 content before and during pentagastrin infusion. J Vet Intern Med 2004;18:545–9.

50. Sykes BW, Sykes KM, Hallowell GD. Efficacy of a combination of apolectol, live yeast (Saccharomyces cerevisiae), and magnesium hydroxide in the management of equine gastric ulcer syndrome in thoroughbred racehorses: a blinded, randomized, placebo-controlled clinical trial. J Equine Vet Sci 2014;34:1274–8.

51. Schumacher J, Edwards JF, Cohen ND. Chronic idiopathic inflammatory bowel diseases of the horse. J Vet Intern Med 2000;14:258–65.

52. Kaikkonen R, Niinistö K, Sykes B, et al. Diagnostic evaluation and short-term outcome as indicators of long-term prognosis in horses with findings suggestive of inflammatory bowel disease treated with corticosteroids and anthelmintics. Acta Vet Scand 2014;56:35.

53. Kemper DL, Perkins GA, Schumacher J, et al. Equine lymphocytic-plasmacytic enterocolitis: a retrospective study of 14 cases. Equine Vet J 2000;108–12.

54. Ponder A, Long MD. A clinical review of recent findings in the epidemiology of inflammatory bowel disease. Clin Epidemiol 2013;2013:237–47.

55. Denson LA, Long MD, McGovern DPB, et al. Challenges in IBD Research: Update on Progress and Prioritization of the CCFA's Research Agenda. Inflamm Bowel Dis 2013;19:677–82.

56. Sartor RB. Microbial influences in inflammatory bowel diseases. United States: Elsevier Sciecne BV Amsterdam; 2008. p. 577–94.

57. van der Kolk JH, van Putten LA, Mulder CJ, et al. Gluten-dependent antibodies in horses with inflammatory small bowel disease (ISBD). Vet Q 2012;32:3–11.

58. Metcalfe LVA, More SJ, Duggan V, et al. A retrospective study of horses investigated for weight loss despite a good appetite (2002-2011). Equine Vet J 2013;45: 340–5.

59. Jacobs G, Collins-Kelly L, Lappin M, et al. Lymphocytic-plasmacytic enteritis in 24 dogs. J Vet Intern Med 1990;4:45–53.

60. Salem PA, Nassar VH, Shahid MJ, et al. Mediterranean abdominal lymphoma," or immunoproliferative small intestinal disease. Part I: clinical aspects. Cancer 1977; 40:2941–7.

61. Jergens AE, Simpson KW. Inflammatory bowel disease in veterinary medicine. Front Biosci (Elite Ed) 2012;4:1404–19.

62. Malewska K, Rychlik A, Nieradka R, et al. Treatment of inflammatory bowel disease (IBD) in dogs and cats. Pol J Vet Sci 2011;14:165–71.

63. Dye TL, Diehl KJ, Wheeler SL, et al. Randomized, Controlled Trial of Budesonide and Prednisone for the Treatment of Idiopathic Inflammatory Bowel Disease in Dogs. J Vet Intern Med 2013;27:1385–91.

64. Vázquez-Baeza Y, Hyde ER, Suchodolski JS, et al. Dog and human inflammatory bowel disease rely on overlapping yet distinct dysbiosis networks. Nature microbiology 2016;1. Article number 16177.

65. Edwards GB, Kelly DF, Proudman CJ. Segmental eosinophilic colitis: a review of 22 cases. Equine Vet J 2000;(Supplement):86–93.

66. Abutarbush SM, Carmalt JL, Shoemaker RW. Causes of gastrointestinal colic in horses in western Canada: 604 cases (1992 to 2002). Can Vet J 2005;46:800–5.

67. Gunes V, Onmaz AC, Pavaloiu A, et al. A retrospective study of gastrointestinal disorders in a predominantly Austrian leisure horse referral hospital population. Equine Vet Educ 2022;34:467–72.

68. Voigt A, Saulez MN, Donnellan CM, et al. Causes of gastrointestinal colic at an equine referral hospital in South Africa (1998-2007). J S Afr Vet Assoc 2009;80: 192–8.

69. Pilorge G, Battail G, Gluntz X, et al. Retrospective study of 75 cases of left dorsal colon displacement in horses. Prat Vet Equine 2002;34:25–35.

70. Weese JS, Holcombe SJ, Embertson RM, et al. Changes in the faecal microbiota of mares precede the development of post partum colic. Equine Vet J 2015;47: 641–9.

71. McGovern KF, Bladon BM, Fraser BSL, et al. Attempted medical management of suspected ascending colon displacement in horses. Vet Surg 2012;41:399–403.

72. Southwood L. Large colon. In: Auer J, Stick J, Kummerle J, et al, editors. *Equine surgery.* 5th edition. St. Louis, MO: Elsevier; 2019. p. 591–621.

73. Cribb NC, Arroyo LG. Techniques and Accuracy of Abdominal Ultrasound in Gastrointestinal Diseases of Horses and Foals. Vet Clin N Am Equine Pract 2018;34:25–38.

74. Beccati F, Pepe M, Gialletti R, et al. Is there a statistical correlation between ultrasonographic findings and definitive diagnosis in horses with acute abdominal pain? Equine Vet J Suppl 2011;98-105.

75. Grenager NS, Durham MG. Ultrasonographic evidence of colonic mesenteric vessels as an indicator of right dorsal displacement of the large colon in 13 horses. Equine Vet J 2011;43:153–5.

76. Gardner RB, Nydam DV, Mohammed HO, et al. Serum gamma glutamyl transferase activity in horses with right or left dorsal displacements of the large colon. J Vet Intern Med 2005;19:761–4.

77. Monreal L, Navarro M, Armengou L, et al. Enteral fluid therapy in 108 horses with large colon impactions and dorsal displacements. Vet Rec 2010;166:259–63.

78. Normand T, Santinelli Y, Carette O, et al. Sixty-eight cases of nephrosplenic attachment treated by rolling under general anaesthesia. Prat Vet Equine 2018; 50:46–51.

79. Gillen A, Kottwitz J, Munsterman A. Meta-analysis of the Effect of Treatment Strategies for Nephrosplenic Entrapment of the Large Colon. J Equine Vet Sci 2020; 92:103169.

80. Khan A, Hallowell GD, Underwood C, et al. Continuous fluid infusion per rectum compared with intravenous and nasogastric fluid administration in horses. Equine Vet J 2019;51:767–73.

81. Schroeder EL, Gardner AK, Mudge MC. How to perform a percutaneous cecal or colonic trocarization in horses with severe abdominal tympany. J Vet Emerg Crit Care 2022;32:57–62.

82. Tadros E. How to perform percutaneous cecal and colonic trocharization in horses with gastrointestinal colic. American Association of Equine Practitioners 61st Annual Conference, December 5-9, 2015, Las Vegas, NV, 2015;169–172.

83. Schoster A, Torgerson PR, Bischofberger AS, et al. Outcome and complications following transrectal and transabdominal large intestinal trocarization in equids with colic: 228 cases (2004-2015). J Am Vet Med Assoc 2020;257:189–95.

84. Frederick J, Giguère S, Butterworth K, et al.: Severe phenylephrine-associated hemorrhage in five aged horses. J Am Vet Med Assoc 2010;237:830-834.

85. Arévalo Rodríguez JM, Grulke S, Salciccia A, et al. Nephrosplenic space closure significantly decreases recurrent colic in horses: a retrospective analysis. Vet Rec 2019;185:657–63.

86. Smith LJ, Mair TS. Are horses that undergo an exploratory laparotomy for correction of a right dorsal displacement of the large colon predisposed to post operative colic, compared to other forms of large colon displacement? Equine Vet J 2010;42:44–6.

87. Whyard J, Brounts S. Post-Operative Complications And Survival In Horses With Right Dorsal Displacement Of The Ascending Colon Compared With Other Non-Strangulating Ascending Colon Lesions. Equine Vet Educ 2017;29:31.

Colic Surgery: Recent Updates

Maia R. Aitken, DVM

KEYWORDS

- Colic surgery • Exploratory celiotomy • Standing flank laparotomy
- Survival outcomes

KEY POINTS

- Colic surgery remains an important focus of study within veterinary medicine as approximately one-quarter of horses that are referred to equine hospitals will require surgical intervention.
- The last several years of research within the field of equine colic surgery have introduced new techniques, new or recently described lesions, methods at prevention of lesion recurrence or postoperative complications, and updates in prognoses following colic surgery.
- Early identification of surgical lesions remains a critical factor in survival of the horse with surgical colic.

INTRODUCTION

Colic has been described as a major medical problem of equids and represents a large proportion, if not the majority, of emergency admissions to referral hospitals.[1] Of the horses that present with colic to a referral hospital, up to 28% will require or will undergo colic surgery.[2] The expense associated with colic surgery or often the perception of "suffering" or putting a horse through it, are some of the major detractors for owners from pursing colic surgery.[3] Current financial costs of colic surgery certainly vary by country, region, and even practice; however, the consensus is that it can be cost-prohibitive for many clients. A recent editorial by Freeman described the improvements made during the previous 50 years of colic surgery.[4] In it, he described early major improvements in intraoperative techniques but also cautioned against the use of postoperative methods and management strategies that do not improve outcome and increase overall cost. The following description provides an overview of the last 5 years of research and innovation within the field of equine colic surgery, focusing on new techniques, new or recently described lesions, prevention of lesion recurrence or postoperative complications, and updates in prognoses.

NEW APPROACHES AND TECHNIQUES

As we move forward toward cost-effective means of treating horses requiring colic surgery, standing laparotomy has become a potentially less expensive option.

Department of Clinical Studies – New Bolton Center, University of Pennsylvania, 382 West Street Road, Kennett Square, PA 19348, USA
E-mail address: maitken@vet.upenn.edu

Vet Clin Equine 39 (2023) 249–262
https://doi.org/10.1016/j.cveq.2023.03.009
0749-0739/23/© 2023 Elsevier Inc. All rights reserved.

Standing procedures avoid expense associated with general anesthesia as well as the risks associated with general anesthesia and recovery. Although standing laparotomy will not replace ventral midline celiotomy, a recent report suggests it can be used successfully to access some parts of the abdomen and the corresponding viscera.[5] The multicenter retrospective case series by Lopes and colleagues describes 37 equids undergoing left flank (n = 31), right flank (n = 2), or bilateral flank (n = 4) approaches for colic. Horses with lesions of the descending colon were excluded from the series because there have been previous reports of treating descending colon lesions via a flank laparotomy.[6] Intraoperative procedures that were performed included examination and decompression of the jejunum and ileum by exteriorizing only a 1 to 1.5-m section at a time, unspecified resection and anastomosis of the small intestine (n = 1), biopsy of the ileum, needle decompression of the small and large intestine, partial typhlectomy (n = 1), pelvic flexure enterotomy, correction of colonic displacements, ablation of the nephrosplenic space (NSS), and a partial large colon resection (pelvic flexure, n = 1). The majority of cases were large intestinal (cecal or large colon, n = 23). No horse with strangulation or infarction of the large or small intestine (n = 4) survived to discharge; 2 out of 4 of these horses were euthanized immediately following surgery based on intraoperative findings. Intraoperative complications that were reported included sudden patient recumbency and subsequent visceral contamination, spontaneous exteriorization of long segments of distended small intestine resulting in mesenteric tearing, and intolerance of visceral manipulation despite repeated sedation. Overall survival to discharge was 54%. In this population of horses,[5] the most common complication was surgical site infection in 20% of cases. Long-term survival (>9 months) was 41% with all surviving equids returning to their intended use. Expense associated with the treatment of the surviving cases was approximately half of the lower end of the estimate for an uncomplicated ventral midline celiotomy within the same hospital.[5] This approach may offer a cost-effective option when a ventral midline approach cannot be performed, paying special attention to case selection based on presumptive diagnosis as well as the patient's signs of discomfort and compliance.

Another alternative approach to the equine abdomen could be a laparoscopic or a laparoscopic-assisted approach. Jones and colleagues described a pilot study evaluating the feasibility of standing laparoscopy for the evaluation of the small intestine.[7] A single portal in the left last intercostal space and 3 portals in the right paralumbar fossa allowed for complete evaluation from the duodenocolic ligament to the ileocecal fold using atraumatic laparoscopic grasping forceps. The laparoscope was inserted through the left-sided portal was used for laparoscope placement and to allow direct observation of the placement of the right-sided portals, which were used for the laparoscope as well as instruments to facilitate the evaluation of the complete length of jejunum and ileum. The procedure, along with a repeat laparoscopy at 2 weeks to assess any iatrogenic damage, was performed successfully and well tolerated in all 5 horses.[7] This procedure may offer an alternative approach to the abdomen, realizing that the evaluation of the entire abdomen is limited. Standing laparoscopy may also be used in combination with a small flank laparotomy as a laparoscopic-assisted approach for small intestinal biopsy or resection-anastomosis.

To facilitate standing laparoscopy and possibly standing laparotomy, Delli-Rocili and colleagues examine the ease and usefulness of the paravertebral block compared with local infiltration of laparoscopic portals.[8] In this randomized clinical trial, 6 horses were randomly assigned to each group: paravertebral (T18-L2) or 3 traditional local portal blocks using 20 mL of 2% lidocaine for each portal. Before administration of local anesthetic, horses in both groups were sedated with a dexmedetomidine and morphine constant rate infusion. No differences were found between the 2 groups in regards to the time needed to perform each technique, nor in the level of anesthesia that was provided.[8] This approach may provide an alternative to the traditional method of anesthesia while allowing for greater flexibility in portal placement or extension of a portal to a flank incision without the need for additional intraoperative local anesthetic administration.

In an effort to reduce the intraoperative time associated with mesenteric vessel ligation, Giusto and Gandini compared sliding knot ligatures to hemostatic clips (Hemoclip Weck, Teleflex Medical, Research Triangle Park, NC) in an ex vivo study.[9] In this study, triple occlusion of 5 mesenteric vessels in a segment of jejunum was performed. The study demonstrated no difference in bursting pressure between the 2 methods of vessel occlusion, whereas a significantly reduced mean time for the application of the 3 hemostatic clips was measured compared with the 3 sliding knot ligature technique (2.40 vs 7.03 min).[9] In the case of a long segment of intestine to be resected, application of hemostatic clips may provide time savings with the added benefit of cost savings compared with a vessel-sealing device. Giusto and colleagues also published a report describing the use of transillumination of the small colon mesentery to aid in the mesenteric vessel identification for surgical planning and vessel ligation.[10] The case series of 6 horses undergoing small colon resection and anastomosis describes the use of either surgical lights (n = 3) or a smartphone with a light-emitting diode (LED) flashlight (n = 3) to backlight the mesocolon, providing a light source behind the mesentery, a technique adapted from human surgery. This allowed the surgeon to easily identify, dissect, ligate, and transect each vessel without complication. A note was made that the use of the smartphone wrapped in a sterile rectal sleeve was easier and decreased assistant fatigue compared with holding the small colon up to the light provided by overhead surgical lights.[10] Both methods allow easy vessel identification and may decrease the risk of intraoperative error and hemorrhage.

There have been several recent studies focused on improving small intestinal surgery, specifically resection-anastomosis and bypass procedures associated with small intestinal strangulating obstructions. Lenoir and colleagues investigated the use of an ultraviolet-polymerizable methacrylate adhesive (UV-PMA) as a second layer of a 2-layer jejunojejunostomy.[11] In their study, cadaver jejunum was used to compare a 2-layer anastomosis comprising of a full thickness simple continuous followed by a Cushing oversew using 2-0 polyglycolic acid (control) to a single layer full thickness simple continuous (2-0 polyglycolic acid) followed by application of UV-PMA that cures with a UV LED lamp for 30 seconds. These 2 constructs were compared with each other along with a length of control jejunum to test luminal diameter and bursting strength pressure (BSP). Investigators found that mean construction time was significantly lower for the UV-PMA group compared with controls (3.02 vs 8.09 minutes); however, the UV-PMA group also had lower BSP compared with controls (mean 170.47 vs 189.93 mm Hg) and shreds of glue were visible on the serosal surface posttesting.[11] The observation of glue material on the serosal surface may make this application of methacrylate adhesive not yet suitable for clinical use.

Another application for small intestinal resection and anastomosis is the use of hyaluronate-carboxymethylcellulose (HA-CMC) membranes to cover anastomosis sites. A recent retrospective study by Troy and colleagues examined the effect of such HA-CMC membranes on anastomosis or enterotomy sites and compared them with control (no HA-CMC membrane) cases with similar intestinal lesions and procedures.[12] In comparing the 2 groups, the volume of preoperative reflux and the duration of lidocaine administration postoperatively were higher in the HA-CMC group. No other differences between the groups were found, suggesting that the use of a HA-CMC membrane did not influence postoperative complications or survival. Although having no positive effect on the postoperative period of the horse, HA-CMC membranes have a relatively short shelf life and can be technically challenging to apply, possibly resulting in a lack of widespread clinical use.[12]

Giusto and colleagues reported a new application of ileocecostomy, where they proposed the use of incomplete ileocecal bypass for varying ileal pathologic conditions in horses.[13] Their study included 21 clinical cases: 13 horses with ileal impactions, 5 with epiploic foramen entrapments (EFEs), and 3 horses with strangulating pedunculated lipomas. Incomplete bypass, whether ileocecal or jejunocecal, was performed as a 2-layer handsewn technique in 19 cases and stapled in 2 cases. The authors reported an overall 92.5% short-term survival. No resections were performed in these cases. The goals of using this technique were to decrease the risk of recurrence of ileal impaction and the development of postoperative reflux (POR) associated with ileal ischemic injury and inflammation.[13] An important consideration for the success of this approach is that the ileum retains viability following lesion correction.

Gandini and Giusto also published a report on the use of a combination of an end-to-end jejunoileostomy and side-to-side incomplete ileocecostomy, or a hybrid jejuno-ileo-cecal anastomosis, for oral ileal strangulation in 7 horses. The authors' rationale for this technique was that the hybrid procedure restored continuity of the small intestine while providing incomplete bypass of the ileocecal valve.[14] All horses survived to discharged; however, one horse was euthanized due to recurrent colic 17 months after surgery (85.7% alive for at least 4 months). The procedure would be an option for horses with lesions where a portion of the ileum is sufficiently viable such that a jejunoileostomy can be performed, and then performing a jejunocecostomy as an adjunct to the jejunoileostomy. The combined technique may improve outcome, given the increased risk of POR associated with jejunoileostomy and long-term colic with jejunocecostomy.[15]

In order to better understand the pathophysiology of POR, Lisowski and colleagues evaluated the use of quantitative real-time PCR to assess the local inflammatory response of the small intestine adjacent to resection sites.[16] The investigators sampled mucosa and muscularis externa from what was deemed healthy margins of resected jejunum or ileum and compared these with midjejunum from control horses euthanized for reasons unrelated to the gastrointestinal tract. Tissue from colic cases showed significant increases in interleukin (IL)1β, IL6, chemokine (C-C motif) ligand 2, and tumor necrosis factor (TNF) compared with controls, despite these areas being deemed apparently "healthy grossly viable" margins.[16] These cytokines and chemokines are released secondary to inflammation and can also represent inflammatory responses to intestinal manipulation.[17] The investigators also found that horses that went on to develop POR had significantly greater relative gene expression of TNF in the mucosa compared with horses that did not develop POR.[16] These results support the notion that both oral and aboral margins demonstrate injury likely secondary to distention, ischemia-reperfusion, and surgical manipulation. These findings underscore the importance of early referral, gentle tissue handling, and adequate resection margins in the prevention of POR.

Although no consensus has been reached regarding the timing and duration of perioperative antimicrobials for horses undergoing colic surgery, antimicrobial drug resistance, expense of treatment, and the potential for antimicrobial-associated complications has led to studies investigating the necessary duration of prophylaxis. Stockle and colleagues compared the use of a short-term prophylaxis regimen with a "standard protocol" in equine colic surgery.[18] This pilot study was a randomized clinical trial that enrolled 67 horses into 2 groups: a "single-shot" group that received a preoperative dose of sodium penicillin and gentamicin (n = 30) and a "5-day lasting" group that received penicillin and gentamicin for 5 days (n = 37). Significant differences were neither found in postoperative complications nor in postoperative clinicopathological data between groups; however, 30 days after surgery, the "single-shot" group had a 23% incisional infection rate compared with a 5% infection rate in the "5-day lasting" group.[18] The sample size was relatively small in this pilot study, leading to a lack of study power to detect a significant difference and an inability to adequately control for confounding variables. Continued research regarding optimal antimicrobial prophylaxis for exploratory celiotomy is warranted, given the expense and potential complications associated with prolonged antimicrobial treatment in at risk patients.

REEMERGING OR NEW DISEASES

In the last 5 years, there have been several reports of reemerging diseases or newly identified disease processes. One alarming problem is the reemergence of *Strongylus vulgaris* within populations of horses maintained with surveillance-based parasite control programs. Pihl and colleagues presented a retrospective case series of 30 horses with nonstrangulating intestinal infarction secondary to *S vulgaris*.[19] Horses in the study presented with a history mild colic of longer than 24 hours duration, dull demeanor, mild pyrexia, leukopenia, high serum amyloid A concentration, and peritonitis (increased peritoneal fluid total protein and nucleated cell count) in 90% of cases. Nine horses were managed medically (0% short-term survival) and 21 horses underwent exploratory laparotomy. Of the surgical cases, 11 were euthanized intraoperatively due to the severity of peritonitis (4 out of 11), ruptured intestine (2 out of 11), or impossibility of resection due to the extent of the infarction (5 out of 11). Nine horses underwent resection and anastomosis, and one had adhesiolysis performed. Infarctions were present within the viscera supplied by the cranial mesenteric artery, most commonly the left dorsal colon/pelvic flexure or the cecum. Only 3 horses survived to hospital discharge, representing 30% of horses recovered from anesthesia. Importantly, these 3 horses underwent intestinal resection within 1 to 4 days of the onset of clinical signs, highlighting the importance of improved recognition and timely surgical intervention. Two horses survived beyond 2 years to compete in their respective disciplines.[19] This report supports the use of peritoneal fluid analysis as part of the diagnostic workup for cases that present with signs of low-grade colic and systemic inflammation as intestinal infarction could be a relevant differential diagnosis, especially in horses from areas where *S vulgaris* is endemic or in horses not effectively treated with anthelmintics.

Lawless and colleagues recently described duodenojejunal mesenteric rents in 37 Thoroughbred broodmares.[20] The study found that rents involving the mesoduodenum caudal to the root of the mesentery were likely associated with parturition and that these specific rents have a better prognosis than previous reports of mesenteric rents.[20,21] Thirty-three horses survived colic surgery and only 9 (27%) of these cases underwent a jejunojejunostomy procedure. The rents were closed in 28 (85%) horses using 0 polypropylene in a simple continuous pattern within the dorsal abdomen without visibility of the affected mesentery (partially blind). Of note is that in only 5 mares, the mesenteric rent was not repaired; 3 of these mares had a repeat surgery to close the rent due to recurrent entrapment (n = 2) or colic (n = 1). Overall survival to hospital discharge was 76% and 74% of mares survived to at least 12 months following surgery. The reported outcome of mares in this study was higher than in previous reports of mesenteric rents reporting a 47% short-term and 40% long-term survival.[20,21] Although the number of mares not undergoing rent closure was small, recurrent colic in 60% of these mares supports closure of the rent, using a partially blind approach, during the initial surgery.[20]

A recent review by Abu-Seida discusses the various types of diaphragmatic hernias in equids, highlighting the challenge of repairing large (>10 cm) tears of the dorsal diaphragm in adult horses.[22] The author underscores perceived improvements in overall survival compared with the previously reported 25% survival.[23] The improved survival was attributed to improvements made in surgical techniques: the use of prosthetic mesh for large defects and thoracoscopic approaches to facilitate visibility and access to the defect. Despite perceived improvement, case selection with respect to location and size of the hernia still plays the largest role in the overall success.

Two congenital abnormalities of the gastrointestinal tract have recently been reported. The first, an unusual presentation of a redundant mesocolon of the ascending colon, was presented by Voss and Dubois.[24] In this case report, a 3-month-old Shire colt was managed surgically for an acute colic episode that was unresponsive to medical management. At surgery, a nonstrangulating volvulus of the ascending colon and cecum at the dorsal mesenteric attachment and pelvic flexure retroversion were encountered and corrected. Examination of the viscera revealed an abnormally wide mesocolon between the dorsal and ventral ascending colon, along with an abnormally long transverse colon mesocolon, allowing exteriorization of the entire ascending and transverse colon. The colt was euthanized based on a high likelihood of recurrence of colic.[24] The second report on congenital abnormalities describes the successful surgical management of a type 3a atresia coli in a 12-hour-old Thoroughbred colt, wherein complete absence of a segment of ascending or descending colon occurs.[25] At the time of surgery, absence of the left and right dorsal colon was found, with a severely distended blind end of the left ventral colon and normal appearance of the descending colon. Based on preoperative contrast radiography and intraoperative findings, a diagnosis of type 3a atresia coli of the dorsal ascending and transverse colon was made. Given the large disparity in luminal size between the left ventral and descending colon, an end-to-side anastomosis was created between the blind end of the left ventral colon and the antimesenteric aspect of the descending colon, at the midpoint of the descending colon. The foal recovered from surgery well without complications associated with surgery and was reportedly growing similarly to his cohorts at 6 months of age.[25]

Although EFE typically affects the distal jejunum and ileum,[26] entrapment of portions or the large intestine have also been documented, including a brief mention of the cecal entrapment within a thesis article.[26–31] Grzeskowiak and colleagues recently described the first complete case report on cecal entrapment within the epiploic foramen.[27] The surgical findings included a 180° large colon volvulus, which was corrected, followed by discovery of the left-to-right entrapped cecal apex. Given the intra-abdominal location of the cecal apex, neither typhlotomy nor typhlectomy could be performed without the risk of gross peritoneal contamination. Following gentle reduction without enlarging the foramen, severe hemorrhage was noted. Palpation of the portal vein revealed a large tear. The mare was euthanized intraoperatively.[27] The authors discussed the options of a partial typhlectomy to facilitate entrapment resolution, similar to the described technique of partial large colon resection to aid in reduction of large colon entrapment.[30] Accessibility to the cecal apex made this option impossible. A recent report by Wanstrath and colleagues describes a technique for surgical enlargement of the epiploic foramen in 14 experimental horses followed by 5 clinical cases.[32] The surgical procedure involved digital dissection of the caudal edge of the foramen to open the fascia and separate the caudate lobe of the liver from the right kidney, pancreas, and right dorsal colon. No hemorrhage was noted throughout the procedure in any horse (n = 19), and necropsy of the 14 experimental cases confirmed the lack of major vessel disruption or damage to adjacent organs. One of the clinical cases had necropsy performed at 30 days that revealed spontaneous closure of the caudal aspect of the foramen.[32] As the authors described, this technique would be applicable for cases of EFE where reduction is difficult and may be especially useful in the rare case of large intestinal entrapment.

TECHNIQUES AIMED AT PREVENTION OR RECURRENCE

The following section will focus on recent techniques that have been developed to prevent recurrence of epiploic foramen and nephrosplenic ligament entrapments (NSLEs), followed by recent studies looking at reducing the risk of surgical site infection.

EFE, as mentioned above, most commonly affects the distal jejunum and ileum. The most recently reported short-term survival rate is 65% of horses recovering from anesthesia with a recurrence rate of 3%.[26] Although spontaneous closure of the epiploic foramen is reported in up to 43% of horses undergoing laparoscopic inspection of the area, cases of EFE recurrence are presumed to occur in horses that do not have closure, warranting the discussion of whether to prophylactically close the foramen.[33] The initial techniques of foramen closure were described via a right flank laparoscopic approach to either obliterate the space with titanium helical coils or insert a diabolo-shaped mesh construct.[34,35] With the successful placement of a mesh via laparoscopy, investigators sought to assess the feasibility of mesh placement via a ventral midline approach. Van Bergen and colleagues piloted this approach using 6 experimental horses to mimic a colic surgery with the horse under general anesthesia and positioned in dorsal recumbency.[36] The horses were recovered from the procedure and follow-up laparoscopy at 1 month confirmed complete mesh-induced closure of the epiploic foramen with dense fibrous tissue with no undesired abdominal adhesions.[36] A similar technique was then pursued on 17 clinical cases by Grulke and colleagues with a modification that included a fan-shaped mesh that was covered with a piece of resected omentum before introduction into the epiploic foramen.[37] Following reduction of the entrapment, 8 horses had some form of open bowel procedure and all survived to discharge: 1 horse had a jejunojejunostomy; 3 had a jejunocecostomy; 2 had a pelvic flexure enterotomy; 1 had a small intestinal enterotomy; and 1 had a typhlotomy.[37] This outcome would suggest that with appropriate adherence to surgical aseptic technique, no additional risk of septic peritonitis exists with the placement of a nonabsorbable mesh.

NSS closure has been encouraged to prevent the recurrence of NSLE of the ascending colon. This procedure has been previously described using laparoscopic techniques, either directly suturing the splenic capsule to the dorsal nephrosplenic ligament or affixing a synthetic mesh into the space.[38–40] A key component to the success of this procedure is case selection because it has been reported to be most effective for surgically confirmed cases of NSLE.[40,41] Colic may still occur, including right dorsal and left dorsal (without entrapment) displacements of the ascending colon.[40,41] Arévalo Rodríguez and colleagues reported on a modification of the Marien and colleagues laparoscopic technique, using only 2 portals (instead of 3) where the single instrument portal uses a larger custom-made 40-mm diameter stainless steel cannula to allow insertion and retrieval of a 48-mm needle, facilitating the direct suturing technique for the closure of the space.[42] This modification provides a simplification of the original technique while allowing for a longer needle to be used, enabling larger bites in the tissue and potentially less risk of suture pull through, reducing the number of portals and potential morbidity associated with standing NSS closure.

Gialletti and colleagues compared the outcomes of horses treated with NSS mesh ablation (n = 9) versus direct suturing with barbed suture (n = 19) following one or more NSLE displacements.[43] In this study, techniques were compared retrospectively between 2 hospitals. Although mean surgery time was significantly shorter in the barbed suture group (mean of 62 vs 78 minutes for mesh), there was no significant difference in complications. Reported complications were postoperative colic, lack of NSS closure/ablation, and adhesion formation. Furthermore, the authors reported lower expense of treatment of the horses undergoing barbed suture closure compared with mesh ablation.[43] Another recent study looking at NSS ablation reported on the feasibility of using homologous pericardium as an alternative to mesh ablation.[44] This pilot study used 6 experimental horses that underwent standing laparoscopic NSS ablation with a 10 × 5 cm homologous pericardium implant that was secured with polydioxanone staples. Horses underwent repeat laparoscopy after 60 days. No intraoperative complications were reported; however, horses developed a significant increase in peritoneal fluid nucleated cell count that peaked on day 3 postoperatively at 137,618 cells/μL, consistent with peritonitis. In comparison, the peritoneal fluid nucleated cell count has been reported to peak at 24 hours postoperatively at values of 32,880 cells/μL and 58,130 cells/μL for horses undergoing standing laparoscopic cryptorchidectomy and ovariectomy, respectively.[45,46] For the horses with pericardial implant, at the time of repeat laparoscopy, the NSS was completely effaced with scar tissue along its length. Four horses developed adhesions without corresponding clinical signs: 2 between the mesocolon and the implant and 2 between the omentum and the implant.[44] Although the procedure was easily performed and may be an alternative to other forms of NSS closure, the pericardial implant was associated with a moderate inflammatory response and potentially unwanted adhesions.

A relatively large body of literature has already been published on surgical site infections (SSIs) after ventral midline celiotomy. A recent review by Shearer and colleagues compiled such studies, including a table with the various risk factors that were found in each study.[47] Some of the protective factors reported in this review included linea alba lavage, use of a stent bandage, and closure with a 2-layer modified subcuticular pattern.[47] Perhaps, the most confounding finding for the veterinary surgeon is the lack of consensus of risk factors for SSIs among studies. To this effect, publication of controlled, multicenter, prospective studies where perioperative factors are standardized and randomized, may provide more useful data and affect prevention strategies. A recent publication by Scharner and colleagues showed that suturing the peritoneum before closing the linea alba significantly decreases the risk of SSI.[48] In this retrospective study, incisional complications were associated with an age of 20 years or older (OR 17.9, 95% CI 4.77–67.2), not suturing the peritoneum (OR 7.68, 95% CI 2.71–21.81), and postoperative fever (OR 7.48 95% CI 2.19–25.58). Three additional studies focus on incisional closure and associations with SSI. Salciccia and colleagues retrospectively describe incisional complications in a population of horses where the body wall is apposed using a combination of interrupted vertical mattress and simple interrupted sutures.[49] Overall 9.52% of cases and 33.3% of relaparotomy cases developed an incisional complication. SSI, defined as purulent drainage with or without positive culture, was reported in 5.31% of cases. Of note, abdominal bandages were maintained for 13 to 15 days, changing every 2 days.[49] This report describes an alternative to other suture patterns for body wall closure; however, with no control group within the same population, direct comparisons to other populations or suture patterns cannot be made. Martinez-Lopez and colleagues presented a retrospective study comparing stainless steel skin staples to *n*-butyl cyanoacrylate for skin apposition and associated incisional complications during a 4-year period.[50] The authors reported no significant difference in development of SSI in the staple compared with the cyanoacrylate groups (19.1% vs 15.9%, respectively), supporting its use as an alternative to skin staples. In a prospective blinded randomized controlled clinical study, Gustafsson and colleagues examined the effects of medical grade honey (MGH) applied to the incision before subcutaneous tissue closure.[51] No adverse effects of MGH application were noted. A significant decrease in SSIs in MGH-treated (8.2%, 4/49) compared with untreated control cases (32.5%, 13/40) was found, supporting further investigation across a larger multicenter population of horses to see whether the beneficial effect can be replicated.

A prospective randomized controlled study by Kilcoyne and colleagues focused on the postoperative management of the incision. The authors compared 3 groups of incisional protection: a sterile cotton towel stent, polyhexamethylene biguanide (PHMB)-impregnated dressing stent, and sterile gauze with iodine-impregnated adhesive drape.[52] Overall SSIs occurred in 15% (11/75) of horses, with 8.3% (2/24) in the sterile towel stent, 0% (0/26) in the PHMB stent bandage, and 36% (9/25) in the iodine adhesive drape. It was reported that the iodine-impregnated drape commonly became displaced during anesthetic recovery, despite adhesive spray being applied to the skin before placement of the drape. Results of this study suggested that SSI risk in this population of horses was lower with either stent bandage compared with the iodine-impregnated adhesive drape.[52] Additional studies or clinical use in other populations is needed to corroborate this finding.

UPDATES ON PROGNOSIS

Although we, as veterinary surgeons, continue to strive for better results, it is incumbent that we document both improvements as well as shortcomings in our outcomes. Both positive and negative results will only improve our collective knowledge. The following recent studies provide updated information on survival or technique-associated outcomes for colic surgery.

A topic that can be a source of frustration for the colic surgeon is client hesitation to pursue surgical treatment of small intestinal strangulating obstructions, especially in the geriatric horse based on client perception of worsening prognosis with age. Often the client and referring veterinarian have concerns regarding the long-term outcome for an older horse, the perspective of the postoperative period and suffering, and the associated expense. To assess whether age plays a factor in the development of POR and survival, Boorman and colleagues compared mature (<16-year-old) to geriatric (≥16-year-old) horses who underwent surgery for small intestinal lesions.[53] Age was associated neither with a high volume of POR nor with nonsurvival. This clinical finding was supported by a recent study by Rudnick and colleagues who reported no differences in survival to discharge between mature and geriatric horses using the same age definitions as Boorman and colleagues.[53,54] This study reported long-term survival of cases that had undergone surgery more than 10 years earlier, a period of time relevant to the potentially long life span of horses.[54] Although geriatric horses had a shorter median long-term survival using Kaplan-Meier statistics compared with mature horses (72 vs 121 months, respectively), each group had the same number of horses die in the long-term period associated with colic. These findings indicate that geriatric horses by nature of their advanced age have fewer years remaining in their normal life span and thus, a shorter long-term survival. The authors also reported that long-term survival was greater for horses managed without a resection compared with those that underwent jejunocecostomy or jejunojejunostomy, highlighting the importance of early referral and surgical intervention of small intestinal strangulating lesions to optimize outcome.[54]

Arndt and colleagues provide an update on cases managed for peritonitis, where peritonitis was defined as nucleated cell counts greater than 25,000 cells/μL in the peritoneal fluid.[55] Similar to previous reports, colic was the most common presenting complaint (47%) followed by fever (24%), and inappetence (18%).[55,56] Interestingly, increased peritoneal fluid volume was apparent in only 11 of 38 (29%) horses undergoing point-of-care targeted transabdominal ultrasonographic examination by the admitting veterinarian and in only 6 of 25 (24%) cases having a complete transabdominal ultrasonographic examination by the hospital ultrasound service. Peritoneal fluid was grossly abnormal in all cases, ranging from serosanguinous to yellow-opaque to brown. All horses were treated with antimicrobials. Five of 8 horses with peritonitis secondary to trauma were treated surgically, including intraoperative abdominal lavage and drain placement (n = 4). Standing abdominal drain placement occurred in an additional 5 horses. This report supports the previous idea that horses with a secondary peritonitis, including those where a definitive diagnosis had been made based on bacterial culture or cytology, have a poorer prognosis than horses with idiopathic peritonitis (25% mortality vs 4% mortality, respectively).[55] Overall survival to discharge was 82%, similar to previous reports where cases were also excluded if they were secondary to abdominal surgery or gastrointestinal rupture.[56]

Another update on survival looked at comparison between large colon resection techniques. Pezzanite and Hackett reported on survival and complications of 26 horses undergoing either sutured end-to-end or stapled functional end-to-end (ie, side-to-side) large colon resection and anastomosis.[57] No significant differences in surgical time, hospitalization, complications, or short-term and long-term survival between the 2 groups was reported. Overall survival to discharge was 81% with long-term survival reported at 67%,[55] supporting either colectomy technique as a good option for horses with large colon lesions, including volvulus and recurrent large colon disease.

In a recent retrospective study examining the outcome of horses undergoing exploratory celiotomy for gastrointestinal disease, van Loon and colleagues reported overall short-term survival at only 59%, with long-term survival of 51%.[58] However, 25% (73 out of 283) of the horses that were taken to surgery were euthanized intraoperatively. Most of these cases had intestinal strangulation of the small intestine (53%) or large intestine (29%). Reasons for euthanasia were poor prognosis based on amount of bowel involved (83%) or financial constraints (17%). Approximately 15% of cases were euthanized between recovery from anesthesia and hospital discharge.[58] As Rudnick and colleagues had underscored in their study, early surgical intervention may improve outcomes.[54] This is especially applicable for horses with strangulating lesions as intervention before bowel necrosis would decrease the number of horses that require intraoperative euthanasia.

SUMMARY

Various improvements in techniques or management strategies have been investigated during the last 5 years. Although no single area of study has had a dramatic change in our outcomes following colic surgery, multiple small changes ultimately contribute to improving survival for equine patients. Across the board, a recurring theme prevails: early identification of strangulating lesions and subsequent surgical treatment improves outcomes. Of the modifications that we have implemented and those yet to be discovered, this concept continues to be one to prioritize.

CLINICS CARE POINTS

- In the last several years, there has been no singular improvement in equine colic surgery as important as early referral.
- Improvements and updates to both surgical technique and postoperative management have occurred.
- However, critical to success in colic surgery is early intervention. This involves clear communication with referring veterinarians and owners of the importance of early referral of horses with potential surgical lesions.

DISCLOSURE

The author does not have a relevant financial interest, arrangement, or affiliation or business entity (including self-employment and sole proprietorship) that could be perceived as a conflict of interest or a source of bias in the context of this publication.

REFERENCES

1. Southwood LL, Dolente BA, Lindborg S, et al. Short-term outcome of equine emergency admissions at a university referral hospital. Equine Vet J 2009;41: 459–64.
2. van der Linden MA, Laffont CM, Sloet van Oldruitenborgh Oosterbaan MM. Prognosis in equine medical and surgical colic. J Vet Intern Med 2003;17:343–8.
3. Archer DC. Colic surgery: keeping it affordable for horse owners. Vet Rec 2019; 185(16):505–7.
4. Freeman DE. Fifty years of colic surgery. Equine Vet J 2018;50:423–35.
5. Lopes MAF, Hardy J, Farnsworth K, et al. Standing flank laparotomy for colic: 37 cases. Equine Vet J 2022;54:934–45.
6. Herbert EW, Lopes MAF, Kelmer G. Standing flank laparotomy for the treatment of small colon impactions in 15 ponies and one horse. Equine Vet Educ 2019; 33:51–6.
7. Jones ARE, Ragle CA, Anderson D, et al. Laparoscopic evaluation of the small intestine in the standing horse: Technique and effects. Vet Surg 2017;46:812–20.
8. Delli-Rocili MM, Cribb NC, Trout DR, et al. Effectiveness of a paraverterbral nerve block versus local portal blocks for laparoscopic closure of the nephrosplenic space: A pilot study. Vet Surg 2020;49:1007–14.
9. Giusto G, Gandini M. Ex vivo comparison of sliding knot ligatures vs. haemostatic clips for equine small intestinal mesenteric vessel occlusion. BMC Vet Res 2020; 16:290.
10. Giusto G, Cerullo A, Gandini M. Transillumination Techniques for Vessel Identification During Small Colon Resection in Six Horses. J Equine Vet Sci 2022;118: 104113.
11. Lenoir A, Perrin BRM, Lepage OM. Ex Vivo Comparison of a UV-Polymerizable Methacrylate Adhesive versus an Inverting Pattern as the Second Layer of a Two-Layer Hand-Sewn Jejunal Anastomosis in Horses: A Pilot Study. Vet Med Int 2021;2021:5545758.
12. Troy JR, Holcombe SJ, Fogle CA, et al. Effects of hyaluronate-carboxymethylcellulose membranes on the clinical outcome of horses undergoing emergency exploratory celiotomy. Vet Surg 2018;47:385–91.

13. Giusto G, Cerullo A, Labate F, et al. Incomplete Ileocecal Bypass for Ileal Pathology in Horses: 21 Cases (2012–2019). Animals 2021;11:403.
14. Gandini M, Giusto G. Combination of end-to-end jejuno-ileal anastomosis and side-to-side incomplete ileocecal bypass (hybrid jejuno-ileo-cecal anastomosis) following subtotal ileal resection in seven horses. J Am Vet Med Assoc 2021; 259(11):1337–43.
15. Stewart S, Southwood LL, Aceto HW. Comparison of short- and long-term complications and survival following jejunojejunostomy, jejunoileostomy and jejunocaecostomy in 112 horses: 2005-2010. Equine Vet J 2014;46(3):333–8.
16. Lisowski ZM, Lefevre L, Mair TS, et al. Use of quantitative real-time PCR to determine the local inflammatory response in the intestinal mucosa and muscularis of horses undergoing small intestinal resection. Equine Vet J 2022;54:52–62.
17. Eskandari MK, Kalff JC, Billiar TR, et al. Lipopolysaccharide activates the muscularis macrophage network and suppresses circular smooth muscle activity. Am J Phys 1997;273:G727–34.
18. Stockle SD, Kannapin DA, Kauter AML, et al. A Pilot Randomised Clinical Trial Comparing a Short-Term Perioperative Prophylaxis Regimen to a Long-Term Standard Protocol in Equine Colic Surgery. Antibiotics 2021;10:587.
19. Pihl TH, Nielsen MK, Olsen SN, et al. Nonstrangulating intestinal infarctions associated with Strongylus vulgaris: Clinical presentation and treatment outcomes of 30 horses (2008-2016). Equine Vet J 2018;50(4):474–80.
20. Lawless SP, Werner LA, Baker WT, et al. Duodenojejunal mesenteric rents: Survival and complications after surgical correction in 38 broodmares (2006-2014). Vet Surg 2017;46(3):367–75.
21. Gayle JM, Blikslager AT, Bowman KF. Mesenteric rents as a source of small intestinal strangulation in horses: 15 cases (1990-1997). J Am Vet Med Assoc 2000; 216:1446–9.
22. Abu-Seida A. Diagnostic and Treatment Challenges for Diaphragmatic Hernia in Equids: A Concise Review of Literature. J Equine Vet Sci 2021;106:103746.
23. Romero AE, Rodgerson DH. Diaphragmatic herniation in the horse: 31 cases from 2001–2006. Can Vet J 2010;51:1247–50.
24. Voss JK, Dubois MS. Redundant mesocolonic mesentery in a Shire colt. Can Vet J 2021;62(2):179–83.
25. Biasutti S, Dart AJ, Dart CM, et al. End-to-side anastomosis of the left ventral colon to the small colon in a neonatal foal with segmental agenesis of the large colon. Aust Vet J 2017;95(6):217–9.
26. van Bergen T, Haspeslagh M, Wiemer P, et al. Surgical treatment of epiploic foramen entrapment in 142 horses (2008–2016). Vet Surg 2019;48:291–8.
27. Grzeskowiak RM, Barrett EJ, Rodgerson DH. Cecal entrapment within the epiploic foramen in a mare. Can Vet J 2017;58(8):842–4.
28. Segura D, Garzon N, Nomen C, et al. Entrapment of large colon through the epiploic foramen in a horse. Equine Vet Educ 1999;11:227–8.
29. Steenhaut M, Vandenreyt I, Van Royt M. Incarceration of the large colon through the epiploic foramen in a horse. Equine Vet J 1993;25:550–1.
30. Foerner JJ, Ringle MJ, Junkins DS, et al. Transection of the pelvic flexure to reduce incarceration of the large colon through the epiploic foramen in a horse. J Am Vet Med Assoc 1993;203:1312–3.
31. Scheidemann W. Beitrag zur diagnostic und therapie der kolik des pferdes die hernia foraminis omentalis. [DVM thesis]. Munich: Ludwig Maximillian University; 1989.

32. Wanstrath MA, Bauck AG, Smith AD, et al. Surgical enlargement of the epiploic foramen in horses. Vet Surg 2023;52(2):308–14.

33. van Bergen T, Wiemer P, Schauvliege S, et al. Laparoscopic evaluation of the epiploic foramen after celiotomy for epiploic foramen entrapment in the horse. Vet Surg 2016;45:596–601.

34. Munsterman AS, Hanson RR, Cattley RC, et al. Surgical technique and short-term outcome for experimental laparoscopic closure of the epiploic foramen in 6 horses. Vet Surg 2014;43(2):105–13.

35. van Bergen T, Wiemer P, Bosseler L, et al. Development of a new laparoscopic Foramen Epiploicum Mesh Closure (FEMC) technique in 6 horses. Equine Vet J 2016;48(3):331–7.

36. van Bergen T, Rötting A, Wiemer P, et al. Foramen epiploicum mesh closure (FEMC) through a ventral midline laparotomy. Equine Vet J 2018;50(2):235–40.

37. Grulke S, Salciccia A, Arévalo Rodríguez JM, et al. Mesh closure of epiploic foramen by ventral laparotomy in 17 horses with entrapment. Vet Rec 2020; 187(6):e43.

38. Mariën T, Adriaenssen A, Hoeck FV, et al. Laparoscopic closure of the renosplenic space in standing horses. Vet Surg 2001;30(6):559–63.

39. Gandini M, Nannarone S, Giusto G, et al. Laparoscopic nephrosplenic space ablation with barbed suture in eight horses. J Am Vet Med Assoc 2017;250(4): 431–6.

40. Burke MJ, Parente EJ. Prosthetic mesh for obliteration of the Nephrosplenic space in horses: 26 clinical cases. Vet Surg 2016;45:201–7.

41. Nelson BB, Ruple-Czerniak AA, Hendrickson DA, et al. Laparoscopic closure of the Nephrosplenic space in horses with Nephrosplenic colonic entrapment: factors associated with survival and colic recurrence. Vet Surg 2016;45. O60–9.

42. Arévalo Rodríguez JM, Grulke S, Salciccia A, et al. Nephrosplenic space closure significantly decreases recurrent colic in horses: a retrospective analysis. Vet Rec 2019;185(21):657.

43. Gialletti R, Nannarone S, Gandini M, et al. Comparison of Mesh and Barbed Suture for Laparoscopic Nephrosplenic Space Ablation in Horses. Animals 2021; 11(4):1096.

44. Spagnolo JD, Castro LM, Corrêa RR, et al. Nephrosplenic Space Ablation in Horses After Homologous Pericardium Implant Using a Laparoscopic Stapler. J Equine Vet Sci 2020;95:103275.

45. Seabaugh KA, Goodrich LR, Bohn AA, et al. A comparison of peritoneal fluid values in mares following bilateral laparoscopic ovariectomy using a vessel sealing and dividing device versus placement of two ligating loops. Vet J 2014; 202(2):297–302.

46. Seabaugh KA, Goodrich LR, Morley PS, et al. Comparison of peritoneal fluid values after laparoscopic cryptorchidectomy using a vessel-sealing device (Ligasure™) versus a ligating loop and removal of the descended testis. Vet Surg 2013;42(5):600–6.

47. Shearer TR, Holcombe SJ, Valberg SJ. Incisional infections associated with ventral midline celiotomy in horses. J Vet Emerg Crit Care 2020;30(2):136–48.

48. Scharner D, Winter K, Brehm W, et al. Incisional complications following ventral median coeliotomy in horses. Does suturing of the peritoneum reduce the risk? Wundheilungsstörungen nach ventraler medianer Laparotomie beim Pferd. Reduziert die Bauchfellnaht Wundheilungsstörungen? Tierarztl Prax Ausg G Grosstiere Nutztiere 2017;45(1):24–32.

49. Salciccia A, de la Rebière de Pouyade G, Gougnard A, et al. Complications associated with closure of the linea alba using a combination of interrupted vertical mattress and simple interrupted sutures in equine laparotomies. Vet Rec 2020; 187(11):e94.

50. Martinez-Lopez J, Brown JA, Werre SR. Incisional complications after skin closure with n-butyl cyanoacrylate or stainless-steel skin staples in horses undergoing colic surgery. Vet Surg 2021;50(1):186–95.

51. Gustafsson K, Tatz AJ, Slavin RA, et al. Intraincisional medical grade honey decreases the prevalence of incisional infection in horses undergoing colic surgery: A prospective randomised controlled study. Equine Vet J 2021;53(6):1112–8.

52. Kilcoyne I, Dechant JE, Kass PH, et al. Evaluation of the risk of incisional infection in horses following application of protective dressings after exploratory celiotomy for treatment of colic. J Am Vet Med Assoc 2019;254(12):1441–7.

53. Boorman S, Stefanovski D, Southwood LL. Clinical findings associated with development of postoperative reflux and short-term survival after small intestinal surgery in geriatric and mature nongeriatric horses. Vet Surg 2019;48(5): 795–802.

54. Rudnick MJ, Denagamage TN, Freeman DE. Effects of age, disease and anastomosis on short- and long-term survival after surgical correction of small intestinal strangulating diseases in 89 horses. Equine Vet J 2022;54(6):1031–8.

55. Arndt S, Kilcoyne I, Vaughan B, et al. Clinical and diagnostic findings, treatment, and short- and long-term survival in horses with peritonitis: 72 cases (2007-2017). Vet Surg 2021;50(2):323–35.

56. Henderson IS, Mair TS, Keen JA, et al. Study of the short- and long-term outcomes of 65 horses with peritonitis. Vet Rec 2008;163:293–7.

57. Pezzanite LM, Hackett ES. Technique-associated outcomes in horses following large colon resection. Vet Surg 2017;46(8):1061–7.

58. van Loon JPAM, Visser EMS, de Mik-van Mourik M, et al. Colic surgery in horses: A retrospective study into short- and long-term survival rate, complications and rehabilitation toward sporting activity. J Equine Vet Sci 2020;90:103012.

Basic Postoperative Care of the Equine Colic Patient

Anje G. Bauck, DVM, PhD

KEYWORDS

- Colic • Equine • Postoperative • Fluids • Surgery

KEY POINTS

- Basic care of the equine postoperative colic patient includes monitoring, fluid therapy, antimicrobials, analgesics, and nutritional support.
- Although standardized protocols can be of benefit to routinizing care, patients should have individualized postoperative diagnostic and therapeutic plans based on their lesion and status.
- Sound, evidence-based decision-making is critical to the successful management of postoperative colic patients and should involve an assessment of the cost–benefit ratio of various diagnostics and therapeutics.
- Careful monitoring of the postoperative colic patient allows for prompt recognition of problems and earlier interventions.
- Acute signs of abdominal pain in a postoperative colic patient are not considered normal and should be investigated fully.

MONITORING

Physical Examination Findings

Routine, careful monitoring of colic patients following surgery allows for prompt recognition of complications, earlier interventions, and better outcomes. Every case must be considered on an individual basis based on the primary disease and expected complications. The surgeon performing the surgery should discuss particular concerns with the care team. Communication with all individuals involved in after-care of the patient allows for a higher standard of care to be provided. Careful documentation is critical in informing all members of the team about the status of the patient, as well as in identifying and tracking trends.

The physical examination (vital parameters, borborygmi, digital pulses, urine/fecal production, and general attitude) is a key component of postoperative monitoring. Frequency of physical examinations will be highest in the immediate postoperative period

Large Animal Surgery, Department of Large Animal Clinical Sciences, University of Florida College of Veterinary Medicine, University of Florida, 2015 Southwest 16th Avenue, Gainesville, FL 32608, USA
E-mail address: baucka@ufl.edu

Vet Clin Equine 39 (2023) 263–286
https://doi.org/10.1016/j.cveq.2023.03.010
0749-0739/23/© 2023 Elsevier Inc. All rights reserved.

(ie, every 4–6 hours) and can then be gradually reduced after the first 72 hours if the patient seems stable. The incidence of recumbency should be carefully recorded, including if the horse lies in sternal or lateral recumbency or is actively rolling. Although the patient is on fluids, the patient should be observed at least once every hour to ensure that fluid administration rates are accurate.

It is not unexpected for postoperative colic patients to be tachycardic (60–70 bpm) for the first 24 hours after surgery, which is unlikely to be caused by anesthesia alone.[1] It can take up to 40 hours for mean heart rate to decrease to normal in most horses following large intestinal procedures.[2] Tachycardia and tachypnea can precede postoperative colic and reflux. Clinicians must consider all reasons for tachycardia including pain, hypovolemia, endotoxemia, certain medications, and primary cardiac disease.

Nonsteroidal anti-inflammatory drugs (NSAIDs) such as flunixin meglumine may mask pyrexia, so interpretations of rectal temperatures must consider the timing of administration of these drugs. Ideally, rectal temperature would be recorded just before administration of any NSAIDs. Mild pyrexia in the early postoperative period is not always associated with infection[3] but should be monitored closely. When considering the cause of a postoperative fever, the following sources should be ruled out: systemic (ie, endotoxemia), lungs (ie, aspiration pneumonia), abdominal cavity (ie, peritonitis), small intestines (ie, enteritis), large intestines (ie, colitis/salmonellosis), catheter site (ie, thrombophlebitis), and surgical site (ie, incisional infection). The nature of the primary disease and physical examination findings should determine what diagnostics to pursue in localizing the source of a fever.

Various numerical pain scales have been developed for use in equine patients that could be of value in postoperative monitoring of the equine colic patient.[1,4–7] Composite pain score is a multifactorial numerical rating scale that includes overt signs of colic.[1,6] The Equine Acute Abdominal Pain Score is another pain scale that was found to be feasible for use in a referral hospital setting.[8] Whether or not a specific pain scale is used, detailed observation of recording of patient's behavior is critical to identify problems early. It is important to consider that adult horses will not typically lie down in the early postoperative period,[9] and persistent periods of recumbency should be considered as a sign of abdominal pain during this time period.

Passage of first feces after colic surgery can vary widely from 1 to 4 hours at the earliest.[2,10] In one study, median time to first defecation was 8 hours following celiotomy in horses that did not develop postoperative ileus.[10] Clinicians should not expect normal fecal production in the postoperative colic patient for many days following surgery. The volume of digesta in the large intestines is reduced by preoperative anorexia, intestinal evacuation at the time of surgery (ie, typhlotomy, pelvic flexure enterotomy, or small colon enema), and gradual refeeding programs following surgery. Reduced fecal output will be observed until the large intestine reestablishes the reservoir of digesta. Palpation per rectum should not be performed on a routine basis after surgery, although it is a valuable tool in any horse experiencing postoperative colic or decreased fecal output, beyond that which is expected. It can be especially critical in horses where the primary disease was either a cecal or a small colon impaction, and clinicians have concerns that lesion may recur. Cases of type II (functional) cecal impactions have a high risk of reoccurrence and should be monitored closely.[11]

Enteral food and water stimulates fecal production, so prolonged periods of fasting as in horses will reduce borborygmi and fecal output.[12] Decreased fecal production and borborygmi is also expected in horses with postoperative reflux.[10]

Physical examination should include careful and frequent monitoring of the incision for heat, pain, swelling, and drainage indicating infection. If the patient has an abdominal or stent bandage in place, it should be noted if there is any slippage or drainage through the bandage. Incisional complications should prompt further diagnostic tests such as sonographic evaluation or bacterial culture and sensitivity testing. Importantly, gloves should be worn when evaluating the incision.

The catheter site should also be examined every 4 to 6 hours for evidence of heat, pain swelling, or drainage at insertion site while the catheter is in place and after removal. Evaluation of the vein from thrombus formation is critical. The catheter's connection to the fluid lines should also be examined to ensure it is not loose and at risk of disconnection. Aspiration of air can occur if the catheter becomes disconnected and can have serious cardiac and neurological effects and even be fatal. If horse is no longer receiving intravenous (IV) fluids, the catheter should be flushed every 4 to 6 hours with heparinized saline, and the catheter should be removed immediately after IV medications are discontinued. Injection caps should be wiped with alcohol before administration of any IV medications, and injection caps changed daily.[13] If prolonged fluid therapy is necessary, IV fluid administration sets should be changed every 72 hours to prevent infection.

Frequent monitoring of digital pulses and as the patient's willingness to walk around the stall allows for early identification of laminitis or other musculoskeletal injuries (ie, injuries incurred during anesthetic recoveries or self-trauma incurred during episodes of colic).

Clinicians should not underestimate the value of the basic physical examination outlined above for an early identification of complications. Laboratory tests and other diagnostic procedures should be chosen selectively and not used if results would not alter decisions on treatment. Repetition of unnecessary diagnostic tests does not improve outcomes and increases cost. Less expensive diagnostic tests combined with a thorough physical examination is sufficient for identifying complications.

Laboratory Tests

The extent and frequency of laboratory tests will depend on disease severity. The following is a general guideline to consider:

Packed cell volume and total solids (PCV/TS) is a quick and inexpensive method to objectively assess hydration and blood volume, anemia (hemorrhage) and hypoproteinemia (protein losing enteropathy), and responses to fluid therapy. If a horse is refluxing, has diarrhea, or evidence of systemic inflammatory response syndrome (SIRS), it is recommended to monitor PCV/TS every 6 hours. If a horse is not refluxing and is otherwise stable, PCV/TS every 12 to 24 hours is sufficient[14] and can be discontinued entirely once IV fluid therapy is discontinued.

In stable patients, blood gas analysis or point-of-care chemistry may be monitored once daily if this modality is available, although some clinicians may think this is unnecessary. In horses with reflux, diarrhea, or endotoxemia, there is a high likelihood of the patient developing hypovolemia and electrolyte disturbances from ongoing fluid losses or maldistribution. More frequent monitoring of these values (ie, every 12 hours) allows fluid therapy to be adjusted to meet the individual patient's needs. Reduced plasma concentrations of K^+, Mg^{++}, and Ca^{++} can be induced by anorexia and/or aggressive fluid therapy deficient in these essential electrolytes. Blood L-lactate concentration provides information on tissue perfusion and can be used to guide the rate of fluid administration[13] and as a prognostic indicator.[15,16] Blood L-lactate concentration should be less than 1 mmol/L on horses receiving IV fluids.

Performing a complete blood count (CBC) every 24 to 48 hours will allow trends in cell counts to be monitored, although this can be misleading due to changes in leukocyte counts depending on the particular phase of inflammation.[17,18] A neutropenia could indicate the onset of endotoxemia or colitis[19] because of extravasation of neutrophils into the surrounding tissues.[20] In one study, there was no difference in neutrophil counts between horses with postoperative infections versus those with noninfectious complications,[21] further questioning the usefulness of these measurements in regards to treatment decisions during this time period. However, persistent leukopenia on serial blood leukocyte count is a negative prognostic indicator for survival following colic surgery.[22] Serial monitoring of CBCs to guide the duration of antimicrobial use, when patient is otherwise doing well, is an expensive approach that lacks evidence-based support. Although some clinicians frequently use hematological evaluations to guide treatment decisions, other clinicians may view CBCs and especially repeated CBCs as an unnecessary cost and only perform these tests when indicated (eg, a horse with a fever of undetermined cause or severe diarrhea).

Frequency of monitoring a patient's serum biochemistry profile will depend on the patient's condition before surgery, the primary disease process and status of the patient postoperatively. Stable patients with no major biochemical abnormalities preoperatively, repeating serum biochemistry profiles every 72 hours or less is likely sufficient, especially if electrolytes are being measured more frequently by blood gas analysis or point-of-care chemistry analyzer. However, prolonged feed deprivation, dehydration, overhydration, metabolic syndrome, and acute kidney injury can all result in changes of a patient's serum biochemistry profile in a postoperative colic patient. Clinicians should consider all these factors, as well as financial factors, in deciding how often to repeat these diagnostics. It may also be less expensive to choose certain variables of interest on a serum biochemistry to analyze, rather than the whole profile. Specific biochemistry values that are important to note in postoperative colic patients:

- Food deprivation leads to hypertriglyceridemia in horses. Transient hypertriglyceridemia is very common in the early postoperative period, although not all horses will experience clinical complications or require specific treatment.[23] In one study of horses undergoing exploratory celiotomy, 58% of horses experienced a mild hypertriglyceridemia (50–250 mg/dL) and 38% experienced moderate hypertriglyceridemia (250–500 mg/dL) in the first 24 to 36 hours postoperatively.[24] However, persistent and severe hypertriglyceridemia (ie, >500 mg/dL) will result in lethargy and inappetence, further exacerbating the metabolic problem. Clinician should aim to reverse the negative energy balance and promote the endogenous release of insulin to help metabolize the triglyceride molecules. In severe cases, supplementation with dextrose and insulin is required. Blood triglyceride concentration should be monitored in miniature horses, ponies, donkeys, and pregnant mares.
- Creatinine concentration is a useful marker of kidney function, specifically glomerular filtration.[25] Many colic patients will present to the hospital with hypovolemia and associated prerenal azotemia. Prerenal azotemia should respond favorably to effective fluid therapy, and a favorable response indicates an improved prognosis compared with persistent azotemia, in horses with colic or colitis.[26] More frequent monitoring of creatinine concentration and urinalysis may be indicated in horses either at risk or with evidence of acute kidney injury, with anecdotal evidence that this may be more common in geriatric patients.
- Hyperglycemia is also common in horses with acute abdominal pain; 45% to 50.2% of horses that present for the treatment of acute abdominal disease will be hyperglycemic on admission.[27,28] Severe hyperglycemia (>195 mg/dL) at the time of admission is associated with poor prognosis.[28] In adult horses with

colic, hypoglycemia is very rare[27] but can occur in foals due to lack of glycogen and fat stores.[29] Critically ill patients or patients at the risk of dysregulation of glucose homeostasis (foals, pregnant mares, horses with preexisting metabolic disease, or horses on partial parenteral nutrition) will require more frequent blood-glucose monitoring.[28] Precise schedule of monitoring will vary patient to patient. For horses receiving dextrose supplementation, the author will routinely check blood glucose levels every 4 hours, then decrease to every 6 or 8 hours if glucose levels seem stable.

Acute-phase proteins are inflammatory markers that can sometimes be useful in postoperative monitoring of colic patients, specifically in determining the risk of complications and prognosis for survival.[18,30–33] Fibrinogen concentration is commonly evaluated on most hematological assessments. However, it is increased as a delayed response to inflammation and is not always useful in distinguishing an active infection.[21,33–35] In horses undergoing exploratory celiotomy for colic, a higher fibrinogen at admission was associated with an increased risk of postoperative complications in one study.[33] Authors in that study postulated that having a high fibrinogen at admission could indicate a chronic underlying inflammatory condition that may have an increased risk of postoperative complications. In contrast, Aitken and colleagues reported that fibrinogen concentrations at days 4 to 6 postoperative were associated with complications such as postoperative colic, diarrhea, IV catheter complications and postoperative reflux,[21] which is more consistent with fibrinogen's usefulness as a delayed marker of inflammation and not necessarily a marker of infection.[21] Other physical examination parameters may more useful than fibrinogen for identifying active infection.

Serum amyloid A (SAA) may be a more useful biomarker than fibrinogen. Healthy animals will have a zero to low (<50 μg/mL) plasma concentration, and then it increases quickly in response to inflammation.[18] It is also a useful biomarker in predicting SIRS in equine colic patients.[36] In a recent study, SAA increased to 568.6 ± 197.7 μg/mL within the first 48 hours after celiotomy and intestinal decompression in healthy horses, and then decreased to 174.4 ± 307.7 μg/mL within the first 7 days following surgery.[37] Hyperfibrinogenemia persisted throughout the study period.[37] These findings should be factored into assessment of SAA in clinical cases. In a clinical study, elevations in SAA and fibrinogen were greater in horses that developed complications, and horses with lower SAA at day 5 postoperatively had better survival to discharge.[33] Despite its usefulness as a predictive marker, clinicians need to consider the cost–benefit analysis of repeated SAA measurements, given that there are significant elevations of this protein even in healthy horses following celiotomy and intestinal decompression.[37] In the author's experience, SAA is more frequently monitored in cases where there is a concern that patient has developed a chronic postoperative infection such as peritonitis or pneumonia, and SAA is one of many tools to assess response to treatment.

Ancillary Tests

Specific assessment of gastrointestinal function may include nasogastric intubation, transabdominal sonographic evaluation, or abdominal examination per rectum. Some clinicians may routinely perform these diagnostics on all postoperative colic cases, regardless of clinical status. However, it is likely unnecessary and may contribute to excessive costs and unnecessary discomfort to the patient. These diagnostics are more commonly reserved for patients that have clinical evidence of abdominal pain (tachycardia, tachypnea, behavioral manifestations of abdominal pain). Any increase in heart rate especially if more than 60 beats/minute, inappetence, or behavioral manifestations of abdominal pain should prompt nasogastric intubation. Horses with more subtle signs such as decreased fecal output or decreased borborygmi require careful monitoring and intervention may or may not be unnecessary (see section on "Physical Examination Findings" for discussion on palpation per rectum).

Early passage of a nasogastric tube following surgery is unlikely to be productive, providing that stomach was adequately decompressed before surgery and patency of the gastrointestinal tract was reestablished during surgery. However, routine placement of an indwelling nasogastric tube following colic surgery is still common practice in 30% to 58% of clinicians, according to recent surveys.[38,39] If a patient is producing reflux following nasogastric intubation, they should be checked every 4 hours, or sooner they are producing large volumes of reflux. If less than 2 L of net reflux is obtained at 2 successive checks, it is reasonable to remove the nasogastric tube or discontinue the repeated intubations. Some clinicians prefer to repass the nasogastric tube at each recheck rather than leaving tube tied in place. The exact protocol used will depend on the comfort and ability of nursing staff to check or repass the nasogastric tube at frequent intervals and the behavior of the patient. The disadvantage of leaving the tube in place is the potential for sinusitis to develop from prolonged blockage of the nasomaxillary opening[40] and aspiration pneumonia. Even if a nasogastric tube is routinely left tied in place between checks, it is prudent to remove and repass a new tube through the opposite nostril every 12 hours while horse is actively refluxing.

Sonographic evaluation is a valuable tool in helping clinicians elucidate the cause and/or progression of postoperative complications such as fever and postoperative colic. Assessment of gastric distension, small intestinal distension, intestinal wall thickening, and volume/consistency of free peritoneal fluid is useful for decision-making in cases where recovery is not as expected. However, the author does not routinely perform abdominal ultrasound on postoperative patients unless physical examination findings or other diagnostics indicate a need for further investigation. Contractility, degree of small intestinal distension and peritoneal fluid undergo minimal changes from normal in the first few days after an exploratory celiotomy.[41] To the author's knowledge, no study has demonstrated that transabdominal sonography is useful in differentiating between functional postoperative ileus and a mechanical obstruction resulting in small intestinal distension. Therefore, in horses with postoperative reflux, sonographic evaluation is unlikely to be useful in determining which cases will respond to medical therapy and which cases will require additional interventions such as repeat celiotomy. Clinicians also have to consider the cost of repeated ultrasound examinations, depending on how the hospital charges for use of the machine.

Monitoring for Biosecurity Purposes

Beyond individual patient outcomes, certain monitoring practice in colic patients are critical to overall hospital biosecurity. Colic surgery has been reported as a risk factor for *Salmonella* shedding when compared with other hospitalized horses.[42,43] The main objective of a biosecurity program is to prevent hospital outbreaks of nosocomial *Salmonella* infection, which can have devastating consequences to patients as well as the hospital at large.[44] Routine *Salmonella* culture or polymerase chain reaction (PCR) following colic surgery is standard practice in many hospitals. Individual protocols should be guided by the hospital's biosecurity officer. It is important to remember that horses can shed *Salmonella* organisms before the development of clinical signs such as diarrhea or pyrexia.[45] Relying on clinical signs alone to identify salmonellosis could result in the spread of *Salmonella* to other hospitalized patients.

At the author's hospital, all horses that are presented for treatment of colic have a fecal sample collected at admission for *Salmonella* testing (culture or PCR). *Salmonella* testing is repeated every 72 hours while the patient is hospitalized.[42] If patient has clinical signs consistent with salmonellosis including diarrhea, fever (>102.5°F without NSAIDs and >102.0°F with NSAIDs), and leukopenia (white cell count <5000 cells/μL),[44] the patient will be moved to isolation and *Salmonella* fecal cultures repeated every 12 hours until 5 samples are collected. However, specific testing requirements will vary hospital to hospital, ideally guided by evidence-based recommendations.[42,44,46,47]

ANTIMICROBIAL USE

Colic surgery is generally classified as clean or clean-contaminated,[48,49] unless a major spillage of gastrointestinal contents is encountered at surgery. Short of major contamination, a single dose of preoperative antimicrobial drugs should be sufficient prophylaxis against surgical site infection (SSI).[50,51] However, there are other factors that need to be considered in determining an appropriate antimicrobial regimen following colic surgery, as discussed below.

A combination of beta-lactam and an aminoglycoside is commonly used in routine colic surgery. Specifically, the most common antimicrobials used in colic surgery are potassium penicillin (22,000 IU/kg IV every 6 hours) and gentamicin (6.6 mg/kg IV every 24 hours) although duration of use varies between surgeons.[3,43,52] Both of these drugs can be administered IV, which is a convenient route of administration while patient has an IV catheter in place. Standard guidelines recommend that antimicrobials should be administered within 1 hour of the start of surgery.[43,53,54] Many equine surgeons will target a 30-minute interval from administration to the first surgical incision in an attempt to maximize antimicrobial efficacy.[43]

The duration and type of antimicrobials used postoperatively will be determined based on the type of procedure performed, the surgeon's perception of intraoperative contamination and postoperative status of the patient (ie, presence of fever or other physical examination findings indicative of infection). Extended prophylaxis beyond a single postoperative dose is common, even in cases with minimal surgical contamination.[43] It should be noted that intraoperative contamination does always result in infection and, therefore, does not warrant prolonged prophylaxis. Thirty-six to 72 hours of antimicrobial prophylaxis is common.[3,43,55] In general, longer duration of antimicrobial administration has not been found to decrease the risk of SSIs or postoperative pyrexia.[3,55] One study found no difference between 3 and 5 days of antimicrobial coverage after colic surgery in preventing SSI.[55] Shorter duration of antimicrobial prophylaxis could, therefore, be more cost effective while decreasing the risk of other negative side effects of these drugs.[56] Preventing or mitigating the risk of SSI in horses that have undergone a celiotomy is a major goal in devising a postoperative antimicrobial plan.[43,55,57–59]

Antimicrobial resistance is common in bacterial organisms routinely cultured from infected abdominal incisions in colic patients. In one study, 92% of organisms isolated from SSIs after colic surgery were penicillin-resistant, whereas 18% were gentamicin-resistant.[57] *Escherichia coli*, a normal commensal organism in the gastrointestinal tract of most mammals, is one of the most commonly isolated organisms from infected incisions after colic surgery.[57] It is, therefore, frequently exposed to antimicrobials and may act as a reservoir for antimicrobial resistance genes.[60,61]

Clinicians must weigh the perceived benefits of antimicrobial use against the risks associated with these drugs including antibiotic resistance,[62] increased risk of

Salmonella shedding,[43] antimicrobial-associated diarrhea,[46,63] and lack of efficacy against treating SSI.[43] Excessive and inappropriate use of antimicrobials will increase the risk of antimicrobial resistance.[64,65] Hospitalization and environmental factors (ie, stress from transport, environmental changes, surgery) can also affect antimicrobial resistance patterns.[60,61] Clinicians should be aware of the prevalence of and risk factors of *Salmonella* shedding, and patterns of antimicrobial resistance, within their own populations.[46,47,60,61]

Guidelines for antimicrobial prophylactic in veterinary patients are few and commonly extrapolated from human medicine.[43,52,54,66] There have been several retrospective studies documenting common antimicrobial practices for the equine colic patient but standardized recommendations for equine patients are still lacking.[3,43,55,67] From these studies, it is evident that incorrect dosing of antimicrobials preoperatively and inadequate timing of administration (ie, more than 60 minutes before the start of surgery) are common occurrences in equine colic surgery.[43] However, incorrect dosing or timing of preoperative antimicrobials is not necessarily associated with an increased risk of infection based on the available literature.[3] Clinicians should adhere to prophylactic antimicrobial use recommendations,[53,56] while also considering the individual patient, when making decisions about antimicrobial use in horses following colic surgery.

ANALGESIA

In devising an appropriate analgesic plan, clinicians need to consider the sources of pain following colic surgery. Common sources of postoperative pain include peritoneal inflammation, the body wall incision, intestinal distention, ongoing intestinal ischemia, or mesenteric tension.[68] Although some degree of pain is expected after colic surgery, careful monitoring for clinical indicators of pain (see "Monitoring" section above) is critical in determining when further interventions are required.

Horses should not show behavioral signs of abdominal pain (ie, abnormal posture, abnormal facial expression, nonresponsive demeanor, pawing, sweating, rolling, and flank-watching) in the immediate postoperative period. Although some horses do take longer than others to return to normal behavior and attitude, acute signs of abdominal pain are not normal and should be investigated fully.[9] Additional analgesics may be helpful in controlling abdominal pain in the short-term but analgesics will not correct an underlying surgical complication. The general approach to pain management in postoperative colic patients should include prophylactic analgesics as well as specific interventions in response to physiological and behavioral manifestations of pain.

Nonsteroidal anti-inflammatory drugs (NSAIDs) are the mainstay of prophylactic, postoperative analgesia in equine colic surgery. In horses with a positive response to surgery, an NSAID alone should provide sufficient analgesia. NSAIDs also have important anti-inflammatory and antiendotoxic effects.[69,70] Flunixin meglumine is the most commonly used NSAID in colic surgery.[38,39,71] Flunixin meglumine is administered at a dose rate of 1.1 mg/kg IV for 3 to 5 days following colic surgery. Lower dose rates (0.25 mg/kg IV) improve cardiovascular function in horses experiencing SIRS.[70]

Nonselective cyclo-oxygenase (COX) inhibitors such as flunixin meglumine and phenylbutazone can cause gastrointestinal ulceration and nephrotoxicity. COX-2 selective NSAIDs, such as meloxicam and firocoxib, may be a useful alternative to the nonselective COX inhibitors due to their reduced negative side effects.[72] However, clinical trials indicate that flunixin meglumine has superior analgesic effects in postoperative colic patients compared with meloxicam.[72] Flunixin meglumine seems to have a similar analgesic effect relative to firocoxib, based on a recent multicenter clinical trial of horses with small intestinal strangulations.[73] The negative side effects of nonselective NSAIDs such as flunixin meglumine (presumably through its COX-1 inhibition) remain controversial, with several experimental and clinical studies failing to demonstrate detrimental effects of flunixin meglumine.[72–75]

Gastric decompression via nasogastric intubation reduces pain in horses with gastric distention and serves as well as a diagnostic tool. Please refer to "Ancillary Tests" section above.

In horses with persistent abdominal pain that is unresponsive to NSAIDs and gastric decompression, additional analgesics (alone or in combination) may be required. By using drugs in combination, lower doses may be sufficient. This decreases some of the negative side effects seen with these drugs, while enhancing the desired effects.[2,76,77] Common ancillary analgesics used in colic surgery include the following:

Alpha-2 agonist
- Alpha-2 agonists such as xylazine (0.5 mg/kg IV or IM)[78] and detomidine (0.0125 mg/kg IV or IM)[78] are effective in providing analgesia and sedation for horses exhibiting acute signs of abdominal pain. The effects of a single IV or IM dose of these drugs are can be short-lived, so they are generally not a long-term solution for horses with persistent signs of pain. Alpha-2 agonists can be administered as a constant-rate infusion (CRI), although these drugs can decrease intestinal motility and, therefore, are less desirable in the postoperative colic patient.[78,79] Detomidine can be used at a loading dose 10 μg/kg, followed by a CRI at 6 μg/kg/h.[80] Xylazine can be used at a loading dose of 0.5 to 1.0 mg/kg, followed by a CRI at 0.69 mg/kg/h.[81]

Butorphanol
- Butorphanol can provide additional analgesia and can be administered IV, IM, or as a CRI.[2,82] Similar to all opioids, butorphanol may have negative effects on intestinal motility. The use of butorphanol in horses is associated with a decreased fecal output.[2] Nevertheless, its use may be warranted in some cases of persistent abdominal pain. Butorphanol can be used at a loading dose of 17.8 μg/kg followed by a CRI of 23.7 μg/kg/h.[2,82]

Lidocaine
- Lidocaine administered as a CRI is commonly used during and after colic surgery, specifically as a prokinetic.[38,39,83] However, the perceived clinical benefits of lidocaine in horses could be attributed to its analgesic properties.[84] It is a drug that is relatively inexpensive, although its administration as a CRI may result in higher nursing fees and disposable costs. Lidocaine has minimal systemic side effects if administered correctly. The recommended dose is 1.3 mg/kg IV (administered slowly over 10–15 minutes), followed by an infusion rate of 0.05 mg/kg/min IV.[85] Lidocaine is highly protein bound and, therefore, should be administered with caution in horses with hypoproteinemia, especially if being treated with other protein-bound drugs that may displace lidocaine and increase the risk of lidocaine toxicity.[86]

Ketamine
- Subanesthetic doses of ketamine can also provide effective analgesia, when administered as a CRI at a rate of 0.55 mg/kg IV over 15 minutes followed by 1.2 mg/kg/h.[87,88] However, this rate of ketamine CRI was associated with decreased fecal passage in one study[89] and should, therefore, not be used as a first-line analgesic in postoperative colic patients.

Repeat celiotomy

- In horses with signs of persistent abdominal pain and/or reflux, repeat celiotomy should be considered.[90] See David E. Freeman and Anje G. Bauck's article, "Repeat Celiotomy – Current Status," in this issue.

FLUID THERAPY

Lack of intake, ongoing fluid loses (reflux or diarrhea), sequestration of fluid within the gastrointestinal tract, and SIRS contribute to water and electrolyte disturbances in postoperative colic patients. Surgical trauma can also increase the secretion of anti-diuretic hormone (ADH), aldosterone, renin, and cortisol,[91–93] which leads to retention of Na^+ and excretion of K^+ through both the renal and intestinal systems.[92] There is a broad range in fluid requirements for the postoperative colic patient ranging from none to maintenance to resuscitation fluid therapy in horses with cardiovascular collapse. An effective fluid plan will require consideration of the individual patient and frequent monitoring to reassess status.

Correction of the underlying lesion, as well as aggressive preoperative and intraoperative fluid supplementation, can often correct any major fluid and electrolyte imbalances that were present at admission. The rate, type of fluid, and the duration of administration following surgery will depend on the degree of derangements preceding surgery, the gastrointestinal lesion present at surgery and recovery process of the horse following surgery. In horses where the primary problem is resolved, and there are no ongoing loses such as reflux or diarrhea, conservative fluid administration is likely sufficient. An example of this would be 12 to 18 hours of a balanced-electrolyte solution administered at maintenance rate (60 mL/kg/d), early access to free-choice water and careful monitoring of physical examination parameters following discontinuation of IV fluids. Overhydration with IV fluids can lead to complications and unnecessary costs.[92,94,95] Increasing costs of IV fluids is one of the biggest contributors to increased costs of hospitalization for the treatment in colic in recent years.[96]

The daily maintenance fluid requirement in adult horses is around 60 mL/kg when on an all-hay diet.[97–99] However, voluntary water consumption is much lower in horses that are feed-deprived, relative to horses on full feed.[100–102] In one study, water needs were reduced by 16% in horses having feed withheld compared with fed horses.[101] Cecal and colonic microbial digestion of fiber requires tremendous volumes of fluid, fluid that is then recovered through the enterosystemic cycle.[102,103] The daily volume of water entering the large intestines in fed horses, either from the small intestines or from fluid secreted across the mucosal surface, is approximately equal to the horse's entire extracellular fluid volume, 95% of which is reabsorbed before defecation.[103] Much less water will be required for normal digestive function in horses that are anorexic or on a restricted diet, as is standard in the immediate postoperative period (see "Postoperative Nutrition" section below). Over hydration can lead to tissue edema and impaired intestinal motility, possibly to the point of exacerbating the postoperative reflux.[94,95] Large volume fluid therapy could increase capillary filtration into the interstitium, causing tissue edema and filtration secretion into the distended small intestine.[104] Fluid overload will exacerbate intestinal edema[105,106] in patients already at risk for intestinal dysfunction.

Prolonged use of IV replacement fluids (ie, Normosol-R) will put horses at risk for complications such as hypernatremia and hypokalemia, unless switched to preparations intended for use as maintenance fluids.[14] A practical problem with this approach is that maintenance fluids are typically not available in the volumes needed for fluid rates required in horses.[107] Therefore, most horses are administered commercial replacement fluids (available in 5 L bags) and the fluids are supplemented as needed with various electrolytes.[102,107] Supplementation of standard replacement fluids with K^+ (additional 20–40 mEq/L) and Ca^{2+} (additional 25 mL/L of 23% calcium gluconate) may be required until horse is back on full-feed.[14] Caution should be used when increasing the fluid rate in preparations with supplemental K^+ and Ca^{2+} due to the risk of electrolyte derangements if administered too quickly. Early transition to free-choice oral fluids over IV replacement fluids is ideal and has the added benefit of decreased expense.[68]

In horses with postoperative reflux, ongoing losses will need to be accounted for, in addition to the maintenance requirements of horse that is not being fed.[101] Matching the exact volume of fluid loss, plus maintenance, in horses refluxing large volumes (>4–5 L/h) is difficult and costly. A more practical approach involves meticulous monitoring of the clinical status of the patient and adjusting fluid rates in response to status changes.[102] For this approach to be successful, careful and frequent monitoring (physical examination, blood gas analysis, point-of-care chemistry analysis, PCV/TS) is critical. Reflux will also contain different concentrations of electrolytes such as Na^+ and K^+ relative to plasma.[108] Routine monitoring of electrolyte values is especially critical in horses that are suffering ongoing loses from postoperative reflux. Supplementation with K^+, Ca^{++}, and Mg^{++} is often required in horses with postoperative reflux.[38,39]

Unlike with postoperative reflux, the total volume of fluid loss may be difficult to quantify in horses with diarrhea. In normal horses, fecal water is approximately 75% but can increase to 90% in cases of acute diarrhea.[97] The fluid needed for replacement in cases of diarrhea is guided by clinical signs and clinical laboratory data, much more so than with postoperative reflux. Loss of bicarbonate and exacerbation of acid–base disturbances is a particular concern in horses with postoperative diarrhea.

Lactating mares will require greater fluid rates that nonlactating adult horses[109] and may increase water consumption by 37% to 74%.[109,110] Ideally, lactating mares will have access to free-choice water as quickly as possible after surgery. Neonates will also have higher maintenance fluid requirements. Special care must be taken with fluid therapy in foals to minimize the risk of overhydration.[102,111]

POSTOPERATIVE NUTRITION

An important goal of postoperative colic care is early return to function for the gastrointestinal system. Postoperative feeding is critical to this process. However, clinicians must balance the benefits of a quick return to enteral nutrition against the risk of impactions and other complications if the surgical sites are challenged too quickly. In general, the aim should be for horses to return to feed quickly but with small, frequent amounts that are very gradually increased over several days.

There is substantial evidence in human and veterinary medicine to support early refeeding in patients undergoing gastrointestinal surgery.[112] Feed deprivation leads to decreased intestinal motility[12] and is a possible risk factor for adhesion formation.[113] Periods of food deprivation associated with colic will also put horses at risk for metabolic disturbances such as hypertriglyceridemia[24] requiring additional monitoring and more intensive management. Feed deprivation can also delay gastric emptying,[114] and decrease jejunal, cecal, and colonic peristaltic activity.[115] Early refeeding may also help prevent postoperative large colon impactions and displacements.[116] Healing of an anastomosis or an enterotomy site will actually be enhanced by the flow of digesta passed it.[117–120]

It is not advisable to use borborygmi and fecal production to guide refeeding. Borborygmi and defecation can require up to 120 hours to return to normal in horses without postoperative reflux[10] and are, therefore, a poor guide for feeding. Horses can tolerate early feeding in the absence of borborygmi and fecal production.[121] Fecal production and borborygmi are both stimulated by feeding through physiological processes such as the gastrocolic reflex.[12,121] As such, delaying the reintroduction of feed until there is fecal passage and improved borborygmi will only slow normal return to function of the gastrointestinal system.

Finally, there are important practical considerations in managing postoperative colic patients. For example, it is recommended to keep horses muzzled between feedings to prevent the ingestion of shavings or straw. Horses are still able to drink water from a bucket when muzzles are in place.

Specific Recommendations

Food and water should be withheld until the horse has completely recovered from general anesthesia and there is no immediate evidence of intestinal obstruction, manifested as postoperative colic or reflux. Water can be offered as early as 3 hours following recovery from anesthesia in horses with large intestinal or small intestinal nonstrangulating lesions.[122] In horses with small intestinal strangulating lesions, reintroduction of water may be delayed until 12 to 24 hours following recovery from anesthesia,[122] although some clinicians may offer water sooner if there is less concern about the potential for postoperative reflux. Horse can initially be offered small sips of tap water and then free choice water within the first 24 hours.[14,102,123]

For most horses with small or large intestinal nonstrangulating lesions, feed can be reintroduced within 6 to 12 hours after recovery from anesthesia.[112,119] In horses with small colon disorders, it is also recommended to administer mineral oil via nasogastric tube postoperatively to help soften fecal material. A lower bulk diet may also be of benefit in horses with small colon disorders, especially in the immediate postoperative period.[112]

For horses with strangulating small intestinal lesions, feeding recommendations are more variable. It is reasonable to start slowly refeeding anywhere from 12 to 24 hours following recovery from anesthesia,[68,122] as long as the horse is comfortable and not refluxing. Horses recovering from a large intestinal strangulation probably should not be refed until signs of SIRS have resolved sufficiently to indicate that colonic mucosa can tolerate refeeding.

It is the author's preference to refeed colic patients on a roughage diet versus any sort of concentrate or extruded feed. Roughage will promote saliva production and gastric secretions compared with pelleted feed or oats,[124] thereby stimulating intestinal propulsive motility.[125] In a recent survey, grass or hay was the most common type of feed offered when food was reintroduced, although many clinicians (7%–24%, depending on specific type of lesion) indicated that they would choose a complete pelleted feed.[122] In cases of large colon resection, a low-bulk diet supplemented with Wel Gel (Purina Animal Nutrition LLC, Arden Hills, MN) or vegetable oil may be more helpful in minimizing colic because horses adjust to feed moving through the stoma in the immediate postoperative period.[112] In the long term, horses with large colon resections may benefit from alfalfa hay in the diet because of the high digestibility of that hay.[126]

If available, fresh grass is a good choice to start any adult horse back on feed after colic surgery.[112] Fresh grass has a high-water content[127] and outside hand grazing provides the added benefit of early ambulation.[128] Small handfuls of good-quality hay can be fed if fresh grass is not available. Legume hays will provide more digestible energy and crude protein compared with the grass hays.[129] Coastal Bermuda hay should be avoided, due to the association with impactions.[130]

Most postoperative colic patients could be started on one handful of hay, or 2 minutes grazing, offered every 4 to 6 hours for the first 24 hours after the start of feeding. If tolerated, feed should gradually be increased during the next 4 to 5 days until back to what is considered "full feed" for that individual. Adult horses require 1.5% to 3.0% of body weight in feed on a dry matter basis,[131] which could be anywhere from 5 to 8 flakes of hay per day, depending on density of flakes and size of the horse. At home, the horse can be gradually transitioned to its routine feeding program during a 5-day to 10-day period. Owners should be counseled that caloric requirements will be decreased due to the exercise restrictions imposed in the first 3 months following surgery. Therefore, it may be advisable to wait longer to reintroduce any concentrate to the diet.

Certain patients will require special nutritional support:

- Neonates and foals: In the neonate (<2 weeks of age), enteral nutrition will be provided through nursing, bottle feeding or tube feeding. Enteral feeding should be delayed if foal continues to show evidence of ileus, enteritis, or colic in the postoperative period and supplemented with parenteral nutrition instead. If the foal does well after surgery, it can be fed every 2 to 4 hours and receive 1% to 2% of its body weight during a 24-hour period, starting at 0.5% to 1% of bodyweight in the immediate postoperative period and slowly increasing.[132] Foals have increased fluid requirements (70–80 mL/kg/d) and have a higher risk of hypoglycemia with prolonged anorexia compared with an adult. Intake can be controlled by muzzling the foal in between feedings if necessary in nursing foals. By 2 weeks of age, the foal will begin supplementing its intake with solid food provided to the mare. By 2 months of age, milk alone will be insufficient to provide all the calories required for a growing foal. Clinicians need to consider all the different sources of fluids and nutrients foals should be receiving at any age in devising postoperative nutrition plans.
- Pregnant and lactating mares: Late gestation and lactating mares will have higher energy and nutritional requirements than other postoperative colic patients.[110,133] In the last 3 months of gestation, pregnant mares will have caloric requirements that are respectively 11%, 13%, and 20% higher than maintenance energy requirements.[112] Supplemental parenteral nutrition will be required if mare cannot obtain all of her nutritional requirements from enteral feed in the postoperative period. Dextrose can be added to IV crystalloid fluids at 2.5% to 5%,[112] or ideally, as a CRI at 1 to 2 mg/kg/min. Supplementing dextrose as a CRI allows the rate to be adjusted independently of the fluid rates. Blood glucose should be monitored every 4 to 6 hours after the start of supplementation to ensure mare is tolerant of the rate, and then decreased to every 8 to 12 hours.[132] If blood glucose increases to more than 180 mg/dL and persists for more than 2 to 4 hours, the CRI should be slowed or even better insulin administered.[132] In lactating mares, the fluid requirements are considerably higher than in a nonlactating horse. The average mare requires an additional 10 to 15 L of water per day,[110] which needs to be accounted for with either IV or enteral fluids.
- Metabolic disturbances: Healthy horses with normal metabolic status can usually tolerate 48 to 72 hours of anorexia without developing complications such as hypertriglyceridemia or other disturbances in lipid metabolism.[112] However, obese horses or breeds such as American miniature horses, ponies, and donkeys are more predisposed to developing such conditions and may develop hypertriglyceridemia after only 24 to 48 hours of fasting.[23,112,134] Horses with metabolic syndrome, including obese horses and those with pituitary pars intermedia dysfunction (equine Cushing syndrome), may be insulin resistant and

have difficulty metabolizing carbohydrates. Careful monitoring of blood glucose and serum triglycerides is required in such cases in order to provide targeted therapies. In horses with mild-to-moderate hypertriglyceridemia (100–500 mg/dL), supplementation with oral Karo syrup (0.15 mL/kg by mouth every 8 hours) may be sufficient, as long as enteral nutrition is also being provided. Horses with plasma triglyceride greater than 500 mg/dL will likely need nutritional support such as IV dextrose supplementation with or without insulin therapy.[23] That degree of hypertriglyceridemia may cause the horse to become even more inappetent, thereby perpetuating the problem. Horses with metabolic disease/insulin resistance will commonly develop hyperglycemia and hyperinsulinemia, which have been associated with laminitis.[131,135,136] These cases should be monitored closely for clinical signs of laminitis including increased digital pulses, weight shifting, and difficulty walking.

MISCELLANEOUS THERAPEUTICS

An in-depth discussion of postoperative complication associated with colic surgery is beyond the scope of this article, including commonly used drugs for the treatment and prevention of postoperative ileus.[38,39] Other common treatments often used in colic surgery are therapies for the prevention and treatment of endotoxemia. This would include medications such as flunixin meglumine, polymyxin-B, hyperimmune plasma, and enteral adsorbents.[9,137] Continuous digital cryotherapy should be performed in any horse with signs of endotoxemia due to the risk of laminitis.[138] These therapies are of value in certain cases but their selection for use should be judicious. Not all horses undergoing colic surgery are at the risk for endotoxemia, and use of these therapies will result in a higher cost of care.

ECONOMICS

The overall cost of colic surgery varies from case to case, and hospital to hospital.[139] Inevitably, there will be horses that undergo premature euthanasia for financial reasons, rather than welfare reasons.[96] It is important that owners are adequately counseled about the cost of colic surgery before the procedure. Decisions about colic surgery often have to be made quickly and with uncertainty. Clinicians should provide owners with a reasonable expectation of cost, outcome, and potential complications, without overwhelming the owners with unnecessary details. If clinicians consistently provide estimates based on the "worst possible outcome," opportunities to perform surgery will decline. Owners should be informed of the average cost of colic surgery at a particular practice, based on the presumptive preoperative diagnosis, while also being warned that there is a certain percentage of horses that develop complications that may put the final cost outside of the estimate range.

In most hospitals, a large portion of the cost following colic surgery can be attributed to consumables such as IV fluids, antimicrobials, analgesics/anti-inflammatory/antiendotoxin therapies, abdominal bandages, replacement IV catheters, and laboratory data. In a recent study, the greatest increase in consumable costs between 2003 and 2012 was attributable to IV fluids, whereas costs of professional fees decreased during that period.[96] In horses with postoperative complication, the additional cost of those consumable items contributes to an even larger proportion of the bill.[140] Clinicians need to carefully weigh the cost–benefit ratio of using different treatments and diagnostics. Therapies with documented, scientific evidence of their benefit should be prioritized over other therapies with anecdotal or weak evidence behind their use.[141] There is also a heavy focus on pharmacological interventions for the treatment and prevention of complications such as postoperative reflux,[142] which should be reconsidered.[143] Diagnostic and monitoring tests should only be used when the results of those tests will substantially change the treatment plan.

Medical insurance for horses is helpful but not widespread enough to cover the majority of horses requiring colic surgery.[139] Utility of the different insurance plans and what is covered in regards to colic surgery varies. In a study performed in the United Kingdom, the mean cost of colic surgery exceeded the maximum insurance coverage for 4 out of 5 insurance companies.[139] The veterinarian plays a key role in counseling owners about the financial costs of colic surgery and the role of insurance policies. Ideally, these conversations happen separate from the emergency situations so decisions can be made quickly when the time comes.

EXPECTATIONS OF NORMAL RECOVERY AND RETURN TO USE

"Normal" recovery from colic surgery will vary greatly depending on patient and primary lesion. This article does not include a complete discussion of postoperative complications. However, understanding the prevalence of common postoperative complications will help guide clinicians' expectations for a normal recovery. Three common and potentially life-threatening postoperative complications of the equine colic patient include postoperative colic, postoperative reflux, and incisional complications, with postoperative reflux being the most common complication.[143]

Average length of hospitalization will vary but certain hallmarks that should be achieved before discharge include the following:

- Ability to maintain hydration status after the discontinuation of IV fluid therapy.
- Normal vital parameters.
- Tolerance of full roughage-based diet (see "Postoperative Nutrition" section above).
- Patient seems comfortable.

The general expectation is for horses to start back in athletic work at around 90 days following colic surgery. The length of time that will be required to return to presurgical athletic potential will vary depending on the horse and athletic discipline. The author recommends the following exercise regimen for most postoperative colic patients:

- Thirty days in a stall (12″ × 12″), starting from the date of discharge from hospital.
- Thirty days of small paddock turn out.
- Thirty days full pasture turn out.
- If no incisional complications, horses can slowly resume athletic activity starting at 90 days from the time of discharge.

It is recommended to have a veterinarian evaluate the incision between each interval of increased activity level. Incisional complications can lead to prolonged convalescence and diminish return to athletic potential.[144] Of horses that survive to discharge, anywhere from 63% to 85% of horses undergoing colic surgery will return to previous athletic potential.[143,145]

CLINICS CARE POINTS

- Careful monitoring of the postoperative colic patient allows for earlier recognition of complications. The value of a basic physical examination should not be underestimated, and the use of more advanced diagnostics should be reserved to situations where those tests are specifically indicated.

- About 36 to 72 hours of broad-spectrum antimicrobial coverage is common following colic surgery. Longer duration of antimicrobial coverage does not decrease the risk of SSIs or pyrexia.
- NSAIDs such as flunixin meglumine remain the mainstay of analgesia in colic surgery. If this drug alone is not sufficient in keeping the patient comfortable following surgery, further investigation may be required in determining the source of pain.
- The maintenance fluid requirements for postoperative colic patients, not yet back on full feed, will be lower relative to horses on full feed. However, ongoing losses from reflux, diarrhea, or maldistribution caused by endotoxemia must be accounted for.
- Early access to oral water and enteral nutrition can help promote return to function for the gastrointestinal system.
- Consumables such as IV fluids contribute to the increasing costs of colic surgery. Clinicians should consider the cost–benefit analysis of various treatments because the level of care should reflect the patient's primary lesion and postoperative status.

DISCLOSURE

The author has no commercial or financial conflicts of interests to disclose, or any funding sources.

REFERENCES

1. Pritchett LC, Ulibarri C, Roberts MC, et al. Identification of potential physiological and behavioral indicators of postoperative pain in horses after exploratory celiotomy for colic. Appl Anim Behav Sci 2003;80(1):31–43.
2. Sellon DC, Roberts MC, Blikslager AT, et al. Effects of continuous rate intravenous infusion of butorphanol on physiologic and outcome variables in horses after celiotomy. J Vet Intern Med 2004;18(4):555–63.
3. Freeman KD, Southwood LL, Lane J, et al. Post operative infection, pyrexia and perioperative antimicrobial drug use in surgical colic patients. Equine Vet J 2012;44(4):476–81.
4. Gleerup KB, Forkman B, Lindegaard C, et al. An equine pain face. Vet Anaesth Analg 2015;42(1):103–14.
5. Sutton GA, Atamna R, Steinman A, et al. Comparison of three acute colic pain scales: Reliability, validity and usability. Vet J 2019;246:71–7.
6. van Loon JPAM, Jonckheer-Sheehy VSM, Back W, et al. Monitoring equine visceral pain with a composite pain scale score and correlation with survival after emergency gastrointestinal surgery. Vet J 2014;200(1):109–15.
7. Costa ED, Pascuzzo R, Leach MC, et al. Can grimace scales estimate the pain status in horses and mice? A statistical approach to identify a classifier. PLoS One 2018;13(8). https://doi.org/10.1371/journal.pone.0200339.
8. Maskato Y, Dugdale AHA, Singer ER, et al. Prospective feasibility and revalidation of the equine acute abdominal pain scale (EAAPS) in clinical cases of colic in horses. Animals 2020;10(12):1–14.
9. Hackett ES, Hassel DM. Colic: Nonsurgical Complications. Vet Clin North Am Equine Pract 2008;24(3):535–55.
10. Cohen ND, Lester GD, Sanchez C, et al. Evaluation of risk factors associated with development of postoperative ileus in horses. J Am Vet Med Assoc 2004; 225(7):1070–8.

11. Smith LCR, Payne RJ, Boys Smith SJ, et al. Outcome and long-term follow-up of 20 horses undergoing surgery for caecal impaction: A retrospective study (2000 2008). Equine Vet J 2010;42(5):388–92.

12. Naylor JM, Poirier KL, Hamilton DL, et al. The effects of feeding and fasting on gastrointestinal sounds in adult horses. J Vet Intern Med 2006;20(6):1408–13.

13. Schoster A, Mitchell K. Fluids, electrolytes, and acid-base therapy. In: Auer JA, Stick JA, editors. Equine surgery. 5th edition. St. Louis, MO: Elsevier; 2019. p. 28–40.

14. Seahorn JL, Seahorn TL. Fluid therapy in horses with gastrointestinal disease. Vet Clin North Am Equine Pract 2003;19(3):665–79.

15. Mccoy AM, Hackett ES, Wagner AE, et al. Pulmonary Gas Exchange and Plasma Lactate in Horses with Gastrointestinal Disease Undergoing Emergency Exploratory Laparotomy: A Comparison with an Elective Surgery Horse Population. Vet Surg 2011;40(5):601–9.

16. Tennent-Brown BS, Wilkins PA, Lindborg S, et al. Sequential plasma lactate concentrations as prognostic indicators in adult equine emergencies. J Vet Intern Med 2010;24(1):198–205.

17. Fessler JF, Bottoms GD, Roesel OF, et al. Endotoxin-induced change in hemograms, plasma enzymes, and blood chemical values in anesthetized ponies: effects of flunixin meglumen. Am J Vet Res 1982;43(1):140–4.

18. Kjelgaard-Hansen M, Jacobsen S. Assay Validation and Diagnostic Applications of Major Acute-phase Protein Testing in Companion Animals. Clin Lab Med 2011;31(1):51–70.

19. Cohen ND, Honnas CM. Risk factors associated with development of diarrhea in horses after celiotomy for colic: 190 cases (1990-1994). J Am Vet Med Assoc 1996;209(4):810–3.

20. Jacobs CC, Holcombe SJ, Cook VL, et al. Ethyl pyruvate diminishes the inflammatory response to lipopolysaccharide infusion in horses. Equine Vet J 2013; 45(3):333–9.

21. Aitken MR, Stefanovski D, Southwood LL. Serum amyloid A concentration in postoperative colic horses and its association with postoperative complications. Vet Surg 2019;48(2):143–51.

22. Salciccia A, Sandersen C, Grulke S, et al. Sensitivity and specificity of blood leukocyte counts as an indicator of mortality in horses after colic surgery. Vet Rec 2013;173(11):267.

23. Dunkel B, McKenzie HC. Severe hypertriglyceridaemia in clinically ill horses: Diagnosis, treatment and outcome. Equine Vet J 2003;35(6):590–5.

24. Underwood C, Southwood LL, Walton RM, et al. Hepatic and metabolic changes in surgical colic patients: a pilot study. J Vet Emerg Crit Care 2010;20(6):578–86.

25. Radcliffe RM, Buchanan BR, Cook VL, et al. The clinical value of whole blood point-of-care biomarkers in large animal emergency and critical care medicine. J Vet Emerg Crit Care 2015;25(1):138–51.

26. Groover ES, Woolums AR, Cole DJ, et al. Risk factors associated with renal insufficiency in horses with primary gastrointestinal disease: 26 Cases (2000-2003). J Am Vet Med Assoc 2006;228(4):572–7.

27. Hollis AR, Boston RC, Corley KTT. Blood Glucose in Horses with Acute Abdominal Disease. J Vet Intern Med 2007;21(5):1099–103.

28. Hassel DM, Hill AE, Rorabeck RA. Association between hyperglycemia and survival in 228 horses with acute gastrointestinal disease. J Vet Intern Med 2009; 23(6):1261–5.

29. Hollis AR, Furr MO, Magdesian KG, et al. Blood glucose concentrations in critically ill neonatal foals. J Vet Intern Med 2008;22(5):1223–7.

30. Borges AS, Divers TJ, Stokol T, et al. Serum iron and plasma fibrinogen concentrations as indicators of systemic inflammatory diseases in horses. J Vet Intern Med 2007;21(3):489–94.

31. Bonelli F, Meucci V, Divers TJ, et al. Plasma Procalcitonin Concentration in Healthy Horses and Horses Affected by Systemic Inflammatory Response Syndrome. J Vet Intern Med 2015;29(6):1689–91.

32. Westerman TL, Foster CM, Tornquist SJ, et al. Evaluation of serum amyloid A and haptoglobin concentrations as prognostic indicators for horses with colic. J Am Vet Med Assoc 2016;248(8):935–40.

33. de Cozar M, Sherlock C, Knowles E, et al. Serum amyloid A and plasma fibrinogen concentrations in horses following emergency exploratory celiotomy. Equine Vet J 2020;52(1):59–66.

34. Crisman Mv, Kent Scarratt W, Zimmerman KL. Blood proteins and inflammation in the horse. Vet Clin North Am Equine Pract 2008;24(2):285–97.

35. Feige K, Kästner SB, Dempfle CE, et al. Changes in coagulation and markers of fibrinolysis in horses undergoing colic surgery. J Vet Med A Physiol Pathol Clin Med 2003;50(1):30–6.

36. Daniel AJ, Leise BS, Burgess BA, et al. Concentrations of serum amyloid A and plasma fibrinogen in horses undergoing emergency abdominal surgery. J Vet Emerg Crit Care (San Antonio) 2016;26(3):344–51.

37. Bowlby C, Mudge M, Schroeder E, et al. Equine inflammatory response to abdominal surgery in the absence of gastrointestinal disease. J Vet Emerg Crit Care 2021;31(5):601–7.

38. Lefebvre D, Pirie RS, Handel IG, et al. Clinical features and management of equine post operative ileus: Survey of diplomates of the European Colleges of Equine Internal Medicine (ECEIM) and Veterinary Surgeons (ECVS). Equine Vet J 2016;48(2):182–7.

39. Lefebvre D, Hudson NPH, Elce YA, et al. Clinical features and management of equine post operative ileus (POI): Survey of Diplomates of the American Colleges of Veterinary Internal Medicine (ACVIM), Veterinary Surgeons (ACVS) and Veterinary Emergency and Critical Care (ACVECC). Equine Vet J 2016; 48(6):714–9.

40. Nieto JE, Yamount S, Dechant JE. Sinusitis associated with nasogastric intubation in 3 horses. Can Vet J 2014;55(6):554–8. Available at: https://pubmed.ncbi.nlm.nih.gov/24891638/.

41. Epstein K, Short D, Parente E, et al. Serial gastrointestinal ultrasonography following exploratory celiotomy in normal adult ponies. Vet Radiol Ultrasound 2008;49(6):584–8.

42. Ernst NS, Hernandez JA, MacKay RJ, et al. Risk factors associated with fecal Salmonella shedding among hospitalized horses with signs of gastrointestinal tract disease. J Am Vet Med Assoc 2004;225(2):275–81.

43. Dallap Schaer BL, Linton JK, Aceto H. Antimicrobial Use in Horses Undergoing Colic Surgery. J Vet Intern Med 2012;26(6):1449–56.

44. Ekiri AB, Morton AJ, Long MT, et al. Review of the epidemiology and infection control aspects of nosocomial Salmonella infections in hospitalised horses. Equine Vet Educ 2010;22(12):631–41.

45. Aceto H, Miller SA, Smith G. Onset of diarrhea and pyrexia and time to detection of Salmonella enterica subsp enterica in feces in experimental studies of cattle,

horses, goats, and sheep after infection per os. J Am Vet Med Assoc 2011; 238(10):1333–9.

46. Ekiri AB, MacKay RJ, Gaskin JM, et al. Epidemiologic analysis of nosocomial Salmonella infections in hospitalized horses. J Am Vet Med Assoc 2009; 234(1):108–19.

47. Kilcoyne I, Magdesian KG, Guerra M, et al. Prevalence of and risk factors associated with Salmonella shedding among equids presented to a veterinary teaching hospital for colic (2013-2018). Equine Vet J 2023;55(3):446–55. https://doi.org/10.1111/EVJ.13864.

48. Brown MP. Perioperative antibiotics in horses. Compend Continuing Educ Pract Vet 1999;21(11):1082–7. Available at: https://agris.fao.org/agris-search/search.do?recordID=US201302940872. Accessed June 19, 2022.

49. Klein WR, Firth EC. Infection rates in contaminated surgical procedures: a comparison of prophylactic treatment for one day or four days. Vet Rec 1988; 123(22):564–6.

50. Esposito S. Is single-dose antibiotic prophylaxis sufficient for any surgical procedure? J Chemother 1999;11(6):556–64.

51. Haven ML, Wichtel J j, Bristol DG, et al. Effects of antibiotic prophylaxis on postoperative complications after rumenotomy in cattle. J Am Vet Med Assoc 1992; 200(9):1332–5. Available at: https://pubmed.ncbi.nlm.nih.gov/1601715/. Accessed June 20, 2022.

52. Traub-Dargatz JL, Dargatz DA, Morley PS. Antimicrobial Resistance: What's the Big Deal? Importance of Antimicrobial Resistance to the Equine Practitioner. In: AAEP Proceedings. ; 2002:138-144. Available at: www.avma.org/scientist/. . Accessed June 24, 2022.

53. Bratzler DW, Houck PM. Antimicrobial prophylaxis for surgery: an advisory statement from the National Surgical Infection Prevention Project. Am J Surg 2005;189(4):395–404.

54. Weese JS, Cruz A. Retrospective study of perioperative antimicrobial use practices in horses undergoing elective arthroscopic surgery at a veterinary teaching hospital. Can Vet J 2009;50(2):185–8. Available at: https://pubmed.ncbi.nlm.nih.gov/19412399/. Accessed June 20, 2022.

55. Durward-Akhurst SA, Mair TS, Boston R, et al. Comparison of two antimicrobial regimens on the prevalence of incisional infections after colic surgery. Vet Rec 2013;172(11):287.

56. Dunkel B, Johns IC. Antimicrobial use in critically ill horses. J Vet Emerg Crit Care 2015;25(1):89–100.

57. Isgren CM, Salem SE, Archer DC, et al. Risk factors for surgical site infection following laparotomy: Effect of season and perioperative variables and reporting of bacterial isolates in 287 horses. Equine Vet J 2017;49(1):39–44.

58. Smith LJ, Mellor DJ, Marr CM, et al. Incisional complications following exploratory celiotomy: Does an abdominal bandage reduce the risk? Equine Vet J 2007;39(3):277–83.

59. WILSON DA, BAKER GJ, BOERO MJ. Complications of Celiotomy Incisions in Horses. Vet Surg 1995;24(6):506–14.

60. Dunowska M, Morley PS, Traub-Dargatz JL, et al. Impact of hospitalization and antimicrobial drug administration on antimicrobial susceptibility patterns of commensal Escherichia coli isolated from the feces of horses. J Am Vet Med Assoc 2006;228(12):1909–17.

61. Maddox TW, Williams NJ, Clegg PD, et al. Longitudinal study of antimicrobial-resistant commensal Escherichia coli in the faeces of horses in an equine hospital. Prev Vet Med 2011;100(2):134–45.

62. Weese JS, Holcombe SJ, Embertson RM, et al. Changes in the faecal microbiota of mares precede the development of post partum colic. Equine Vet J 2015; 47(6):641–9.

63. Cohen ND, Woods AM. Characteristics and risk factors for failure of horses with acute diarrhea to survive: 122 cases (1990-1996). J Am Vet Med Assoc 1999; 214(3):382–90. Available at: https://pubmed.ncbi.nlm.nih.gov/10023402/. Accessed June 20, 2022.

64. Southwood LL. Principles of Antimicrobial Therapy: What Should We Be Using? Vet Clin North Am Equine Pract 2006;22(2):279–96.

65. Johns IC, Adams EL. Trends in antimicrobial resistance in equine bacterial isolates: 1999-2012. Vet Rec 2015;176(13):334.

66. Morley PS, Apley MD, Besser TE, et al. Antimicrobial drug use in veterinary medicine. J Vet Intern Med 2005;19:617–29. https://doi.org/10.1892/0891-6640 (2005)19[617:ADUIVM]2.0.CO;2.

67. Traub-Dargatz JL, George JL, Dargatz DA, et al. Survey of complications and antimicrobial use in equine patients at veterinary teaching hospitals that underwent surgery because of colic. J Am Vet Med Assoc 2002;220(9):1359–65.

68. Fogle C. Postoperative Care, Complications, and Reoperation of the Colic Patient. In: Auer JA, Stick JA, editors. Equine Surgery. Philadelphia, PA: Elsevier; 2019. p. 660–77. https://doi.org/10.1016/b978-0-323-48420-6.00041-7.

69. Semrad SD, Moore JN. Effects of multiple low doses of flunixin meglumine on repeated endotoxin challenge in the horse. Prostaglandins Leukot Med 1987; 27(2–3):169–81.

70. Semrad SD, Hardee GE, Hardee MM, et al. Low dose flunixin meglumine: Effects on eicosanoid production and clinical signs induced by experimental endotoxaemia in horses. Equine Vet J 1987;19(3):201–6.

71. Gibbs R, Duz M, Shipman E. A survey of non-steroidal anti-inflammatory drug use in the post-operative period following equine colic surgery. Equine Vet Educ 2022. https://doi.org/10.1111/eve.13660.

72. Naylor RJ, Taylor AH, Knowles EJ, et al. Comparison of flunixin meglumine and meloxicam for post operative management of horses with strangulating small intestinal lesions. Equine Vet J 2014;46(4):427–34.

73. Ziegler AL, Freeman CK, Fogle CA, et al. Multicentre, blinded, randomised clinical trial comparing the use of flunixin meglumine with firocoxib in horses with small intestinal strangulating obstruction. Equine Vet J 2019;51(3):329–35.

74. Matyjaszek SA, Morton AJ, Freeman DE, et al. Effects of flunixin meglumine on recovery of colonic mucosa from ischemia in horses. Am J Vet Res 2009;70(2): 236–46.

75. Morton AJ, Grosche A, Matyjaszek SA, et al. Effects of flunixin meglumine on the recovery of ischaemic equine colonic mucosa in vitro. Equine Vet J 2011; 43(SUPPL.39):112–6.

76. van Loon JPAM. Multimodal analgesia, a fashionable term or evidence-based medicine? Equine Vet Educ 2019;31(7):363–4.

77. Muir WW. Pain: Mechanisms and Management in Horses. Vet Clin North Am Equine Pract 2010;26(3):467–80.

78. Merritt AM, Burrow JA, Hartless CS. Effect of xylazine, detomidine, and a combination of xylazine and butorphanol on equine duodenal motility. Am J Vet Res 1998;59(5):619–23.

79. Zullian C, Menozzi A, Pozzoli C, et al. Effects of α2-adrenergic drugs on small intestinal motility in the horse: An in vitro study. Vet J 2011;187(3):342–6.

80. Hollis AR, Pascal M, van Dijk J, et al. Behavioural and cardiovascular effects of medetomidine constant rate infusion compared with detomidine for standing sedation in horses. Vet Anaesth Analg 2020;47(1):76–81.

81. Ringer SK, Schwarzwald CC, Portier KG, et al. Effects on cardiopulmonary function and oxygen delivery of doses of romifidine and xylazine followed by constant rate infusions in standing horses. Vet J 2013;195(2):228–34.

82. Sellon DC, Monroe VL, Roberts MC, et al. Pharmacokinetics and adverse effects of butorphanol administered by single intravenous injection or continuous intravenous infusion in horses. Am J Vet Res 2001;62(2):183–9.

83. van Hoogmoed LM, Nieto JE, Snyder JR, et al. Survey of prokinetic use in horses with gastrointestinal injury. Vet Surg 2004;33(3):279–85.

84. Vigani A, Garcia-Pereira FL. Anesthesia and analgesia for standing equine surgery. Vet Clin North Am Equine Pract 2014;30(1):1–17.

85. Malone E, Ensink J, Turner T, et al. Intravenous continuous infusion of lidocaine for treatment of equine ileus. Vet Surg 2006;35(1):60–6.

86. Milligan M, KuKanich B, Beard W, et al. The disposition of lidocaine during a 12-hour intravenous infusion to postoperative horses. J Vet Pharmacol Ther 2006;29(6):495–9.

87. Valverde A, Gunkel CI. Pain management in horses and farm animals. J Vet Emerg Crit Care 2005;15(4):295–307.

88. Muir WW. NMDA Receptor Antagonists and Pain: Ketamine. Vet Clin N Am Equine Pract 2010;26(3):565–78.

89. Elfenbein JR, Robertson SA, Corser AA, et al. Systemic Effects of a Prolonged Continuous Infusion of Ketamine in Healthy Horses. J Vet Intern Med 2011;25(5):1134–7.

90. Bauck AG, Easley JT, Cleary OB, et al. Response to early repeat celiotomy in horses after a surgical treatment of jejunal strangulation. Vet Surg 2017;46(6):843–50.

91. Hoffis GF, Murdick PW, Tharp VL, et al. Plasma concentrations of cortisol and corticosterone in the normal horse. Am J Vet Res 1970;31(8):1379–87. Available at: https://www.cabdirect.org/cabdirect/abstract/19712200404. Accessed June 21, 2022.

92. Holte K, Sharrock NE, Kehlet H. Pathophysiology and clinical implications of perioperative fluid excess. Br J Anaesth 2002;89(4):622–32.

93. Hinchcliff KW, Rush BR, Farris JW. Evaluation of plasma catecholamine and serum cortisol concentrations in horses with colic. J Am Vet Med Assoc 2005;227(2):276–80.

94. Shah SK, Moore-Olufemi SD, Uray KS, et al. A murine model for the study of edema induced intestinal contractile dysfunction. Neuro Gastroenterol Motil 2010;22(10). https://doi.org/10.1111/j.1365-2982.2010.01546.x.

95. Brandstrup B, Tønnesen H, Beier-Holgersen R, et al. Effects of intravenous fluid restriction on postoperative complications: comparison of two perioperative fluid regimens: a randomized assessor-blinded multicenter trial. Ann Surg 2003;238(5):641–8.

96. Bates A, Whiting M, Witte TH. The Changing Costs of Hospital Treatment for Colic: A Preliminary Audit. Equine Vet J 2014;46:22.

97. Tasker JB. Fluid and electrolyte studies in the horse. 5. The effects of diarrhea. Cornell Vet 1967;57:668–77. Available at: https://www.cabdirect.org/cabdirect/abstract/19681408833. Accessed June 21, 2022.

98. Groenendyk S, English PB, Abetz I. External balance of water and electrolytes in the horse. Equine Vet J 1988;20(3):189–93.

99. Lester GD, Merritt AM, Kuck Hv, et al. Systemic, renal, and colonic effects of intravenous and enteral rehydration in horses. J Vet Intern Med 2013;27(3): 554–66.

100. Norris ML, Houpt KA, Houpt TR. Effect of Food Availability on the Physiological Responses to Water Deprivation in Ponies. J Equine Vet Sci 2013;33(4):250–6.

101. Freeman DE, Mooney A, Giguère S, et al. Effect of feed deprivation on daily water consumption in healthy horses. Equine Vet J 2021;53(1):117–24.

102. Freeman DE. Effect of Feed Intake on Water Consumption in Horses: Relevance to Maintenance Fluid Therapy. Front Vet Sci 2021;8:79.

103. Argenzio RA, Lowe JE, Pickard DW, et al. Digesta passage and water exchange in the equine large intestine. Am J Physiol 1974;226(5):1035–42.

104. Allen D, Kvietys PR, Granger DN. Crystalloids versus colloids: implications in fluid therapy of dogs with intestinal obstruction. Am J Vet Res 1986;47(8): 1751–5. Available at: https://pubmed.ncbi.nlm.nih.gov/3752685/. Accessed June 21, 2022.

105. Chan STF, Kapadia CR, Johnson AW, et al. Extracellular fluid volume expansion and third space sequestration at the site of small bowel anastomoses. Br J Surg 1983;70(1):36–9.

106. Shah SK, Uray KS, Stewart RH, et al. Resuscitation-induced intestinal edema and related dysfunction: State of the science. J Surg Res 2011;166(1):120–30.

107. Schott H.C. II, Wüger C., Rossetto J.R., et al., Intravenous fluid therapy: can we do it better? In: 53rd Annual Convention of the American Association of Equine Practitioners. American Association of Equine Practitioners (AAEP); Dec. 1-5, 2007, Orlando, FL. p86.

108. Schott HC. Volume of distended small intestine and ionic composition of gastric reflux and small intestinal fluid in horses. In: ACVIM Proceedings. May 30- June 2. New Orleans, LA; 2012.

109. Lewis LD. Broodmare feeding and care. In: Lewis LD, editor. Equine Clinical Nutrition. 1st edition. Media, PA: Williams & Wilkins; 1995. p. 286–306.

110. Dolente BA. Critical peripartum disease in the mare. Vet Clin North Am Equine Pract 2004;20(1):151–65.

111. Palmer JE. Fluid therapy in the neonate: not your mother's fluid space. Vet Clin Equine Pract 2004;20(1):63–75.

112. Practice KMVCE, 2003 undefined. Nutrition for critical gastrointestinal illness: feeding horses with diarrhea or colic. vetequine.theclinics.com. . Available at: https://www.vetequine.theclinics.com/article/S0749-0739(03)00050-6/abstract. Accessed July 24, 2022.

113. Murphy DJ, Peck LS, Detrisac CJ, et al. Use of a high-molecular-weight carboxymethylcellulose in a tissue protective solution for prevention of postoperative abdominal adhesions in ponies. Am J Vet Res 2002;63(10):1448–54.

114. Freeman DE, Ferrante PL, Kronfeld DS, et al. Effect of food deprivation on D-xylose absorption test results in mares. Am J Vet Res 1989;50(9):1609–12. Available at: https://europepmc.org/article/med/2802339. Accessed July 24, 2022.

115. Mitchell CF, Malone ED, Sage AM, et al. Evaluation of gastrointestinal activity patterns in healthy horses using B mode and Doppler ultrasonography. Can Vet J 2005;46(2):134–40.

116. jones RS, Edwards GB, Brearley JC. Commentary on prolonged starvation as a factor associated with post operative colic. Equine Vet Educ 1991;3(1):16–8.

117. Basse L, Jakobsen DH, Billesbølle P, et al. A clinical pathway to accelerate recovery after colonic resection. Ann Surg 2000;232(1):51–7.

118. Kiyama T, Onda M, Tokunaga A, et al. Effect of early postoperative feeding on the healing of colonic anastomoses in the presence of intra-abdominal sepsis in rats. Dis Colon Rectum 2000;43(10 SUPPL). https://doi.org/10.1007/bf02237227.

119. Fukuzawa J, Terashima H, Ohkohchi N. Early postoperative oral feeding accelerates upper gastrointestinal anastomotic healing in the rat model. World J Surg 2007;31(6):1234–9.

120. Tadano S, Terashima H, Fukuzawa J, et al. Early postoperative oral intake accelerates upper gastrointestinal anastomotic healing in the rat model. J Surg Res 2011;169(2):202–8.

121. Freeman DE, Ferrante PL, Palmer JE. Comparison of the effects of intragastric infusions of equal volumes of water, dioctyl sodium sulfosuccinate, and magnesium sulfate on fecal composition and output in clinically normal horses. Am J Vet Res 1992;53(8):1347–53. Available at: https://pubmed.ncbi.nlm.nih.gov/1380786/. Accessed June 21, 2022.

122. Lawson AL, Sherlock CE, Ireland JL, et al. Equine nutrition in the post-operative colic: Survey of Diplomates of the American Colleges of Veterinary Internal Medicine and Veterinary Surgeons, and European Colleges of Equine Internal Medicine and Veterinary Surgeons. Equine Vet J 2021;53(5):1015–24.

123. Sufit E, Houpt KA, Sweeting M. Physiological stimuli of thirst and drinking patterns in ponies. Equine Vet J 1985;17(1):12–6.

124. Meyer H. Influence of feed intake and composition, feed and water restriction, and exercise on gastrointestinal fill in horses. 1. Equine Pract 1997;18(7):26–9. Available at: https://agris.fao.org/agris-search/search.do?recordID=US9629105. Accessed June 21, 2022.

125. Ruckebusch Y. Motor functions of the large intestine. Adv Vet Sci Comp Med 1981;25:345–69.

126. Bertone AL, Ralston SL, Stashak TS. Fiber digestion and voluntary intake in horses after adaptation to extensive large-colon resection. Am J Vet Res 1989;50(9):1628–32.

127. Lewis LD. Diet evaluation, formulation, and preparation for horses. In: Lew LD, editor. Equine clinical nutrition. 1st edition. Media, PA: Williams & Wilkins; 1995. p. A.147–174.

128. Williams S, Horner J, Orton E, et al. Water intake, faecal output and intestinal motility in horses moved from pasture to a stabled management regime with controlled exercise. Equine Vet J 2015;47(1):96–100.

129. Lewis LD. Nutrient content of horse feeds (Appendix Table 7). In: Lewis LD, editor. Equine clinical nutrition. 1st edition. Media: Williams & Wilkins; 1995. p. A.558–560.

130. Fleming K, Mueller EPO. Ileal impaction in 245 horses: 1995-2007. Can Vet J 2011;52(7):759–63. Available at: https://pubmed.ncbi.nlm.nih.gov/22210940/. Accessed June 25, 2022.

131. Magdesian KG. Parenteral nutrition in the mature horse. Equine Vet Educ 2010; 22(7):364–71. https://doi.org/10.1111/j.2042-3292.2010.00092.x.

132. Carr EA, Fecteau ME, Linton M. Nutrition of the Sick.... In: Smith BP, van Metre DC, Pusterla N, eds Large Animal Internal Medicine. 6th edition ; 2020:1694-1702. Available at: https://expertconsult.inkling.com/read/smith-large-animal-internal-medicine-6e/chapter-50/chapter50-reader-0. Accessed June 22, 2022.

133. Council NR. Nutrient Requirements of Horses,: Fifth Revised Edition, 1989. Nutrient Requirements of Horses,. Published online January 1, 1AD. doi:10.17226/1213.
134. Moore BR–, Abood SK, Hinchcliff KW. Hyperlipemia in 9 Miniature Horses and Miniature Donkeys. J Vet Intern Med 1994;8(5):376–81.
135. Asplin KE, Sillence MN, Pollitt CC, et al. Induction of laminitis by prolonged hyperinsulinaemia in clinically normal ponies. Vet J 2007;174(3):530–5.
136. de Laat MA, McGowan CM, Sillence MN, et al. Equine laminitis: Induced by 48 h hyperinsulinaemia in Standardbred horses. Equine Vet J 2010;42(2):129–35.
137. Kelmer G. Update on Treatments for Endotoxemia. Vet Clin North Am Equine Pract 2009;25(2):259–70.
138. van Eps AW, Pollitt CC, Underwood C, et al. Continuous digital hypothermia initiated after the onset of lameness prevents lamellar failure in the oligofructose laminitis model. Equine Vet J 2014;46(5):625–30.
139. Barker I, Freeman SL. Assessment of costs and insurance policies for referral treatment of equine colic. Vet Rec 2019;185(16):508.
140. Archer DC. Colic surgery: Keeping it affordable for horse owners. Vet Rec 2019; 185(16):505–7.
141. Meyer JC. Evaluating evidence for new therapies in equine medicine. Equine Vet Educ 2020;32(1):6–7.
142. Blikslager A. Advances in management of small intestinal diseases causing colic. Proceedings of the 55th Annual Convention of the American Association of Equine Practitioners, Las Vegas, Nevada, USA, 5-9 December 2009. Published online 2009:207-211.
143. Freeman DE. Fifty years of colic surgery. Equine Vet J 2018;50(4):423–35.
144. Shearer TR, Holcombe SJ, Valberg SJ. Incisional infections associated with ventral midline celiotomy in horses. J Vet Emerg Crit Care (San Antonio) 2020; 30(2):136–48.
145. Salem SE, Proudman CJ, Archer DC. Prevention of post operative complications following surgical treatment of equine colic: Current evidence. Equine Vet J 2016;48(2):143–51.

Critical Care of the Colic Patient
Monitoring, Fluid Therapy, and More

Charlie Barton, DVM, Diana M. Hassel, DVM, PhD, DACVS, DACVECC*

KEYWORDS

• Horse • Colic • Diagnostic tests • Critical care • Monitoring • Fluid therapy

KEY POINTS

- Serial monitoring of the horse with colic allows for an early identification of high-risk cases that require either more intensive medical or surgical intervention.
- Blood values such as serum amyloid A, lactate, and glucose concentrations, when assessed serially, can provide valuable insight into the risk of complications and help to direct appropriate therapy.
- Current fluid therapy guidelines should consider the impact of high-volume rapid fluid resuscitation on endothelial health and consider altered fluid needs in states of stall rest and anorexia.
- An aggressive multimodal approach to monitoring, pain control, and treatment during the early postoperative period may be effective in reducing the risk of complications and improving outcomes.

ADVANCES IN MONITORING

Serial monitoring of patients with colic is a critical piece for an early identification of developing problems. Palpation per rectum, transabdominal sonography, and a wide variety of blood values, including serum amyloid A (SAA), lactate, creatinine, electrolyte, glucose and triglyceride concentrations, and blood gases, can provide helpful guidelines to direct therapy in critical colic patients.

Physical Examination and Palpation per Rectum

Physical examination forms the mainstay of monitoring the critical colic patient because it enables crude assessment of hydration and cardiovascular status. The discriminant use of palpation per rectum may be a key component of the physical examination in many circumstances. For medically treated colic patients, it may provide

Department of Clinical Sciences, Colorado State University, College of Veterinary Medicine & Biological Sciences, 300 West Drake Road, Fort Collins, CO 80523, USA
* Corresponding author.
E-mail address: Diana.Hassel@ColoState.EDU

Vet Clin Equine 39 (2023) 287–305
https://doi.org/10.1016/j.cveq.2023.03.011
0749-0739/23/© 2023 Elsevier Inc. All rights reserved.

evidence for or against the need for surgical intervention by determining resolution or worsening of visceral distension and displacement, or provide information on the effectiveness of medical therapy on an impaction. Postoperative palpation per rectum is less commonly used but is indicated for horses displaying signs of postoperative pain or increasing abdominal distension.

Transabdominal Sonography

Transabdominal sonography is a well-established diagnostic tool for the initial assessment of the colic patient and has a critical role in monitoring the medically managed colic patient with the progression of clinical signs to aid in determining the need for surgery. In the postoperative colic patient, sonography is invaluable for an early detection of impending postoperative reflux from gastric fluid accumulation, small intestinal distension from ileus or obstruction, peritonitis, hemoperitoneum, colonic wall edema resolution after large colon volvulus (LCV), and assessment of the pulmonary parenchymal surface for evidence of postoperative pneumonia. Detection of persistent edema within the colonic wall following correction of an LCV is associated with increased morbidity.[1]

Inflammatory Biomarkers

Serial monitoring of the inflammatory response through serum biomarkers can aid in the assessment of treatment in addition to enabling early detection of possible complications. SAA has been shown as a useful marker for acute inflammation associated with both infectious and noninfectious origins.[2] In horses presenting for acute abdominal pain, SAA was significantly higher in horses that did not survive the colic episode, and for horses with inflammatory lesions such as enteritis, colitis, and peritonitis.[3] Additionally, SAA was accurate in differentiating between horses with a surgical lesion or an inflammatory lesion requiring medical management.[4] SAA increases 60 to 80 fold within 72 hours of abdominal exploration and then decreases rapidly nearing normal values within 168 hours postoperatively.[5] Horses that do not survive to hospital discharge, because they develop complications following abdominal surgery, have SAA increases of higher magnitudes and duration.[6]

Although SAA is a more sensitive indicator of inflammation in the preoperative and postoperative period, hyperfibrinogenemia is also seen in horses with postoperative complications or preoperative systemic inflammatory response syndrome (SIRS).[7] Fibrinogen is also upregulated in inflammatory conditions in response to bleeding or clotting, and to support wound healing. In the intestine, fibrinogen has been shown to be deposited within the basement membrane where it contributes to epithelial cell healing and within the colon and small intestine in both normal and pathologic conditions requiring rapid epithelial repair.[8] Fibrinogen concentration has a slower and less dramatic increase in response to abdominal surgery, taking 120 hours to reach peak values of approximately twice the values detected on admission.[5]

Monitoring of Blood Parameters

Blood parameters can be useful prognostic indicators in horses presenting with abdominal pain; however, no individual parameter can accurately provide the complete clinical picture of the patient. Therefore, all findings of the diagnostic workup must be considered alongside one another to give an accurate assessment of the horse's condition. In addition to packed cell volume (PCV)/total plasma protein (TP) (see Anje G. Bauck's article, "Basic Post-operative Care of the Equine Colic Patient," in this issue), the following blood parameters are most commonly assessed in the critical colic patient.

- Blood and peritoneal fluid lactate
- Creatinine
- Electrolytes (calcium, magnesium, potassium, and chloride)
- Blood gases (acid/base)
- Triglycerides
- Glucose

Lactate: Blood lactate concentration can be rapidly measured point-of-care, and increases are seen with hypoxia, hypovolemia, or SIRS. High blood lactate concentrations have been associated with outcome in colic patients. Previous studies have investigated the use of plasma and peripheral lactate values in predicting prognosis in specific gastrointestinal disorders. Peritoneal fluid lactate concentration is a better predictor of a horse having a strangulating lesion than peripheral blood lactate concentration, with a peritoneal lactate concentration of greater than 3.75 mmol/L being 81% sensitive and 92% specific for a strangulating lesion.[9] When looking specifically at horses presenting with LCV, the peripheral blood lactate concentration on admission and after manual correction of the LCV were an accurate predictor of nonsurvival. A horse with a venous lactate of greater than 5 mmol/L after correction of the LCV had 27 times higher odds of dying in the postoperative period than those with blood lactate less than 5 mmol/L (CI 2.1–348; P = .01).[10] Additionally, horses with arterial lactate values of greater than 5 mmol/L in recovery had a 2.25 times greater relative risk to develop postoperative complications, and those with recovery lactate greater than 7 mmol/L had a 10.5 times higher relative risk of death.[11] However, the lactate concentration must be considered alongside the entire clinical picture of the horse. In a study looking at the outcome of horses following colic, a peritoneal lactate value of more than 6 mmol/L was the most accurate predictor of outcome, being correct 73% of the time. Importantly, if the blood lactate concentration is assessed alone, more than one-fourth of all patients would be incorrectly categorized as survivors or nonsurvivors.[12]

Creatinine: Plasma creatinine concentration is useful for evaluating renal perfusion and many horses with colic will present with a high creatinine concentration due to hypovolemia. It is not always possible to evaluate renal function before fluid therapy. Evaluating the plasma creatinine concentration in combination with urine specific gravity and urine output can help to identify horses with renal dysfunction. Additionally, creatinine values that do not decrease to reference ranges following complete restoration of fluid deficits may indicate acute kidney injury. Early assessment of the plasma creatinine concentration is critical to avoid permanent renal insult with commonly used perioperative nephrotoxic drugs such as flunixin meglumine and gentamicin sulfate.

Electrolytes: The most common electrolyte derangements seen in horses presenting with colic are hypocalcemia, hypokalemia, hypomagnesemia, and hypochloremia.[13] Calcium is essential for intestinal motility; therefore, where present, hypocalcemia should be addressed due to its role in ileus, particularly in postsurgical colic cases.[14] Horses with strangulating lesions had significantly lower preoperative serum ionized calcium concentrations than those with nonstrangulating lesions.[15] It is important to note that the ionized calcium is a more accurate measure to assess the severity of hypocalcemia because total calcium is affected by the total protein concentration and acid–base balance. Horses with gastrointestinal disease, and particularly those undergoing colic surgery, may benefit from supplemental calcium as part of fluid therapy; 125 mL of 23% calcium gluconate added to 5L of balance isotonic crystalloids administered at maintenance rates, will aid correction of hypocalcemia. Keep in mind that calcium supplementation in laboratory rats subjected to endotoxemia increases mortality,[16] and calcium supplementation in septic human intensive care unit (ICU) patients has mixed results, demonstrating potential benefits in the most critically ill patients, and possible harmful effects on outcome in those ICU patients with lower morbidity scores.[17]

Hypomagnesemia is frequently seen in horses with gastrointestinal disease and was documented in 50% of horses with obstructive gastrointestinal lesions, compared with approximately 30% of horses with ischemic or inflammatory lesions.[18] Hypomagnesemia has been associated with a poorer outcome, and horses that developed postoperative ileus had significantly lower serum ionized magnesium concentrations following surgical correction of the lesion.[15] Supplemental magnesium can be provided by the addition of 4 g of magnesium sulfate to 5L of balanced isotonic crystalloid fluid, administered at maintenance rates.

Hypokalemia is seen in horses with gastrointestinal dysfunction, especially those with metabolic acidosis. Additionally, hypokalemia has been associated with hypomagnesemia; therefore, horses that are unresponsive to potassium supplementation should have their magnesium status assessed.[19] In severe hypokalemia (<2.0 mEq/L), cardiac changes can occur; however, in mild-to-moderate cases muscle, weakness is the most common clinical sign. Supplemental potassium can be administered at a rate of 100 mEq of potassium chloride in 5L of fluids. Rates should never exceed 0.5 mEq KCl/kg/h.

Acid base status: Acid–base imbalances are an important manifestation of underlying disease. Metabolic acidosis is the primary derangement seen in the colic patient, which is often a result of hyperlactatemia secondary to hypoperfusion or hypoxemia. Hypochloremic metabolic alkalosis can also be observed when large volume gastric reflux is present. Hyperlactatemia can also occur in horses with sepsis in the presence of normal tissue oxygenation because leukocytes produce a large amount of lactate when activated and metabolic derangements may result in cellular and mitochondrial dysfunction, negatively influencing lactate clearance.[20] Correction of the underlying disease process and hypovolemia will also correct acid–base imbalances. Bicarbonate administration in lactic acidosis is generally contraindicated and has been shown to be detrimental in humans and other species, causing increased carbon dioxide production in addition to increasing the pH.[21,22] However, in cases of severe metabolic acidosis with a pH of 7 or less in a volume-resuscitated patient, bicarbonate therapy may be beneficial. This may be most commonly observed in horses and foals with persistent and voluminous diarrhea. The bicarbonate deficit in mEq = base deficit × 0.3 × body weight in kg. The first half of the deficit can be administered over 1 hour, and the remainder during the following 12 to 24 hours, with frequent reassessments to guide therapy.

Glucose: Hyperglycemia is common in horses presenting with colic. At one referral facility, 45% of horses presenting for abdominal pain had values above the reference range.[23] Elevations may be due to a stress response or endotoxemia, and severe hyperglycemia of greater than 195 mg/dL was shown to be associated with a worse prognosis for survival.[23]

Triglycerides: It is important to monitor serum triglyceride concentrations in any horse with reduced feed intake as triglyceride concentrations increase within as little as 48 hours of fasting.[24] Miniature horses, ponies, donkeys, and pregnant or lactating mares, especially those with a high body condition score and SIRS, are at increased risk of developing hyperlipemia. Most postoperative colics exhibit increases in triglycerides up to 300 mg/dL but most will rapidly respond favorably to reintroduction of feed.[25] The clinical signs of hyperlipemia (TG > 500 mg/dL) can be similar to those of the primary gastrointestinal disorder and include anorexia, lethargy, and weakness; when untreated, the disease can progress rapidly in susceptible patients. Early or mild hypertriglyceridemia (100–400 mg/dL) can be managed with oral Karo syrup (60 mL every 4–6 hours) in an adult horse, whereas more severe or prolonged elevations must be managed with intravenous (IV) dextrose and potentially, insulin administration. In these horses, blood glucose should also be closely monitored. It is important to note the relationship of insulin administration and laminitis as exogenous insulin administration has been reliably used as a model for the development of laminitis.[26] Consider concurrent cryotherapy of the limbs if insulin administration is considered. Published guidelines suggest regular insulin be administered as a continuous rate infusion at 0.07 U/kg/h[27] or intermittently IV (0.2 U/kg) q4 to 6 h with frequent monitoring of blood glucose levels.

Current methods for monitoring critical patients with gastrointestinal disease in human medicine:

Basic principles in modern perioperative management of gastrointestinal surgical patients include the following.[28]

- Preoperatively: risk assessment, optimization of physical condition and medication, and routine laboratory assessment of complete blood count, International normalized ratio (a method to assess clotting times), activated partial thromboplastin time, and serum electrolytes and creatinine.
- Intraoperatively: thoracic epidural anesthesia, glucose control, optimized fluid management, and control of hypothermia.
- Postoperatively: opioid-sparing analgesia, early mobilization for the prevention of venous thromboembolism, extended lung expansion exercises, early removal of tubes, catheters and drains, early enteral nutrition and early detection of complications.

Many of the procedures performed in human gastrointestinal surgical patients are less relevant to horses with surgical colic because they have fewer comorbidities. There are, however, areas that are universally applicable including the optimization of the patient before induction (eg, fluid volume support and hypertonic saline), attention to preoperative serum creatinine concentration to optimize antimicrobial choice and avoid nephrotoxicity, advanced analgesia for both recovery and the postoperative period inclusive of local/regional anesthesia, control of hypothermia, diligence with early removal of catheters, monitoring for the development of complications, and early enteral nutrition.

ADVANCES IN FLUID THERAPY

The primary goals of fluid therapy in the critically ill colic patient are to rapidly expand circulating blood volume to restore tissue perfusion and total body water deficits from dehydration. In the most critical surgical colic patients, rapid fluid expansion before general anesthesia at fluid rates of 200 mL/min through a 14-gauge IV catheter may be accomplished. In the past decade, a more critical evaluation of resuscitative fluid therapy practices has ensued, initiated by data acquired in the human medical field. Rapid fluid bolus administration is associated with adverse effects on the microcirculation and the endothelial surface layer (ESL), which contains a structural scaffold called the endothelial glycocalyx. The ESL is the protective barrier that regulates transvascular fluid movement, vasomotor tone, coagulation, and inflammation.[29] Thinning or shedding of this critically important layer through rapid intravascular volume expansion may promote interstitial edema, inflammation, and promote microcirculatory dysfunction.[29] With the size of equine patients and the need for large volumes of fluid to correct deficits, this presents difficulties with respect to preservation of the ESL. A patient-specific, goal-directed approach may be prudent to limit endothelial injury.

The distinction between hypovolemia and dehydration is important because the conditions have different physiologic mechanisms and, therefore, require different approaches to treatment. Hypovolemia is an emergency and describes an acute loss of circulating volume requiring rapid volume expansion. Crystalloid fluid boluses with the addition of hypertonic saline or colloid support are used to restore the intravascular volume. Conversely, dehydration is a loss of total body water without a loss of circulating volume; it can be gradually corrected during 12 to 24 hours with either enteral or IV fluid therapy.

As discussed above, careful monitoring of the PCV and total plasma protein/solids (TS), as well as cardiovascular parameters, is essential to evaluate the effectiveness of fluid therapy in hydrating the horse as well as ensuring adequate cardiovascular support is provided. Horses presenting with reduced intravascular volume and concurrent protein loss often have more severe gastrointestinal disease. Hypoproteinemia, in combination with an elevated PCV, is associated with an increased risk of death in horses with small intestinal surgical lesions.[30]

When developing a fluid therapy plan, it is essential to consider ongoing losses due to the primary gastrointestinal disease in addition to preexisting dehydration and maintenance needs. The methods of fluid therapy differ depending on the underlying lesion.

Enteral Fluid Therapy

Enteral fluids are more effective than IV systemic overhydration for hydrating colonic ingesta. Enterally administered fluids have the additional benefit of stimulating colonic motility through the gastrocolic reflex. Enteral fluid therapy alone was found to resolve 99% of large colon impactions in one case series.[31] Additionally, rapid IV fluid infusions were shown to be less effective than enteral fluids in promoting colonic hydration and were also associated with hemodilution and electrolyte derangement.[32] Continuous flow enteral fluid therapy at 15 mg/kg/h was recently shown to be a safe and effective alternative to IV fluid therapy for the treatment of dehydrated horses. Continuous rate enteral fluids successfully corrected electrolyte and acid–base imbalanced caused by dehydration.[33]

Aggressive fluid therapy consisting of frequent administration of 8 to 10L of water, in horses with preexisting gastric or colon impactions, was thought to potentially predispose 4 horses to LCV in one case series.[34] Studies support the administration of 5 to 8L of isotonic enteral fluids every 1 to 2 hours for horses with nonstrangulating large colon.[31,35,36] Enteral fluid therapy is contraindicated for horses with gastric distention and reflux on nasogastric intubation, and in some cases enteral fluid therapy may not be tolerated due to extensive large colon distention. Care must be taken with long-term enteral fluid administration if water is used without the addition of electrolytes as sodium depletion can occur.

Fluid Therapy Administered per Rectum

Tap water administered per rectum has been shown to be a safe and well-tolerated alternative, or adjunct, to enteral fluid or intravascular fluid therapy, providing comparable hemodilution to isotonic enteral fluids at a rate of 5 mL/kg/h[37] This represents an inexpensive alternative in cases with economic constraints. More research is needed to assess its effects on intestinal motility, colonic content hydration, and systemic electrolyte balance.

Correction of Hypovolemia

In horses presenting with severe gastrointestinal disease and hypovolemia, emergency restoration of the circulating volume is required. These horses often have a strangulating obstruction requiring surgical correction; therefore, cardiovascular stabilization before anesthesia is critical. Intravascular fluid expansion can be provided by the administration of 2 to 6 mL/kg of hypertonic saline, which increases intravascular volume by drawing water from the intracellular and interstitial compartments. Hypertonic saline increases the circulating volume by between 4 and 5 times the volume administered; however, this effect only lasts approximately 60 minutes. Subsequent large-volume isotonic fluid administration (10 L of crystalloid fluids per 1 L of 7.2% hypertonic saline administered) is needed to restore fluid to all vascular compartments. This approach may reduce the need for a high rate of fluid administration (eg, 200 mL/min) in the hypovolemic patient, with the goal of preserving the ESL and reducing endothelial injury. Synthetic colloids may be indicated to maintain plasma oncotic pressures in horses losing protein, and when used in combination with hypertonic saline in endotoxic horses, it was shown to offer some protection against endotoxin-mediated hypocalcemia.[38] Although the use of synthetic colloids has been controversial in human and small animal critical care medicine, there is little evidence that colloid use in horses has a negative impact on survival.

Replacement of Ongoing Losses

In horses presenting with abdominal disease, the most common ongoing fluid losses are gastric reflux or diarrhea. It is important that the fluid administration rate is adjusted to account for the volume lost, which can be recorded in horses with nasogastric reflux but must be estimated when direct measurement is not possible. It is, therefore, important to regularly evaluate the effectiveness of fluid therapy using the clinical parameters mentioned previously. A goal-directed approach may be prudent to avoid complications associated with fluid overload and edema formation.

Maintenance Requirements

Maintenance fluid requirements in healthy horses are 2 mL/kg/h; however, it has recently been shown that the fluid requirements of horses with restricted feed intake are reduced to approximately 16% of normal fed values.[39] Horses with abdominal disease normally have a period of restricted feed intake, and so may require lower IV fluid rates. This is particularly important in surgical cases that are at increased risk of developing postoperative ileus, gastric dilation, and reflux. There are currently no recommended fluid requirements for these cases; however, goal-directed fluid therapy using clinical parameters such as heart rate, PCV, TS, and blood lactate to discontinue fluid administration earlier may result in reduced expenses to the client and perhaps shorten the period of hospitalization.[40] In addition, electrolyte supplementation is required either in horses receiving long-term fluid support or in those with electrolyte derangements at presentation.

ADVANCES IN NUTRITION MANAGEMENT

Recent research suggests that early feeding may be associated with a shorter recovery period in horses undergoing exploratory laparotomy.[41] Feeding induces motility due to stimulation of the gastrocolic reflex and may reduce ileus.[42] Feeding horses with gastric dilation and reflux on nasogastric intubation is contraindicated; however, sham feeding with an apple-flavored bit shortened the gastrointestinal total transit time and augmented motility.[43]

In human surgical patients, supplementation with the amino acid, glutamine, has been shown to be associated with reduced infection rates and shorter hospital stays,[44] and limited study in horses suggests a positive effect on reducing mucosal permeability in a model of ischemic and reperfused large colon.[45] Glutamine plays a central role in nitrogen transport within the body, is a fuel for rapidly dividing cells such as in the gut and immune system, and has many other essential metabolic functions.[44]

There are few studies specifically looking at nutrition in horses; however, in humans, early enteral nutrition may enhance wound healing and increase anastomotic strength in addition to reducing the incidence of postoperative complications.[46] Several biochemical indicators of starvation including increases in triglycerides, total bilirubin, albumin, and urea were found in horses withheld from feed following small intestinal resection and anastomosis compared with horses receiving parental nutrition.[47] This state of negative energy balance could have detrimental effects on wound healing and increase the risk of complications. Additionally, there is little evidence assessing the ideal postoperative feeding protocol to aid restoration of a normal colonic microbiome and colon function.

Adult horses with a preexisting compromised nutritional state that require a period of starvation may need earlier nutritional supplementation in the form of IV dextrose or partial parenteral nutrition consisting of dextrose, amino acids, B-vitamins and electrolytes. Early nutritional intervention may also be required in obese horses, pregnant mares, and donkeys, due to concerns of hyperlipidemia following short periods of negative energy balance. Plasma triglyceride concentrations should be closely monitored in these cases, and the addition of lipid to parenteral nutrition is typically contraindicated due to the high prevalence of hyperlipidemia in critically ill patients who are not consuming enteral nutrition. A negative energy balance has been shown to compromise the immune system and wound healing, as well as being a cause of muscle mass loss. Therefore, it is important to accurately calculate the caloric needs of the patient to ensure they are being met. Nutritional needs for the critically ill horse have not been established but basal energy requirements of a horse on stall rest is estimated to be between 20 and 24 kcal/kg BW/d. The authors employ early supplementation of 1.25% to 2.5% dextrose in isotonic fluids (if not hyperglycemic) or Karo Syrup (see above) in patients intended to be feed restricted for 24 hours or more, although this only meets between 10% and 30% of basal energy requirements depending on the percentage dextrose (3.4 kcal/gm) and rate of fluid administration. In hyperglycemic patients with concurrent hyperlipidemia, insulin supplementation may be considered, although administration of high concentrations of exogenous insulin is a reliable model for laminitis[26] and, therefore, used infrequently by the authors, and used in combination with limb cryotherapy.

PHARMACOTHERAPEUTICS
Analgesics and Recognition of Pain

Analgesia is a critical component of management for medically managed and postoperative colic patients. Pain, in addition to negatively influencing the welfare of the horse, causes a stress response resulting in the stimulation of the neuroendocrine system leading to alterations in hormone release, a reduction in the horse's feed intake and reduction in gastrointestinal motility.

Assessment of pain, along with defining its origin, is the first and most important step in determining the appropriateness of analgesia. In addition to overt colic signs such as pawing, rolling, circling, kicking the abdomen and sweating, more subtle signs of pain manifest as reduced activity, reduced engagement when approached, and inappetence. The Equine Acute Abdominal Pain Score is the only pain score that has been tested within the referral hospital setting, and has found to be feasible and reliable in practice.[48]

The most commonly used analgesics in colic patients include nonsteroidal anti-inflammatory drugs (NSAIDs), opioids, the alpha-2 agonists, and lidocaine. **Table 1** provides a list of the currently available analgesic agents suitable for management of visceral or postoperative pain in colic patients. Please refer to article on "Basic post-operative care" for a summary of the more commonly used analgesic drugs including NSAIDs and lidocaine.

Opioid Analgesics: Opioids bind to the mu, kappa, or delta receptors in the spinal cord and brain, producing analgesia. When used alone, opioids can cause central nervous system excitation and dysphoria, and so they are often administered in combination with an alpha-2-adrenoceptor agonists. Opioids are potent depressors of the respiratory system, with minimal effects on cardiovascular function. They also have detrimental effects on motility.

Morphine is a potent analgesic; however, its use in horses with colic is largely contraindicated. It has been shown to reduce the number of contractions in the duodenum, caecum, left and right ventral colons, and increase locomotor activity. The size of the stomach was increased significantly with a cumulative effect after repeated doses.[49] Morphine is commonly used in the epidural space, often in combination with alpha-2 agonists but its utility in colic patients is limited, perhaps with the exception of some distal colorectal surgical procedures (eg, colostomy). A similarly acting pure μ-opioid receptor agonist, hydromorphone, has shown promise for pain control[50] in horses with fewer locomotor activity side effects at single doses of (0.025 and 0.05 mg/kg IV),[51] but further work on pharmacokinetics of multidosing, visceral analgesia, and impact on motility is indicated before advocating its use in the critical colic patient.

Butorphanol is a partial μ-opioid receptor agonist and is 7 times more potent than morphine. It is often used in combination with an alpha-2-agonist at a dose of 0.01 to 0.05 mg/kg intravenously for sedation, and 0.1 mg/kg for analgesia. Butorphanol has the fewest side effects when compared with the other opioids; however, it has been shown to delay gastric emptying and gastrointestinal transit time.[52,53] Due to the short duration of action for analgesia (30–60 minutes), a constant rate effusion (CRI) is recommended. A CRI of 13 μg/kg/h in the immediate postoperative period, when compared with a bolus of 0.13 mg/kg, had less effect on gastrointestinal motility.[54] Additionally, horses receiving a butorphanol CRI in the immediate postoperative period had a lower plasma cortisol level, lost less weight during hospitalization, and had a shorter time to hospital discharge when compared with controls. It was also found that horses receiving the butorphanol CRI were significantly delayed in their median time to first defecation.[54]

Alpha-2 adrenoreceptor agonists: These drugs have both central and peripheral mechanisms of producing dose-dependent sedation, as well as being effective analgesics in horses with colic. A side effect is reduced motility for the duration of sedation.

Xylazine has a recommended dose of 0.2 to 1.1 mg/kg intravenously. Although xylazine provides very effective visceral analgesia, similar to that of flunixin meglumine and opioids, the cardiovascular side effects including bradycardia, decreased cardiac output, and sustained hypotension, makes the use of xylazine challenging with horses in shock, although an initial bout of hypertension precedes its depressant effects.[55]

Table 1
Doses and mechanisms of action of commonly used analgesic medications for the management of visceral pain in horses

Drug	Dosage	Mechanism of Action
Xylazine	0.25–1.0 mg/kg IV PRN	α-2 agonist
Butorphanol	0.01–0.02 mg/kg IV or IM PRN or 13 μg/kg/h IV	Opioid agonist-antagonist
Detomidine	0.01–0.02 mg/kg IV or IM	α-2 agonist
Flunixin Meglumine	0.25–1.0 mg/kg IV q8–12 h	NSAID—nonspecific COX inhibitor
Firocoxib	0.3 mg/kg (loading), then 0.1 mg/kg PO q24 h	NSAID—COX-1 sparing
Meloxicam	0.6 mg/kg IV q24 h	NSAID—COX-1 sparing
Lidocaine	50 μg/kg/min IV	Anti-inflammatory, analgesic, sympathoadrenal inhibition
Romifidine	0.04 mg/kg IV	α-2 agonist

Other side effects include ileus and reduced intestinal blood flow, which can be prolonged, lasting beyond the period of analgesia and sedation.

Detomidine has a recommended dose of 4 to 20 μg/kg intravenously. The duration of effect is longer than that of xylazine, between 60 and 120 minutes. If the horse becomes painful within 1 hour of administering detomidine, it may be an indication that a more severe lesion is present, potentially requiring surgical correction or relaparotomy in the case of a horse with postoperative colic.

Prokinetic Medications

There is an abundance of prokinetic medications that have been studied for use in horses but the availability of these medications is variable. The 3 most commonly used agents beyond lidocaine will be described with a more comprehensive list, including recommended dosages and targeted regions to enhance motility available in **Table 2**.

Metoclopramide is the second most commonly used promotility agent following lidocaine.[56] It increases motility through agonistic action on serotonin receptors, increasing the cholinergic transmission in the enteric nervous system.[57] Metoclopramide may also be an antagonist of dopamine receptors, preventing the inhibitory effects of dopamine on intestinal smooth muscle.[58] In healthy horses, metoclopramide improves cecal and colonic contractions, with a longer duration of action and less side effects than neostigmine.[59] Metoclopramide increases smooth muscle contractility at the pyloric antrum, duodenum, and jejunum.[60] Metoclopramide can be administered at 0.5 mg/kg subcutaneously every 3 hours, or as a CRI at 0.04 mg/kg/h. Extrapyramidal side effects observed with CRI administration include excitement, restlessness, and abdominal pain. Adverse extrapyramidal side effects following subcutaneous administration of 0.25 mg/kg metoclopramide at 6-hour intervals have also been reported.[61]

Bethanechol hydrochloride is a muscarinic cholinergic agonist that causes smooth muscle contraction within the gastrointestinal tract via stimulation of the acetylcholine receptors. There is evidence that bethanechol produces a concentration-dependent increase in circular muscle of the intestine, most notable within the jejunum[62] in addition to increasing the rate of gastric emptying.[63] The recommended dose is 0.025 mg/kg IV or SQ q4 to 6 h. It is most readily available as an oral formulation but its use would be limited in actively refluxing horses.

Erythromycin is a macrolide antimicrobial, with side effects involving the gastrointestinal tract through motilin receptor agonist activity. A single dose of erythromycin was found to increase the contractility of longitudinal smooth muscle but decrease contractility of circular smooth muscle in vitro, with an overall improvement of jejunal motility.[60] Erythromycin also altered the myoelectric activity of the ileum, cecum, and pelvic flexure in clinically normal ponies; however, the same effect was not appreciated in the postoperative patient.[64] This highlights the different effect of prokinetic agents in normal horses and those with gastrointestinal dysfunction. Erythromycin is administered at a subtherapeutic dose for antimicrobial use of 0.5 to 1.0 mg/kg administered in saline over 60 minutes, every 6 hours. The beneficial effects of erythromycin diminish with repeated use as the drug can downregulate the motilin receptors. Notably, there have been reports of severe colitis associated with usage.

Therapeutics Targeting Systemic Inflammatory Response Syndrome and Endotoxemia

SIRS is often present in the critical colic with intestinal wall compromise and is associated with prolongation of prothrombin time (PT), activated partial thromboplastin time (aPTT) and disseminated intravascular coagulation, all of which are associated

Table 2
Prokinetic agents, recommended dosages, and most common clinical uses

Drug	Dosage	Clinical Applications in Order of Common Use
Lidocaine	1.3 mg/kg IV bolus, then 0.05 mg/kg/min IV as a CRI	Adjunct to anesthesia = general pain = small intestinal ileus > large colon inflammation
Metoclopramide	CRI at 0.01–0.05 mg/kg/h; 0.25 mg/kg SQ; 0.04 mg/kg SQ q3 (author protocol)	Gastric emptying = small intestinal ileus > cecum/large colon
Erythromycin	1.0 mg/kg in 1 L saline over 1 h q6h	Small intestine > cecum/large colon
Cisapride	0.1 mg/kg IM or IV q8h (compounding required due to poor oral bioavailability)	All parts of GI tract
Neostigmine	0.0044–0.022 mg/kg IM or SQ q20–60 min	Cecum/large colon > small intestine
Bethanechol	0.025 mg/kg IV or SQ q4–6h	Gastric emptying = small intestine
Domperidone	5 mg/kg PO	Stomach, jejunum, ileum, colon

with nonsurvival in horses with acute gastrointestinal disease.[65] Increased mucosal permeability during gastrointestinal obstruction leads to the absorption of bacterial toxins including endotoxin, causing a dysregulated host systemic inflammatory response to infection.[66] The treatment of SIRS or endotoxemia largely involves treatment of the secondary inflammatory response. There are a handful of therapeutic interventions with evidence supporting their use. The importance of fluid therapy to provide cardiovascular support should not be overlooked.

NSAIDs may be of benefit once the inflammatory cascade has been initiated. They act by inhibiting the enzyme cyclooxygenase (COX), thus preventing the production of prostaglandins from the arachidonic acid pathway.[67] Prostanoids are important mediators of shock as thromboxane A2 has potent aggregatory and vasoconstrictive effects[68]; therefore, inhibiting this pathway may reduce the clinical signs of endotoxemia. A recent randomized clinical trial demonstrated equivocal effects of firocoxib and flunixin on postoperative pain following small intestinal strangulating obstruction along with more effective reduction of a common biomarker of endotoxemia (sCD14) along with a trend toward reduction in mortality in horses treated with firocoxib versus flunixin meglumine.[69]

Polymyxin B binds to the lipid-A portion of lipopolysaccharide (LPS), also called endotoxin, aiding in the removal of endotoxin from the circulation, as evidenced by a reduction in the endotoxin-induced tumor necrosis factor alpha (TNF-α) activity.[70] Treatment with polymyxin B in endotoxic horses significantly reduced fever, tachycardia, and serum TNF-α activity when compared with those receiving saline.[71] In foals challenged with LPS, those treated with polymyxin B had significantly lower blood lactate concentration, serum TNF-α, and plasma thromboxane B2.[72] The recommended dose of 6000 IU/kg given in 1 L of saline IV every 8 hours was shown to be safe for the treatment of endotoxemia with no side effects noted.[73] Polymyxin B has known side effects including severe nephrotoxicity and neurotoxicity, limiting its use in human medicine. Although many studies investigating the effect of polymyxin B in endotoxic horses have not identified any detrimental side effects, a recent study demonstrated that administration of polymyxin B at the recommended dose to healthy horses caused transient ataxia, worsening with cumulative doses.[74] Nephrotoxicity was appreciated when polymyxin B was administered with gentamicin in healthy horses.[74] Additionally, polymyxin B has been shown to have little benefit in the prevention of sepsis-related laminitis.[75] The use of antimicrobial agents such as polymyxin B at subtherapeutic dosages for nonantimicrobial purposes is undesirable from an antimicrobial stewardship perspective.

Di-tri-octahedral (DTO) smectite (Biosponge, Platinum Performance, Los Olivos, CA, USA) is an adsorbent used in the treatment of diarrhea. Horses treated with DTO smectite had a significant reduction in postoperative diarrhea following abdominal surgery when compared with untreated controls.[76] DTO smectite (Biosponge) effectively adsorbed *Clostridium perfringens* exotoxins and had a dose-dependent effect on the availability of equine colostral antibodies in foals, so the use of Biosponge should be avoided in neonates younger than 24 hours of age.[77] Biosponge can be easily administered directly into the colon via an enterotomy during surgery, reducing the risk of postoperative diarrhea and may aid in the prevention of endotoxemia postoperatively. The authors recommend administering 1 lb of DTO smectite in 1 L of water into the right ventral colon via pelvic flexure enterotomy followed by 1 to 2 lbs via nasogastric tube daily in patients at risk for SIRS or postoperative fever such as horses with LCV and surgically managed sand and feed impactions.

Pentoxifylline is a methylxanthine derivative that has both anti-inflammatory and rheologic properties. The anti-inflammatory effects are brought about predominantly by the downregulation of proinflammatory cytokine production and inhibition of phosphodiesterase.[78] In a model of endotoxemia, the administration of pentoxifylline was shown to reduce the plasma activity of matrix metalloproteinase 2 and 9.[79] An additional benefit of pentoxifylline is its ability to induce vasodilation of equine digital veins, which may have a vasculoprotective effect in laminitic horses.[80] The current recommended oral dosage for pentoxifylline in horses is 10 mg/kg every 12 hours.

Management of the Hypercoagulable State

As coagulopathies occur commonly in postoperative horses with strangulating gastrointestinal obstruction, a brief discussion of therapeutic agents to combat thrombosis is relevant. Clopidogrel (2 mg/kg PO q24 h) has been shown to be superior to a low dose of aspirin (5 mg/kg) on ADP-induced platelet aggregation and may have therapeutic potential.[81] A loading dose (6–6.5 mg/kg) followed by 1.2 to 1.4 mg/kg per os q24 h has been shown to provide a rapid onset and sustain platelet inhibition.[82] Heparin therapy is generally considered an effective and safe treatment of the hypercoagulable state in horses[83] but unfractioned heparin (40 IU/kg q12 h SQ) has side effects including anemia and prolongation of clotting times.[84,85] Low molecular weight heparin (LMWH) has fewer reported side effects and is more effective than unfractioned heparin, with limited impact on clotting times.[85] Recommended dosages for Dalteparin (Kabi Pharmacia AB, Stockholm, Sweden) and Enoxaparin (Sanofi-Aventis US, Bridgewater, NJ) are 50 IU/kg subcutaneously every 24 hours and 0.5 mg/kg subcutaneously every 24 hours, respectively.[83] An added reported benefit of LMWH is prophylaxis for laminitis prevention.[86] The use of hyperimmune or J5 plasma may have benefits in the management of endotoxemia.

SUMMARY

Advances in monitoring and treatment have improved outcomes of critically ill horses with signs of colic. Some evidence-based practices have failed to become mainstream in management of these cases but larger, multicenter studies will help to consolidate the efficacy of both new and old treatments that may prove to be superior to current methods commonly in use. With data derived from human medicine and veterinary research, we can strive to optimize outcomes of our critically ill colic patients. An early and aggressive multimodal approach to monitoring, pain control, and treatment may help to reduce the risk of complications and improve outcomes.

CLINICS CARE POINTS

- Vigilance in the early detection and treatment of pain, fluid deficits, coagulopathies and motility disturbances is critical to reduce morbidity in the post-operative colic patient.

- There is little evidence of efficacy of prokinetic medications for treatment of ileus in adult equine clinical patients with gastrointestinal disease, so a focus on prevention is prudent. Early detection and proactive treatment prior to development of ileus may be a more effective approach.

- Routine assessment of select point of care parameters in the immediate post-operative period such as lactate, creatinine and electrolytes may help guide early therapy to optimize outcomes.

DISCLOSURES

None.

FUNDING SOURCES

Dr C. Barton: None, Dr D.M. Hassel: None.

CONFLICT OF INTEREST

The authors declare no competing interests.

REFERENCES

1. Sheats MK, Cook VL, Jones SL, et al. Use of ultrasound to evaluate outcome following colic surgery for equine large colon volvulus. Equine Vet J 2010;42: 47–52.
2. Jacobsen S, Anderson PH. The acute phase protein serum amyloid A (SAA) as a marker of inflammation in horses. Equine Vet Educ 2007;19:38–46.
3. Vandenplas ML, Moore JN, Barton MH, et al. Concentrations of serum amyloid A and lipopolysaccharide-binding protein in horses with colic. Am J Vet Res 2005; 66:1509–16.
4. Pihl TH, Scheepers E, Sanz M, et al. Acute-phase proteins as diagnostic markers in horses with colic. J Vet Emerg Crit Care 2016;26:664–74.
5. Bowlby C, Mudge M, Schroeder E, et al. Equine inflammatory response to abdominal surgery in the absence of gastrointestinal disease. J Vet Emerg Crit Care 2021;31:601–7.
6. De Cozar M, Sherlock C, Knowles E, et al. Serum amyloid A and plasma fibrinogen concentrations in horses following emergency exploratory celiotomy. Equine Vet J 2020;52:59–66.
7. Daniel AJ, Leise BS, Burgess BA, et al. Concentrations of serum amyloid A and plasma fibrinogen in horses undergoing emergency abdominal surgery. J Vet Emerg Crit Care 2016;26:344–51.
8. Seltana A, Cloutier G, Reyes Nicolas V, et al. Fibrin(ogen) Is Constitutively Expressed by Differentiated Intestinal Epithelial Cells and Mediates Wound Healing. Front Immunol 2022;13:916187.
9. Kilcoyne I, Nieto JE, Dechant JE. Predictive value of plasma and peritoneal creatine kinase in horses with strangulating intestinal lesions. Vet Surg 2019;48: 152–8.
10. Orr KE, Baker WT, Lynch TM, et al. Prognostic value of colonic and peripheral venous lactate measurements in horses with large colon volvulus. Vet Surg 2020;49:472–9.
11. McCoy AM, Hackett ES, Wagner AE, et al. Pulmonary gas exchange and plasma lactate in horses with gastrointestinal disease undergoing emergency exploratory laparotomy: a comparison with an elective surgery horse population. Vet Surg 2011;40:601–9.
12. Bishop RC, Gutierrez-Nibeyro SD, Stewart MC, et al. Performance of predictive models of survival in horses undergoing emergency exploratory laparotomy for colic. Vet Surg 2022;51:891–902.
13. Hesselkilde EZ, Almind ME, Petersen J, et al. Cardiac arrhythmias and electrolyte disturbances in colic horses. Acta Vet Scand 2014;56:58.
14. Toribio RE. Disorders of calcium and phosphate metabolism in horses. Vet Clin North Am Equine Pract 2011;27:129–47.
15. Garcia-Lopez JM, Provost PJ, Rush JE, et al. Prevalence and prognostic importance of hypomagnesemia and hypocalcemia in horses that have colic surgery. Am J Vet Res 2001;62:7–12.

16. Malcolm DS, Zaloga GP, Holaday JW. Calcium administration increases the mortality of endotoxic shock in rats. Crit Care Med 1989;17:900–3.

17. He W, Huang L, Luo H, et al. The Positive and Negative Effects of Calcium Supplementation on Mortality in Septic ICU Patients Depend on Disease Severity: A Retrospective Study from the MIMIC-III. Crit Care Res Pract 2022;2520695.

18. Sanmarti J, Armengou L, Troya-Portillo L, et al. Plasma-Ionized Magnesium in Hospitalized Horses with Gastrointestinal Disorders and Systemic Inflammatory Response Syndrome. Animals (Basel) 2022;12.

19. Stewart AJ. Magnesium disorders in horses. Vet Clin North Am Equine Pract 2011;27:149–63.

20. Vernon C, Letourneau JL. Lactic acidosis: recognition, kinetics, and associated prognosis. Crit Care Clin 2010;26:255–83, table of contents.

21. Boyd JH, Walley KR. Is there a role for sodium bicarbonate in treating lactic acidosis from shock? Curr Opin Crit Care 2008;14:379–83.

22. Rachoin JS, Weisberg LS, McFadden CB. Treatment of lactic acidosis: appropriate confusion. J Hosp Med 2010;5:E1–7.

23. Hassel DM, Hill AE, Rorabeck RA. Association between hyperglycemia and survival in 228 horses with acute gastrointestinal disease. J Vet Intern Med 2009;23: 1261–5.

24. Filippo PAD, Duarte BR, Albernaz AP, et al. Effects of feed deprivation on physical and blood parameters of horses. Rev Bras Med Vet 2021;22:e000321.

25. Underwood C, Southwood LL, Walton RM, et al. Hepatic and metabolic changes in surgical colic patients: a pilot study. J Vet Emerg Crit Care 2010;20:578–86.

26. de Laat MA, McGowan CM, Sillence MN, et al. Equine laminitis: induced by 48 h hyperinsulinaemia in Standardbred horses. Equine Vet J 2010;42:129–35.

27. Han JH, McKenzie HC, McCutcheon LJ, et al. Glucose and insulin dynamics associated with continuous rate infusion of dextrose solution or dextrose solution and insulin in healthy and endotoxin-exposed horses. Am J Vet Res 2011;72: 522–9.

28. Grade M, Quintel M, Ghadimi BM. Standard perioperative management in gastrointestinal surgery. Langenbeck's Arch Surg 2011;396:591–606.

29. Smart L, Hughes D. The effects of resuscitative fluid therapy on the endothelial surface layer. Front Vet Sci 2021;8.

30. Proudman CJ, Edwards GB, Barnes J, et al. Factors affecting long-term survival of horses recovering from surgery of the small intestine. Equine Vet J 2005;37: 360–5.

31. Monreal L, Navarro M, Armengou L, et al. Enteral fluid therapy in 108 horses with large colon impactions and dorsal displacements. Vet Rec 2010;166:259–63.

32. Lopes MA, Walker BL, White NA 2nd, et al. Treatments to promote colonic hydration: enteral fluid therapy versus intravenous fluid therapy and magnesium sulphate. Equine Vet J 2002;34:505–9.

33. Dias DCR, Filho JDR, Viana RB, et al. Comparative Trial of Continuous Flow Enteral and Intravenous Fluid Therapy in Horses. Front Vet Sci 2021;6.

34. Gessica G, Anna C, Marco G. Gastric and large colon impactions combined with aggressive enteral fluid therapy may predispose to large colon volvulus: 4 cases. J Equine Vet Sci 2021;102.

35. Hallowell GD. Retrospective study assessing efficacy of treatment of large colonic impactions. Equine Vet J 2008;40:411–3.

36. Lester GD, Merritt AM, Kuck HV, et al. Systemic, renal, and colonic effects of intravenous and enteral rehydration in horses. J Vet Intern Med 2013;27:554–66.

37. Khan A, Hallowell GD, Underwood C, et al. Continuous fluid infusion per rectum compared with intravenous and nasogastric fluid administration in horses. Equine Vet J 2019;51:767–73.
38. Pantaleon LG, Furr MO, McKenzie HC, et al. Effects of small- and large-volume resuscitation on coagulation and electrolytes during experimental endotoxemia in anesthetized horses. J Vet Intern Med 2007;21:1374–9.
39. Freeman DE. Effect of Feed Intake on Water Consumption in Horses: Relevance to Maintenance Fluid Therapy. Front Vet Sci 2021;8:626081.
40. Giusto G, Vercelli C, Gandini M. Comparison of liberal and goal-directed fluid therapy after small intestinal surgery for strangulating lesions in horses. Vet Rec 2021;188(e5).
41. Valle E, Giusto G, Penazzi L, et al. Preliminary results on the association with feeding and recovery length in equine colic patients after laparotomy. J Anim Physiol Anim Nutr 2019;103:1233–41.
42. Hellstrom EA, Ziegler AL, Blikslager AT. Postoperative Ileus: Comparative Pathophysiology and Future Therapies. Front Vet Sci 2021;8:714800.
43. Patton ME, Leise BS, Baker RE, et al. The effects of bit chewing on borborygmi, duodenal motility, and gastrointestinal transit time in clinically normal horses. Vet Surg 2022;51:88–96.
44. Novak F, Heyland DK, Avenell A, et al. Glutamine supplementation in serious illness: a systematic review of the evidence. Crit Care Med 2002;30:2022–9.
45. Rotting AK, Freeman DE, Constable PD, et al. Effects of phenylbutazone, indomethacin, prostaglandin E2, butyrate, and glutamine on restitution of oxidant-injured right dorsal colon of horses in vitro. Am J Vet Res 2004;65:1589–95.
46. Silk DB, Gow NM. Postoperative starvation after gastrointestinal surgery. Early feeding is beneficial. BMJ 2001;323:761–2.
47. Durham AE, Phillips TJ, Walmsley JP, et al. Nutritional and clinicopathological effects of post operative parenteral nutrition following small intestinal resection and anastomosis in the mature horse. Equine Vet J 2004;36:390–6.
48. Maskato Y, Dugdale AHA, Singer ER, et al. Prospective Feasibility and Revalidation of the Equine Acute Abdominal Pain Scale (EAAPS) in Clinical Cases of Colic in Horses. Animals (Basel) 2020;10.
49. Tessier C, Pitaud JP, Thorin C, et al. Systemic morphine administration causes gastric distention and hyperphagia in healthy horses. Equine Vet J 2019;51:653–7.
50. Reed R, Barletta M, Mitchell K, et al. The pharmacokinetics and pharmacodynamics of intravenous hydromorphone in horses. Vet Anaesth Analg 2019;46:395–404.
51. Reed RA, Knych HK, Barletta M, et al. Pharmacokinetics and pharmacodynamics of hydromorphone after intravenous and intramuscular administration in horses. Vet Anaesth Analg 2020;47:210–8.
52. Merritt AM, Burrow JA, Hartless CS. Effect of xylazine, detomidine, and a combination of xylazine and butorphanol on equine duodenal motility. Am J Vet Res 1998;59:619–23.
53. Sutton DG, Preston T, Christley RM, et al. The effects of xylazine, detomidine, acepromazine and butorphanol on equine solid phase gastric emptying rate. Equine Vet J 2002;34:486–92.
54. Sellon DC, Roberts MC, Blikslager AT, et al. Effects of continuous rate intravenous infusion of butorphanol on physiologic and outcome variables in horses after celiotomy. J Vet Intern Med 2004;18:555–63.

55. Morton AJ, Varney CR, Ekiri AB, et al. Cardiovascular effects of N-butylscopolammonium bromide and xylazine in horses. Equine Vet J 2011;Suppl:117–22.
56. Lefebvre D, Hudson NP, Elce YA, et al. Clinical features and management of equine post operative ileus (POI): Survey of Diplomates of the American Colleges of Veterinary Internal Medicine (ACVIM), Veterinary Surgeons (ACVS) and Veterinary Emergency and Critical Care (ACVECC). Equine Vet J 2016;48:714–9.
57. Doherty TJ, Frazier DL. Effect of intravenous lidocaine on halothane minimum alveolar concentration in ponies. Equine Vet J 1998;30:300–3.
58. Tonini M, De Ponti F, Di Nucci A, et al. Review article: cardiac adverse effects of gastrointestinal prokinetics. Aliment Pharmacol Ther 1999;13:1585–91.
59. Beder NA, Mourad AA, Aly MA. Ultrasonographic evaluation of the effects of the administration of neostigmine and metoclopramide on duodenal, cecal, and colonic contractility in Arabian horses: A comparative study. Vet World 2020;13:2447–51.
60. Nieto JE, Rakestraw PC, Snyder JR, et al. In vitro effects of erythromycin, lidocaine, and metoclopramide on smooth muscle from the pyloric antrum, proximal portion of the duodenum, and middle portion of the jejunum of horses. Am J Vet Res 2000;61:413–9.
61. Agass RF, Brennan M, Rendle DI. Extrapyramidal side effects following subcutaneous metoclopramide injection for the treatment of post operative ileus. Equine Vet Educ 2017;29:564–8.
62. Marti M, Mevissen M, Althaus H, et al. In vitro effects of bethanechol on equine gastrointestinal contractility and functional characterization of involved muscarinic receptor subtypes. J Vet Pharmacol Ther 2005;28:565–74.
63. Ringger NC, Lester GD, Neuwirth L, et al. Effect of bethanechol or erythromycin on gastric emptying in horses. Am J Vet Res 1996;57:1771–5.
64. Roussel AJ, Hooper RN, Cohen ND, et al. Prokinetic effects of erythromycin on the ileum, cecum, and pelvic flexure of horses during the postoperative period. Am J Vet Res 2000;61:420–4.
65. Epstein KL, Brainard BM, Gomez-Ibanez SE, et al. Thrombelastography in horses with acute gastrointestinal disease. J Vet Intern Med 2011;25:307–14.
66. Sheats MK. A Comparative Review of Equine SIRS, Sepsis, and Neutrophils. Front Vet Sci 2019;6(69).
67. Marshall JF, Blikslager AT. The effect of nonsteroidal anti-inflammatory drugs on the equine intestine. Equine Vet J 2011;Suppl:140–4.
68. Wise WC, Cook JA, Halushka PV. Implications for thromboxane A2 in the pathogenesis of endotoxic shock. Adv Shock Res 1981;6:83–91.
69. Ziegler AL, Freeman CK, Fogle CA, et al. Multicentre, blinded, randomised clinical trial comparing the use of flunixin meglumine with firocoxib in horses with small intestinal strangulating obstruction. Equine Vet J 2019;51:329–35.
70. Parviainen AK, Barton MH, Norton NN. Evaluation of polymyxin B in an ex vivo model of endotoxemia in horses. Am J Vet Res 2001;62:72–6.
71. Barton MH, Parviainen A, Norton N. Polymyxin B protects horses against induced endotoxaemia in vivo. Equine Vet J 2004;36:397–401.
72. Wong DM, Sponseller BA, Alcott CJ, et al. Effects of intravenous administration of polymyxin B in neonatal foals with experimental endotoxemia. J Am Vet Med Assoc 2013;243:874–81.
73. Morresey PR, Mackay RJ. Endotoxin-neutralizing activity of polymyxin B in blood after IV administration in horses. Am J Vet Res 2006;67:642–7.
74. van Spijk JN, Beckmann K, Wehrli Eser M, et al. Adverse effects of polymyxin B administration to healthy horses. J Vet Intern Med 2022;36:1525–34.

75. Raisbeck MF, Garner HE, Osweiler GD. Effects of polymyxin B on selected features of equine carbohydrate overload. Vet Hum Toxicol 1989;31:422–6.

76. Hassel DM, Smith PA, Nieto JE, et al. Di-tri-octahedral smectite for the prevention of post-operative diarrhea in equids with surgical disease of the large intestine: results of a randomized clinical trial. Vet J 2009;182:210–4.

77. Lawler JB, Hassel DM, Magnuson RJ, et al. Adsorptive effects of di-tri-octahedral smectite on Clostridium perfringens alpha, beta, and beta-2 exotoxins and equine colostral antibodies. Am J Vet Res 2008;69:233–9.

78. Coimbra R, Loomis W, Melbostad H, et al. Role of hypertonic saline and pentoxifylline on neutrophil activation and tumor necrosis factor-alpha synthesis: a novel resuscitation strategy. J Trauma 2005;59:257–64 [discussion: 264-255].

79. Fugler LA, Eades SC, Moore RM, et al. Plasma matrix metalloproteinase activity in horses after intravenous infusion of lipopolysaccharide and treatment with matrix metalloproteinase inhibitors. Am J Vet Res 2013;74:473–80.

80. Kabbesh N, Gogny M, Chatagnon G, et al. Vasodilatory effect of pentoxifylline in isolated equine digital veins. Vet J 2012;192:368–73.

81. Brainard BM, Epstein KL, LoBato D, et al. Effects of clopidogrel and aspirin on platelet aggregation, thromboxane production, and serotonin secretion in horses. J Vet Intern Med 2011;25:116–22.

82. Roscher KA, Failing K, Moritz A. Inhibition of platelet function with clopidogrel, as measured with a novel whole blood impedance aggregometer in horses. Vet J 2015;203:332–6.

83. Monreal L, Cesarini C. Coagulopathies in horses with colic. Vet Clin North Am Equine Pract 2009;25:247–58.

84. Monreal L, Villatoro AJ, Monreal M, et al. Comparison of the effects of low-molecular-weight and unfractioned heparin in horses. Am J Vet Res 1995;56:1281–5.

85. Feige K, Schwarzwald CC, Bombeli T. Comparison of unfractioned and low molecular weight heparin for prophylaxis of coagulopathies in 52 horses with colic: a randomised double-blind clinical trial. Equine Vet J 2003;35:506–13.

86. de la Rebiere de Pouyade G, Grulke S, Detilleux J, et al. Evaluation of low-molecular-weight heparin for the prevention of equine laminitis after colic surgery. J Vet Emerg Crit Care 2009;19:113–9.

When Things Do Not Go As Planned

Update on Complications and Impact on Outcome

Isabelle Kilcoyne, MVB, Diplomate ACVS

KEYWORDS

- Equine • Colic • Surgery • Complication • Infection

KEY POINTS

- Substantial improvements in early referral, surgical techniques, anesthesia, and post-operative care have led to reductions in mortality and morbidity in colic patients over the last number of years. However, post-operative complications still occur with some frequency.
- Although the goal is to prevent complications, strategies to identify these complications as early as possible and institute appropriate treatment are paramount in managing these cases.
- Regardless of what complication is being considered, the use of common terminology and uniform definitions should be used by researchers to allow more meaningful comparisons between studies.

Colic is an economically important disease of the horse and a major cause of morbidity and mortality in the equine population. Over the last number of years substantial improvements in outcomes of horses undergoing colic surgery have been made, however, post-operative complications still occur. The purpose of this article is to review the literature and determine best practices to prevent these complications and strategies to identify them as early as possible to institute appropriate treatment when they do occur.

INTRODUCTION

Colic is an economically important disease of the horse and a major cause of morbidity and mortality in the equine population and constitutes one of the most common medical conditions necessitating veterinary intervention.[1–3] Of these cases, up to 17% will require surgical intervention.[4–10] Over the last number of years substantial

---

Department of Surgical and Radiological Sciences, UC Davis School of Veterinary Medicine, One Shields Avenue, Davis, CA 95616, USA
E-mail address: ikilcoyne@ucdavis.edu

Vet Clin Equine 39 (2023) 307–323
https://doi.org/10.1016/j.cveq.2023.03.002
0749-0739/23/© 2023 Elsevier Inc. All rights reserved.

improvements in outcomes of horses undergoing colic surgery have been made, much of which can be attributed to earlier referral and expedited diagnosis, safer anesthetic protocols, improved surgical techniques, and post-operative care. In the recent literature, survival to discharge following colic surgery is reported to range from 76% to 88%[11–14] with 69% to 85%[15–17] reported to return to athletic function.

Despite these considerable improvements, post-operative complications still commonly occur[4,18] and can have substantial consequences with regard to the horse's recovery, survival, and return to athletic performance. The additional economic burden for the owner can be substantial, and can have huge implications in the decision-making process in ongoing care for these cases. Strategies to identify these complications as early as possible and institute appropriate treatment are paramount in managing these cases. However, protocols to prevent, or at least minimize, these complications based on the available scientific literature would be ideal.

The purpose of this article is to review the more common post-operative complications following colic surgery and summarize the most recent literature pertaining to these topics with an emphasis on diagnosis, treatment, and prevention.

POST-OPERATIVE ILEUS

Post-operative ileus (POI) is commonly encountered after colic surgery, with a higher incidence noted after small intestinal surgery. It can be a common reason for euthanasia or re-laparotomy in post-operative patients and results in a major increase in cost to the client. Prevalence and predisposing factors have been discussed extensively in the literature.[18–21] However, the criteria to define POI differ between studies which can make comparisons difficult. More recently, the term post-operative reflux (POR) has been used[12,18] to describe >2 L reflux after passage of a nasogastric tube any time in the post-operative period in horses who have not undergone repeat laparotomy to determine the exact cause of the reflux. Although any horse undergoing colic surgery can develop POR, horses with small intestinal lesions, particularly those undergoing resection and anastomosis seem to be more at risk. This is likely due to systemic inflammation as a consequence of ischemia, manipulation of the intestine at the time of surgery, and disturbances in the normal neural signals.[19,22] POR may be caused by a functional or mechanical obstruction and differential diagnoses such as ileus, obstruction at an anastomosis site due to kinking, hematoma formation or volvulus at the anastomosis site, intestinal ischemia, intestinal leakage resulting in septic peritonitis, and adhesions should all be considered.[23] A definitive diagnosis can only be made during repeat laparotomy or at necropsy. One of the most difficult decisions facing a surgeon managing this condition is whether a re-laparotomy is necessary, and when is the optimum time for re-laparotomy to be performed. Repeat laparotomy increases the expense associated with treatment and patient morbidity. Prolonged medical management, however, can also result in substantial expense and is obviously unlikely to be successful in cases requiring surgical intervention, that is, in cases with ischemic bowel or problems with an anastomosis. Limited studies investigating clinical variables associated with POR caused by ileus versus a surgical problem necessitating repeat laparotomy are available in the literature. One study[24] did identify horses with POR after small intestinal surgery, in conjunction with pyrexia and persistent colic to be more likely to have a surgical reason for POR. Typically, horses exhibiting persistent or recurrent pain with POR that is not resolving within 48 to 72 hours should be considered strong candidates for repeat laparotomy. Serious conversations with the client should be undertaken as early as possible in the post-operative period, if complications are arising, regarding clinical and financial expectations to ascertain if re-laparotomy is an option and what budgetary con-straints, if any, exist. Other factors to consider are timing, that is, increased expense if a repeat laparotomy is to be performed on an after-hours basis, and availability of more experienced surgical personnel if needed to assist.

Although multiple therapies have been proposed to prevent and decrease the dura-tion of POR in horses, no specific treatment to date has been considered completely effective. For this reason, a multimodal approach, including surgical intervention, appropriate non-steroidal anti-inflammatory, pro-kinetic and anti-endotoxin therapy, gastric decompression as needed, and appropriate fluid administration, is currently used in attempts to prevent and treat POR with varying success. Early initiation of management strategies in these cases can, we hope, prevent, or at least, reduce the duration of POR.

Supportive care including intravenous (IV) fluid therapy and electrolyte supplemen-tation is a mainstay in the management of most post-operative colic patients. Overhy-dration can result in bowel edema, which can impair the correct functioning of the gastrointestinal tract and slow healing of surgical lesions and is theorized to contribute to POR in human patients.[22,25] Subsequently, the current protocols in human medi-cine are to avoid fluid excess using restricted IV fluid therapy regimens.[20,26] However, one recent study[22] in horses that aimed to evaluate the role of IV fluid volume admin-istration and electrolyte supplementation on the development of POR in horses under-going celiotomy for colic found that fluid overload was not a contributing factor for POR in horses and inadequate fluid resuscitation in the perioperative period seemed to be more detrimental. However, it should be noted that fluid rates in horses are more typical of a "restricted" fluid regimen in people. It should also be noted that acute kid-ney injury can occur in horses who are receiving insufficient fluid replacement therapy, particularly older horses and horses concurrently treated with a non-steroidal anti-in-flammatory drug. Close monitoring of physical examination findings, packed cell vol-ume, plasma lactate, and creatinine concentrations in the peri-anesthetic period should be performed to monitor hydration and perfusion, and the fluid therapy regimen adjusted accordingly.

There is a paucity in the literature regarding refeeding and nutrition after gastroin-testinal surgery in horses, although this is a critical component of patient care, particularly regarding POR. Gum chewing, a form of sham feeding, has been shown to decrease the time from surgery to the first fecal passage in people.[27] In horses, one study[28] showed that sham feeding in the form of bit chewing resulted in increased right upper quadrant intestinal borborygmi. More recently, a study by Patton and colleagues[29] was performed to determine if bit chewing would shorten gastrointestinal total transit time (GI TTT) in horses who are being fasted and refed. As part of this study, the horses were randomly assigned to treatment (apple-flavored bit) and control (no bit) groups. Bit chewing was found to be safe, inexpensive, and well-tolerated (**Fig. 1**). There was evidence that the bit chewing group demonstrated shorter GI TTT at the 80% bead passage time point, however, there was no significant difference at the 50% bead pas-sage time point. Further studies in clinical cases are warranted to ascertain if this sim-ple and inexpensive technique might be useful to augment progressive GI motility in clinical cases affected by POR.

The principal pharmacologic targets in the treatment of POR include anti-inflammatories drugs and the use of prokinetics. The most commonly used prokinetics include IV lidocaine, metoclopramide, and neostigmine. Although IV lidocaine is one of the most commonly used, evidence of the pro-kinetic properties of IV lidocaine in the literature is contradictory. A 2019 meta-analysis[30] of the effects of IV lidocaine on POR in horses found that the use of IV lidocaine was significantly associated with the

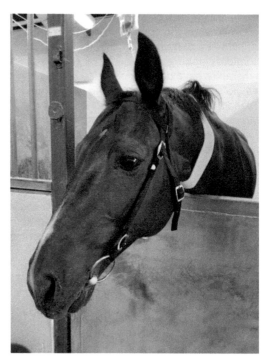

Fig. 1. Placement of a flavored snaffle bit for treatment of POR. The bit was placed for 10 to 15 minutes up to four times a day. (*Photo courtesy of* Dr. Julie Dechant DVM, MS, DACVS, DACVECC.).

development of POR (likely due to its common use in the treatment of POR) and that use of prophylactic IV lidocaine had no effect on the occurrence of POR. It did, however, find that IV lidocaine was significantly associated with an increased survival rate in horses undoing exploratory celiotomy for small intestinal disease, thereby, supporting its administration to improve survival rather than preventing POR. Factors associated with the development of POR can be multifactorial rather than a simple functional obstruction and factors such as mechanical obstruction should be taken into consideration as to why medical management might not work.[4,30] Previous studies[31] had reported that improved survival in horses treated with IV lidocaine was the result of anti-inflammatory effects on ischemia-injured intestine and that coadministration of IV lidocaine with flunixin meglumine ameliorated the flunixin meglumine-induced increase in mucosal neutrophil count. However, other studies[32] have not found such benefits. Given its potential anti-inflammatory properties, use as part of a multi-model analgesia protocol in post-operative patients, and relative inexpensive cost in North America, it is routinely used at the author's institution. The commonly used dose rate is 1.3 mg/kg bolus given over 15 minutes, followed by 0.05 mg/kg/minute continuous rate infusion (CRI). At the author's institution, it is usually administered for 24 hours in the immediate post-operative period but may be extended depending on case progression.

The use of metoclopramide to treat POR was reported to significantly decrease the rate and volume of gastric reflux in one older study,[33] when used as a continuous IV infusion compared with intermittent administration or no use at all. However, other studies regarding its use as a pro-kinetic in the literature are lacking. At the author's institution, the dose for CRI typically starts at 0.02 mg/kg/hour and it is increased gradually over 6 to 12 hours to 0.04 mg/kg/hour if no significant side effects are seen. Due to the fact metoclopramide can cross the blood–brain barrier and suppress dopamine D2 receptors, extrapyramidal side effects can be seen such as agitation, aggression, and/or excitement. Metoclopramide is routinely used by the author in cases of POR following small intestinal surgery and started in the presence of gastric reflux and distended or amotile small intestine on ultrasonographic monitoring.

Neostigmine methylsulfate is a cholinesterase inhibitor that prolongs acetylcholine activity at the synaptic junction by delaying its metabolism. Neostigmine was previously shown[34] to delay gastric emptying and decrease propulsive motility in the stomach and jejunum, but to increase propulsive motility in the pelvic flexure suggesting this drug would be more appropriate for large intestinal motility dysfunction. However, one other study[35] did show a neostigmine CRI at a dose of 0.008 mg/kg/hour did not decrease gastric emptying and neostigmine stimulated the contractile activity of jejunum and pelvic flexure smooth muscle strips in vitro, indicating it may potentially have some beneficial effects on the small intestine.

Unfortunately, there have been relatively few clinical trials undertaken to determine the efficacy of a lot of these drugs. There is a stark need for prospective randomized clinical trials to be performed on therapies used routinely to treat POR. Additionally, a consensus on the criteria used to define POI and POR is needed so there is consistency between studies moving forward.

ADHESIONS

The true prevalence of clinical adhesions is hard to enumerate; however, the current rate of adhesions is estimated to be 6% to 13% after small intestinal surgery, and although more commonly encountered after small intestinal surgery, they have been reported after large intestinal surgery.[4,23,36–38] Fibrinous or fibrous bands extending between bowel, mesentery, omentum, and body wall have all been reported. Multiple risk factors have been identified in the literature with foals and horses undergoing small intestinal surgery being over-represented and endotoxemia, POR, intra- or post-operative hemorrhage, and peritonitis all possibly contributing to adhesion formation.

Clinical signs as a result of adhesion formation typically result in colic which can vary in severity. Although some adhesions in the caudal abdomen may be palpated per rectum, transabdominal ultrasonographic evaluation can be used to diagnose their presence on occasion, particularly adhesions associated with the ventral abdomen. More commonly, pathologic adhesions are identified during repeat laparotomy. Therapies to combat adhesions are currently focused on prevention. Adherence to Halstead's principles of surgery including aseptic and atraumatic surgical technique, adequate hemostasis, and reduced surgery time is critical. Additionally, pharmacologic modulation of the coagulation and fibrinolysis pathways, and physical barriers can all help reduce the incidence of adhesions.[39] Prompt recognition and treatment of horses suffering from POI is also paramount to stimulate motility and reduce the time bowel may be static to facilitate adhesion formation. IV dimethylsulphoxide (DMSO) and flunixin meglumine administered with antimicrobial drugs (potassium penicillin and gentamicin) were found to reduce adhesions in an ischemia/reperfusion model in foals.[40] At the author's institution, DMSO is typically administered intraoperatively (20 mg/kg IV) and then post-operatively twice daily for 3 days in at-risk cases. In cases with previous adhesions or at risk for septic peritonitis, placement of an abdominal drain to facilitate post-operative abdominal lavage may be used to try and reduce the incidence of adhesions.[41]

Adhesion barriers act by providing a physical barrier between serosal surfaces and preventing fibrin deposition that might link serosal or peritoneal surfaces. Different barriers reported in the literature include sodium carboxymethylcellulose (CMC) solutions, sodium hyaluronate/carboxymethylcellulose membranes (HA/CMC), oxidized regenerated cellulose, hyaluronate (HA) and fucoidan solutions. Although some researchers[4,42] might argue the development of adhesions is a more global issue and application of a membrane at the site of resection is likely not beneficial, strategic placement at a damaged area may help reduce the incidence of adhesions at that site (**Fig. 2**). It should be noted, however, that these membranes were reported to impair anastomotic healing in human intestinal surgery.[43] A recent meta-analysis looking at the effects of adhesion barriers on adhesion formation in horses found the odds of adhesions in horses treated with an adhesion barrier was significantly lower than untreated controls (OR = 0.102; 95% CI [0.041, 0.254]; $P < .001$). Additionally, horses treated with HA/CMC membranes (Seprafilm, Genzyme Corp, Cambridge, MA) and CMC solutions specifically had significant OR for fewer adhesions (OR = 0.061; 95% CI [0.013, 0.292]; OR = 0.119; 95%CI [0.034,0.415], respectively; $P < .001$).[39] It should be noted that most of the studies included in the meta-analysis used experimental models of adhesion formation rather than clinical cases. Sodium carboxymethylcellulose is a lubricating agent that is typically used during surgery to facilitate handling of the bowel and then placed directly on the bowel at the end of surgery. Some studies[39,44] have shown a benefit of this treatment and anecdotally it seems to be effective in reducing adhesions.

Fucoidans are a class of broad molecular weight, sulfated polysaccharides extracted from the extracellular matrix of various brown seaweeds with potential anti-adhesive and anticoagulant properties. A purified solution, PERIDAN, was evaluated in an adult horse jejunojejunostomy model and was found to be safely administered intraperitoneally to healthy horses. No significant differences between treatment and control (LRS) groups, with regard to tissue healing, inflammation, or infection were noted but a significant effect on reducing adhesions was not apparent.[45] Unfortunately, PERIDAN is currently unavailable and to the author's knowledge, there is no replacement product at this time.

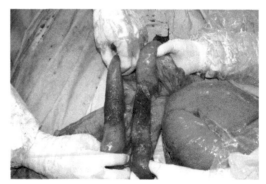

Fig. 2. Picture taken at re-laparotomy following jejunal resection and anastomosis in a case of small intestinal strangulating lesion. At re-laparotomy, bowel-to-bowel adhesions were noted involving the area just oral to the previous anastomosis site and another segment of jejunum. Following separation of the bowel loops a sodium hyaluronate/carboxymethylcellulose membrane (Seprefilm) was applied to the affected bowel in an attempt to prevent further adhesions forming in this area. (*Photo courtesy of* Dr. Jorge Nieto MVZ, PhD, DACVS, DACVSMR.)

Intraperitoneal heparin therapy was reported to reduce adhesions in one study[46]; however, this was a retrospective study where treatments were not allocated on random basis. Doses reported for intraperitoneal heparin use include administration of 30,000 IU diluted in 4 L LRS into the abdomen before closure.[47]

Omentectomy for adhesion prevention is controversial but has been advocated by some to prevent adhesions.[37] However, reports of omental adhesions resulting in colic are rare and the potential absence of the omentum may actually increase the incidence of bowel-to-bowel or bowel-to-mesentery adhesions.[4,47] It is not commonly performed in adult horses at the author's institution undergoing colic surgery.

Adhesions, and their associated recurrent colic episodes, can sometimes be managed through dietary modification and transitions to a more digestible pelleted diet. If a repeat surgery is performed, resection of the adhesion is executed in the most atraumatic manner possible and every effort is made to prevent recurrence using the aforementioned methods. Alternatively, complete en-bloc resection of the adhered portion of bowel and anastomosis of healthier adjacent segments of bowel can be performed. The prognosis for a post-operative patient with adhesion formation has generally been guarded.[48] One study[42] did find the mortality in horses with or without adhesions was similar, indicating that the presence of adhesions at second surgery did not influence long-term survival; however, many of the horses included had large intestinal lesions and adhesions. Location of the adhesion, that is, small versus large intestine, the underlying cause, and options for re-laparotomy based on the owner's financial constraints and the surgeon's ability to treat, all likely play a role in the outcome.

INCISIONAL COMPLICATIONS

Equine colic surgery poses several challenges in the post-operative period relative to the actual incision and healing. The sheer size of the equine patient and the activity they are expected to perform are but a few of the factors that can increase the post-operative morbidity in our colic patients.

Incisional Infections

Recent incidences of incision infections have been reported to vary from 15% to 28%[49–51] with factors such as suture pattern,[49] suture material,[52] degree of trauma to the surgical site and incisional length greater than 27 cm,[53] experience level of the surgeon,[54] and increased body weight[55] or body mass index (BMI)[56] predisposing to an increased or decreased rate of incisional complications. Incisional infections tend to occur to a greater extent with repeated laparotomy, with the reported risk of incisional infections being as high as 76.5% in a recent study.[57] Although many studies have reported on different risk factors associated with surgical site infection following laparotomy, varying definitions and descriptive terms between studies make direct comparisons difficult. Additionally, most studies lack adequate follow-up and only report incidences up to the point of discharge. Two recent studies[50,58] found that most of the cases were diagnosed with incisional infection after discharge from the hospital, which emphasizes the need for long-term follow-up and good communication with referring veterinarians and owners in identifying these cases. It is possible that previous studies where follow-up was limited to a shorter period of time may actually underestimate their incisional complication rate based on these findings.

Regardless, some studies have identified potential strategies to help reduce the incidence of surgical site infection following laparotomy. The use of a protective dressing to cover the incision in the initial recovery period has been evaluated recently in the literature. In one study[50] which looked at the use of an antimicrobial impregnated (0.2% polyhexamethylene biguanide [PHMB]) dressing, only 2/50 (4%) horses who had some type of stent bandage placed, either PHMB impregnated or sterile towel, went on to develop an incisional infection compared with 9/25 (36%) of those who did not have one placed (**Fig. 3**). These findings mirror those of another study[51] where the application of stent bandage reduced the incisional infection rate to 2.7% compared with 21.8% in those without a stent. A recent prospective randomized control study[58] that examined the effect of intra-incisional medical grade honey (MGH) on the prevalence of incisional infection in horses undergoing colic surgery found horses in the treatment group (4/49; 8.3%) had a significantly lower rate of incisional infection compared with the control group 13/40; 32.5%). No adverse effected were seen associated with the application of the MGH.

Diagnosis of incisional infection is typically based on clinical signs such as fever, heat, pain, redness, swelling, or excessive edema around the incision and wound drainage. Ultrasonographic evaluation can also be a helpful tool to diagnosis the presence of infection in the early stages[59] by identifying areas of fluid accumulation, particularly if there is no wound drainage. Ultrasonography can be used to monitor body wall healing and the response to treatment. Definitive diagnosis is based on a positive bacterial culture of an aseptically-obtained sample from the subcutaneous tissues in the area of fluid accumulation. If antimicrobial therapy is deemed necessary, decisions on antimicrobial choice should be based on these culture results and susceptibility profiles. The most common bacteria isolated in one study[55] were *Escherichia coli*, *Enterococcus* spp. and *Staphylococcus* spp. In that same study, mixed bacterial infections were common and present in 63% of cases with only 37% of cases growing a single isolate. Although antimicrobials might not be necessary to treat every case, bacterial culture and sensitivity testing is prudent, not only for patient treatment, but also for

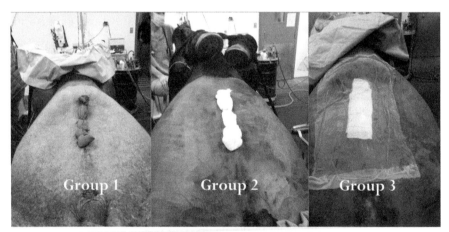

Fig. 3. One study[50] looked at the placement of a 0.2% polyhexamethylene biguanide-impregnated rolled gauze over a laparotomy incision at the end of surgery (Group 2) and secured in place using 3 to 4 interrupted sutures using size 2 polypropylene suture. Using this antimicrobial-impregnated dressing 0/26 developed an incisional discharge, compared with 2/24 horses who had a sterile towel secured using 3 to 4 interrupted sutures using size 2 polypropylene suture (Group 1) and 9/25 who had sterile gauze placed over the incision and secured in place with an iodine impregnated adhesive drape (Group 3). Stents are typically left in place for 24 to 48 hours post-operatively at the author's institution, but may be removed sooner if they are soiled or dislodged at recovery.

hospital biosecurity monitoring as the emergence of multi-drug resistant organisms may be responsible for nosocomial infections.

Currently, there are little data presented in the literature regarding the treatment of these cases and most strategies revolve around the establishment of drainage by removing some staples or sutures and appropriate antimicrobial therapy based on the results of bacterial culture and sensitivity testing. Application of an abdominal bandage to protect the area and possibly facilitate the application of a topical antimicrobial dressing is also commonplace. At the author's institution, it is current practice to recommend application of a hernia belt in all cases that develop incisional infection in an attempt to reduce the risk for acute dehiscence or hernia development. Additionally, prolonged stall rest is recommended for up to 4 weeks after resolution of the infection. Although little objective data are present in the literature regarding rehabilitation for these types of cases, there is some evidence to suggest core abdominal muscle rehabilitation exercises may facilitate faster convalesce and improved performance in horses after colic surgery.[60] It would be reasonable to assume that these types of exercises could also be beneficial and may help prevent or reduce hernia formation in cases with known predisposing factors, that is, surgical site infection. As previously outlined, prolonged rest is recommended in such cases; therefore, it would be prudent to delay the institution of these exercises in cases of incisional infection.

Strategies to minimize the incidence of infection include strict adherence to Halstead's principles of surgery and appropriate antimicrobial prophylaxis. Despite published recommendations regarding antimicrobial prophylaxis in horses undergoing colic surgery, studies have found that compliance is poor. Administration of a first-line broad-spectrum parenteral antimicrobial within 30 to 60 minutes of the initial incision is recommended. Although re-dosing of potassium penicillin intra-operatively if the surgery exceeds two half-lives of the pre-operative dose has been recommended,[59,61] recent research suggests that re-dosing of potassium penicillin within 4 to 5 hours of the pre-operative dose is not necessary because of the longer half-life and slower clearance in anesthetized horses.[62] Although there are differing reports in the literature regarding the length of perioperative antimicrobial prophylaxis, one study found no benefit in administering antimicrobials for 120 hours versus 72 hours in terms of preventing surgical site infection (SSI) after colic surgery.[63] Based on recommendations for antimicrobial prophylaxis in human patients undergoing abdominal surgery, antimicrobials should not be administered beyond 24 hours or even beyond the operative period[64] and prolonged prophylaxis may be detrimental.

Body Wall Hernia Formation

Typically, infection localized to the skin and subcutaneous tissue heals without additional complication; however, if there is involvement of underlying linea alba, disruption of the normal healing process may result in acute incisional dehiscence or hernia formation. Incisional herniation has been reported in 6% to 16% of horses following laparotomy,[16,65] with surgical site infection being identified as a risk factor for the development of incisional herniation. Horses with incisional infection were 17.8 to 62.5 times more likely to develop a hernia compared with those without incisional drainage.[65,66]

The use of a commercial hernia belt (CM Equine Hernia Belt, CM Equine Products, Downey, CA) has been reported to reduce the incidence of hernia development in horses who have developed other incisional complications and is typically used as part of the treatment protocol after hernia formation too. The size of the defect will typically dictate the treatment pursued with smaller defects often not requiring intervention if no adverse effects on the horses' health or athletic pursuits are observed.

Conservative management of larger defects consisting of dietary modification to a low bulk pelleted feed, application of a supportive hernia belt, and gradual increase in exercise and rehabilitation exercises can often decrease the diameter of even larger hernias. Surgical management, including primary repair or using mesh placement,[59,67,68] can also be pursued for larger defects for functional or cosmetic reasons, but should be delayed until a firm fibrous hernia ring has formed which may take up to 4 to 6 months after surgery. Additionally, any infection should be completely resolved to reduce the risk of mesh infection post-operatively.

Acute Incisional Dehiscence

Acute incisional dehiscence is an uncommonly reported complication but has potentially catastrophic consequences. In a recent multicenter study[69] that examined cases reported from nine hospitals in the United Kingdom, Ireland, and the United States over 10 years, only 63 cases were identified. Acute abdominal dehiscence (AAD) occurred early in the post-operative period in most cases at a median of 5 days post-operatively, and broodmares accounted for 25% of the cases. Contrary to previous reports,[68] leakage of peritoneal fluid from the incision was not a consistent sign of impending AAD. In this study, infection developed in 44% of the horses before ADD, which is a higher rate compared with other studies. It would seem that infection is a risk factor for AAD and careful ultrasonographic assessment of the incision, including linea alba integrity, is warranted in cases where the infection is identified. In this study, conservative treatment, consisting of supportive bandages and antimicrobial treatment, was instituted in 10 cases where there was no evisceration of abdominal contents, and surgical repair was performed in 27 horses. Overall survival to hospital discharge was 38%, with 55% of those treated surgically and 90% of those treated conservatively surviving to discharge. Although the overall prognosis was poor, many horses (40%) were euthanized immediately which may have biased survival rates as some horses may have survived if surgery had been performed.

POST-OPERATIVE DIARRHEA

Development of diarrhea in a post-operative colic patient is another frequently encountered complication and can similarly be a source of substantial expense for the owner, particularly if an infectious agent is identified. Diarrhea is usually defined as the passage of unformed feces for more than 24 hours, or on more than two occasions, and has previously been more frequently associated with large intestinal lesions.[70] Colitis, however, refers to inflammation of the colon with or without diarrhea and can occur in horses with any type of lesion and is often associated with an infectious agent. Damage to the gastrointestinal tract and mucosal barrier, administration of perioperative antibiotics, surgical evacuation of the colonic contents, stress of anesthesia, and reduced feed intake can all contribute to the development of diarrhea/colitis.

Salmonellosis is probably the most recognized disease associated with diarrhea/colitis post-colic surgery and a serious concern for the clinician with regard to nosocomial infection and biosecurity. Salmonellosis in horses has typically been associated with diarrhea/colitis, fever, and leukopenia; however, more recently, it has been shown that other predictors, such as the presence of reflux, can also be an indicator of infection.[71,72] Although abdominal surgery has been previously associated with an increased incidence of *Salmonella* shedding,[71,73,74] a recent study[72] did not find a significant effect of abdominal surgery on the subsequent shedding of *Salmonella*. Although post-operative colic patients who develop *Salmonella* may experience more complications and longer hospitalization, there does not seem to be a significant effect on subsequent survival to discharge or long-term survival and return to function.[72,75] Other infectious agents frequently implicated include *Clostridium difficile* and *Clostridium perfringens*.

Ideally, the focus should be on prevention, and lacking that, early recognition. Di-tri-octahedral (DTO) smectite (Bio-Sponge, Platinum Performance, Buellton, CA) has been shown to adsorb substances like endotoxins and exotoxins. In one study, DTO smectite (0.5 kg in 4 L water administered via a nasogastric tube every 24 hours for 3 days beginning 4 hours after surgery) reduced the occurrence of post-operative diarrhea in horses with large colon disease compared with placebo (4 L water administered via a nasogastric tube every 24 hours for 3 days), with the prevalence being 10.8% in the treated and 41.4% in the placebo group.[76] At the author's institution, 0.5 kg is typically administered into the ventral colon at the time of surgery after the evacuation of colonic contents through a pelvic flexure enterotomy, if performed. Due to the potential for impaction, not more than 0.5 kg (1lb) is administered. Another study[77] investigating the use of probiotics for prevention of *Salmonella* shedding in the post-operative period did not find a significant effect, however, a more recent study[78] did find a beneficial effect in administering *Saccharomyces boulardii* for treatment of acute enterocolitis.

Investigation into intestinal microbiota and the changes that may occur perioperatively are ongoing and we hope in the future results of this research may help further our understanding of equine gastrointestinal health and help to minimize complications like colitis and diarrhea post-operatively.

OTHER COMPLICATIONS

Although respiratory diseases post-colic surgery are not the most common complications encountered, the development of sinusitis or pneumonia post-operatively should not be discounted by the clinician, particularly in cases that develop a fever post-operatively. The development of sinusitis in horses being treated for colic and associated with nasogastric intubation has been previously reported.[79] Another recent report[80] found that compared with control horses, peri-anesthetic reflux was more common in horses with sinusitis, pneumonia, and respiratory complications. Although these horses were associated with longer duration of antimicrobial therapy and longer periods of hospitalization, all horses survived to discharge. Care should always be taken with nasogastric intubation and extubation particularly if the horse is badly behaved or sedated and the horse should have nil by mouth if a nasogastric tube is in place.

IV catheter-associated complications are not uncommon in the post-operative colic patient. Although thrombophlebitis is likely the most common of these, air embolism, regional cellulitis, or even catheter fragmentation (**Fig. 4**) can be encountered. Horses with signs of shock and systemic inflammatory response syndrome, fever at the time of catheterization, diarrhea, and administration of parenteral nutrition have been associated with an increased risk of thrombophlebitis.[81,82] Use of polyurethane or silastic catheters, ideally inserted using an over-the-wire (Seldinger) technique should be used in any case where prolonged catheterization might be required.[23,83] Additionally, treatment with low-molecular-weight heparin (enoxaparin; 40 U/kg subcutaneously q24 hours) or clopidogrel (loading dose 4 mg/kg followed by 2 mg/kg orally q24 hours) in cases where oral meds are tolerated (ie, not refluxing) may be helpful in reducing catheter-associated complications. Aside from the typical clinical signs associated with thrombophlebitis such as heat, swelling, pain over the catheter site,

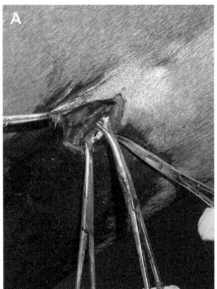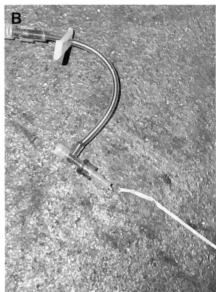

Fig. 4. (*A*) Removal of a 14 g 5.25″ fragmented IV catheter which was discovered following anesthetic recovery of a post-operative colic patient who underwent exploratory laparotomy for enterolithiasis. An incision was made directly over the vein using ultrasound guidance to identify the exact location of the proximal portion of the catheter, while an assistant held off the jugular vein to prevent displacement of the portion of the catheter. A hemostat was used to grasp the proximal tip within the vein, and it was removed intact. (*B*) Location of the fragmented piece of catheter.

and potentially fever, ultrasound can be a useful diagnostic to confirm and subsequently monitor the response to treatment.[84]

Other commonly encountered complications in patients recovering from gastrointestinal surgery include endotoxemia and laminitis. Clinical manifestations of endotoxemia have been found to be an important factor in the development of acute laminitis.[70,85] Treatment of these conditions has been reported extensively elsewhere,[86] but supportive care and aggressive antiendotoxic and anti-inflammatory therapy should be instituted rapidly for horses who have an ischemic lesion, placing them at risk for endotoxemia and subsequent laminitis. Digital cryotherapy for at-risk patients (eg, febrile, enteritis/colitis, previous history of laminitis) should be considered.[86]

SUMMARY

Early diagnosis and expedited treatment remain the cornerstones of reducing many complications in post-operative colic patients. Unfortunately, there is a lack of evidence-based data as to the efficacy of a lot of treatments proposed to help reduce or treat complications. Much of the evidence on how complications can be prevented is inconclusive due to relatively few studies and their largely retrospective, single-hospital design, and small sample size with resulting inherent bias. Moving forward, standardization of definitions to allow more direct comparisons between studies of risk factors, prevention, and treatment strategies is paramount. Additionally, multicenter, randomized controlled studies to gain better evidence and identify trends are needed to further our understanding of the pathophysiology of these complications and also to gain better insights into prevention and treatment.

DISCLOSURE

The author has no relationship with a commercial company that has a direct financial interest in the subject matter or materials discussed in the article or with a company making a competing product.

REFERENCES

1. Bowden A, Boynova P, Brennan ML, et al. Retrospective case series to identify the most common conditions seen 'out-of-hours' by first-opinion equine veterinary practitioners. Vet Rec 2020;187:404.
2. Bowden A, England GCW, Brennan ML, et al. Indicators of 'critical' outcomes in 941 horses seen 'out-of-hours' for colic. Vet Rec 2020;187:492.
3. Traub-Dargatz JL, Salman MD, Voss JL. Medical problems of adult horses, as ranked by equine practitioners. J Am Vet Med Assoc 1991;198:1745–7.
4. Freeman DE. Fifty years of colic surgery. Equine Vet J 2018;50:423–35.
5. Tinker MK, White NA, Lessard P, et al. Prospective study of equine colic incidence and mortality. Equine Vet J 1997;29:448–53.
6. Archer DC, Proudman CJ. Epidemiological clues to preventing colic. Vet J 2006; 172:29–39.
7. Proudman CJ. A two year, prospective survey of equine colic in general practice. Equine Vet J 1992;24:90–3.
8. Curtis L, Burford JH, Thomas JS, et al. Prospective study of the primary evaluation of 1016 horses with clinical signs of abdominal pain by veterinary practitioners, and the differentiation of critical and non-critical cases. Acta Vet Scand 2015;57:69.
9. Hillyer MH, Taylor FG, French NP. A cross-sectional study of colic in horses on thoroughbred training premises in the British Isles in 1997. Equine Vet J 2001; 33:380–5.
10. Kaneene JB, Miller R, Ross WA, et al. Risk factors for colic in the Michigan (USA) equine population. Prev Vet Med 1997;30:23–36.
11. Mair TS, Smith LJ. Survival and complication rates in 300 horses undergoing surgical treatment of colic. Part 1: Short-term survival following a single laparotomy. Equine Vet J 2005;37:296–302.
12. Stewart S, Southwood LL, Aceto HW. Comparison of short- and long-term complications and survival following jejunojejunostomy, jejunoileostomy and jejunocaecostomy in 112 horses: 2005-2010. Equine Vet J 2014;46:333–8.
13. Morton AJ, Blikslager AT. Surgical and postoperative factors influencing short-term survival of horses following small intestinal resection: 92 cases (1994-2001). Equine Vet J 2002;34:450–4.
14. Kilcoyne I, Dechant JE, Nieto JE. Comparison of clinical findings and short-term survival between horses with intestinal entrapment in the gastrosplenic ligament and horses with intestinal entrapment in the epiploic foramen. J Am Vet Med Assoc 2016;249:660–7.
15. Tomlinson JE, Boston RC, Brauer T. Evaluation of racing performance after colic surgery in Thoroughbreds: 85 cases (1996-2010). J Am Vet Med Assoc 2013; 243:532–7.

16. Davis W, Fogle CA, Gerard MP, et al. Return to use and performance following exploratory celiotomy for colic in horses: 195 cases (2003-2010). Equine Vet J 2013;45:224–8.

17. Hart SK, Southwood LL, Aceto HW. Impact of colic surgery on return to function in racing Thoroughbreds: 59 cases (1996-2009). J Am Vet Med Assoc 2014;244: 205–11.

18. Salem SE, Proudman CJ, Archer DC. Prevention of post operative complications following surgical treatment of equine colic: Current evidence. Equine Vet J 2016; 48:143–51.

19. Torfs S, Delesalle C, Dewulf J, et al. Risk factors for equine postoperative ileus and effectiveness of prophylactic lidocaine. J Vet Intern Med 2009;23:606–11.

20. Lisowski ZM, Pirie RS, Blikslager AT, et al. An update on equine post-operative ileus: Definitions, pathophysiology and management. Equine Vet J 2018;50: 292–303.

21. Mair TS, Smith LJ. Survival and complication rates in 300 horses undergoing surgical treatment of colic. Part 2: Short-term complications. Equine Vet J 2005;37: 303–9.

22. Hoaglund EL, Hess AM, Hassel DM. Retrospective evaluation of the effect of intravenous fluid administration on development of postoperative reflux in horses with colic (2004-2012): 194 horses. J Vet Emerg Crit Care 2018;28:566–72.

23. Southwood LL. Complications of the Postoperative Colic Patient. In: Rubio-Martinez LM, Hendrickson DA, editors. Complications in equine surgery. Hoboken, NJ: John Wiley & Sons, Inc.; 2021. p. 310–73.

24. Jacobs CC, Stefanovski D, Southwood LL. Use of perioperative variables to determine the requirement for repeat celiotomy in horses with postoperative reflux after small intestinal surgery. Vet Surg 2019;48:1204–10.

25. Nisanevich V, Felsenstein I, Almogy G, et al. Effect of intraoperative fluid management on outcome after intraabdominal surgery. Anesthesiology 2005;103:25–32.

26. Lassen K, Soop M, Nygren J, et al. Consensus review of optimal perioperative care in colorectal surgery: Enhanced Recovery After Surgery (ERAS) Group recommendations. Arch Surg 2009;144:961–9.

27. Liu Q, Jiang H, Xu D, et al. Effect of gum chewing on ameliorating ileus following colorectal surgery: A meta-analysis of 18 randomized controlled trials. Int J Surg 2017;47:107–15.

28. Giusto G, Pagliara E, Gandini M. Effects of bit chewing on right upper quadrant intestinal sound frequency in adult horses. J Equine Vet Sci 2014;34:520–3.

29. Patton ME, Leise BS, Baker RE, et al. The effects of bit chewing on borborygmi, duodenal motility, and gastrointestinal transit time in clinically normal horses. Vet Surg 2022;51:88–96.

30. Durket E, Gillen A, Kottwitz J, et al. Meta-analysis of the effects of lidocaine on postoperative reflux in the horse. Vet Surg 2020;49:44–52.

31. Cook VL, Jones Shults J, McDowell M, et al. Attenuation of ischaemic injury in the equine jejunum by administration of systemic lidocaine. Equine Vet J 2008;40: 353–7.

32. Bauck AG, Grosche A, Morton AJ, et al. Effect of lidocaine on inflammation in equine jejunum subjected to manipulation only and remote to intestinal segments subjected to ischemia. Am J Vet Res 2017;78:977–89.

33. Dart AJ, Peauroi JR, Hodgson DR, et al. Efficacy of metoclopramide for treatment of ileus in horses following small intestinal surgery: 70 cases (1989-1992). Aust Vet J 1996;74:280–4.

34. Adams SB, MacHarg MA. Neostigmine methylsulfate delays gastric emptying of particulate markers in horses. Am J Vet Res 1985;46:2498–9.

35. Nieto JE, Morales B, Yamout SZ, et al. In vivo and in vitro effects of neostigmine on gastrointestinal tract motility of horses. Am J Vet Res 2013;74:579–88.

36. Baxter GM, Broome TE, Moore JN. Abdominal adhesions after small intestinal surgery in the horse. Vet Surg 1989;18:409–14.

37. Kuebelbeck KL, Slone DE, May KA. Effect of omentectomy on adhesion formation in horses. Vet Surg 1998;27:132–7.

38. Phillips TJ, Walmsley JP. Retrospective analysis of the results of 151 exploratory laparotomies in horses with gastrointestinal disease. Equine Vet J 1993;25:427–31.

39. Munsterman AS, Kottwitz JJ, Reid Hanson R. Meta-Analysis of the Effects of Adhesion Barriers on Adhesion Formation in the Horse. Vet Surg 2016;45:587–95.

40. Sullins KE, White NA, Lundin CS, et al. Prevention of ischaemia-induced small intestinal adhesions in foals. Equine Vet J 2004;36:370–5.

41. Hague BA, Honnas CM, Berridge BR, et al. Evaluation of postoperative peritoneal lavage in standing horses for prevention of experimentally induced abdominal adhesions. Vet Surg 1998;27:122–6.

42. Gorvy DA, Barrie Edwards G, Proudman CJ. Intra-abdominal adhesions in horses: a retrospective evaluation of repeat laparotomy in 99 horses with acute gastrointestinal disease. Vet J 2008;175:194–201.

43. Ten Broek RPG, Stommel MWJ, Strik C, et al. Benefits and harms of adhesion barriers for abdominal surgery: a systematic review and meta-analysis. Lancet 2014;383:48–59.

44. Mueller PO, Hunt RJ, Allen D, et al. Intraperitoneal use of sodium carboxymethylcellulose in horses undergoing exploratory celiotomy. Vet Surg 1995;24:112–7.

45. Morello S, Southwood LL, Engiles J, et al. Effect of intraperitoneal PERIDAN concentrate adhesion reduction device on clinical findings, infection, and tissue healing in an adult horse jejunojejunostomy model. Vet Surg 2012;41:568–81.

46. Mair TS, Smith LJ. Survival and complication rates in 300 horses undergoing surgical treatment of colic. Part 3: Long-term complications and survival. Equine Vet J 2005;37:310–4.

47. Eggleston RB, Mueller PO. Prevention and treatment of gastrointestinal adhesions. Vet Clin North Am Equine Pract 2003;19:741–63.

48. Findley JA, Salem S, Burgess R, et al. Factors associated with survival of horses following relaparotomy. Equine Vet J 2017;49:448–53.

49. Colbath AC, Patipa L, Berghaus RD, et al. The influence of suture pattern on the incidence of incisional drainage following exploratory laparotomy. Equine Vet J 2014;46:156–60.

50. Kilcoyne I, Dechant JE, Kass PH, et al. Evaluation of the risk of incisional infection in horses following application of protective dressings after exploratory celiotomy for treatment of colic. J Am Vet Med Assoc 2019;254:1441–7.

51. Tnibar A, Grubbe Lin K, Thuroe Nielsen K, et al. Effect of a stent bandage on the likelihood of incisional infection following exploratory coeliotomy for colic in horses: a comparative retrospective study. Equine Vet J 2013;45:564–9.

52. Anderson SL, Devick I, Bracamonte JL, et al. Occurrence of Incisional Complications After Closure of Equine Celiotomies With USP 7 Polydioxanone. Vet Surg 2015;44:521–6.

53. Darnaud SJ, Southwood LL, Aceto HW, et al. Are horse age and incision length associated with surgical site infection following equine colic surgery? Vet J 2016;217:3–7.

54. Torfs S, Levet T, Delesalle C, et al. Risk factors for incisional complications after exploratory celiotomy in horses: do skin staples increase the risk? Vet Surg 2010; 39:616–20.

55. Isgren CM, Salem SE, Archer DC, et al. Risk factors for surgical site infection following laparotomy; effect of season and perioperative variables and reporting of bacterial isolates in 287 horses. Equine Vet J 2015;49:39–44.

56. Hill JA, Tyma JF, Hayes GM, et al. Higher body mass index may increase the risk for the development of incisional complications in horses following emergency ventral midline celiotomy. Equine Vet J 2020;52:799–804.

57. Bauck AG, Easley JT, Cleary OB, et al. Response to early repeat celiotomy in horses after a surgical treatment of jejunal strangulation. Vet Surg 2017;46: 843–50.

58. Gustafsson K, Tatz AJ, Slavin RA, et al. Intraincisional medical grade honey decreases the prevalence of incisional infection in horses undergoing colic surgery: A prospective randomised controlled study. Equine Vet J 2021;53:1112–8.

59. Shearer TR, Holcombe SJ, Valberg SJ. Incisional infections associated with ventral midline celiotomy in horses. J Vet Emerg Crit Care 2020;30:136–48.

60. Holcombe SJ, Shearer TR, Valberg SJ. The Effect of Core Abdominal Muscle Rehabilitation Exercises on Return to Training and Performance in Horses After Colic Surgery. J Equine Vet Sci 2019;75:14–8.

61. Dallap Schaer BL, Linton JK, Aceto H. Antimicrobial use in horses undergoing colic surgery. J Vet Intern Med 2012;26:1449–56.

62. Wilson KE, Bogers SH, Council-Troche RM, et al. Potassium penicillin and gentamicin pharmacokinetics in healthy conscious and anesthetized horses. Vet Surg 2023;52(1):87–97.

63. Durward-Akhurst SA, Mair TS, Boston R, et al. Comparison of two antimicrobial regimens on the prevalence of incisional infections after colic surgery. Vet Rec 2013;172:287.

64. Bratzler DW, Patchen Dellinger E, Olsen KM, et al. Clinical practice guidelines for antimicrobial prophylaxis in surgery. Am J Health Syst Pharm 2013;70(3): 195–283.

65. Gibson KT, Curtis CR, Turner AS, et al. Incisional hernias in the horse. Incidence and predisposing factors. Vet Surg 1989;18:360–6.

66. Ingle-Fehr JE, Baxter GM, Howard RD, et al. Bacterial culturing of ventral median celiotomies for prediction of postoperative incisional complications in horses. Vet Surg 1997;26:7–13.

67. Kelmer G, Schumacher J. Repair of abdominal wall hernias in horses using primary closure and subcutaneous implantation of mesh. Vet Rec 2008;163:677–9.

68. Toth F, Schumacher J. Abdominal Hernias. In: Auer JA, Stick JA, Kummerle JM, Prange T, editors. Equine surgery. 5th edition. St Louis, (MO): Elsevier Inc; 2018. p. 645–59.

69. Hann MJ, Mair TS, Gardner A, et al. Acute abdominal dehiscence following laparotomy: A multicentre, international retrospective study. Equine Vet J 2021. https://doi.org/10.1111/evj.13498.

70. Cohen ND, Honnas CM. Risk factors associated with development of diarrhea in horses after celiotomy for colic: 190 cases (1990-1994). J Am Vet Med Assoc 1996;209:810–3.

71. Schaer BLD, Aceto H, Caruso MA, et al. Identification of Predictors of Salmonella Shedding in Adult Horses Presented for Acute Colic. J Vet Intern Med 2012;26: 1177–85.

72. Kilcoyne I, Magdesian KG, Guerra M, et al. Prevalence of and risk factors associated with Salmonella shedding among equids presented to a veterinary teaching hospital for colic (2013-2018). Equine Vet J 2022. https://doi.org/10.1111/evj.13864.

73. Ernst NS, Hernandez JA, MacKay RJ, et al. Risk factors associated with fecal Salmonella shedding among hospitalized horses with signs of gastrointestinal tract disease. J Am Vet Med A 2004;225:275–81.

74. Hird DW, Pappaioanou M, Smith BP. Case-Control Study of Risk-Factors Associated with Isolation of Salmonella-Saintpaul in Hospitalized Horses. Am J Epidemiol 1984;120:852–64.

75. Southwood LL, Lindborg S, Aceto HW. Influence of Salmonella status on the long-term outcome of horses after colic surgery. Vet Surg 2017;46:780–8.

76. Hassel DM, Smith PA, Nieto JE, et al. Di-tri-octahedral smectite for the prevention of post-operative diarrhea in equids with surgical disease of the large intestine: results of a randomized clinical trial. Vet J 2009;182:210–4.

77. Parraga ME, Spier SJ, Thurmond M, et al. A clinical trial of probiotic administration for prevention of Salmonella shedding in the postoperative period in horses with colic. J Vet Intern Med 1997;11:36–41.

78. Desrochers AM, Dolente BA, Roy MF, et al. Efficacy of Saccharomyces boulardii for treatment of horses with acute enterocolitis. J Am Vet Med Assoc 2005;227:954–9.

79. Nieto JE, Yamout S, Dechant JE. Sinusitis associated with nasogastric intubation in 3 horses. Can Vet J 2014;55:554–8.

80. Tyma JF, Epstein, K.L. Post-operative respiratory complications following colic surgery. 13th International Equine Colic Research Symposium 2021;6-53.

81. Dolente BA, Beech J, Lindborg S, et al. Evaluation of risk factors for development of catheter-associated jugular thrombophlebitis in horses: 50 cases (1993-1998). J Am Vet Med Assoc 2005;227:1134–41.

82. Traub-Dargatz JL, Dargatz DA. A retrospective study of vein thrombosis in horses treated with intravenous fluids in a veterinary teaching hospital. J Vet Intern Med 1994;8:264–6.

83. Spurlock SL, Spurlock GH, Parker G, et al. Long-term jugular vein catheterization in horses. J Am Vet Med Assoc 1990;196:425–30.

84. Gardner SY, Reef VB, Spencer PA. Ultrasonographic evaluation of horses with thrombophlebitis of the jugular vein: 46 cases (1985-1988). J Am Vet Med Assoc 1991;199:370–3.

85. Parsons CS, Orsini JA, Krafty R, et al. Risk factors for development of acute laminitis in horses during hospitalization: 73 cases (1997-2004). J Am Vet Med Assoc 2007;230:885–9.

86. Leise BS, Fugler LA. Laminitis Updates: Sepsis/Systemic Inflammatory Response Syndrome-Associated Laminitis. Vet Clin North Am Equine Pract 2021;37(3):639–56.

Repeat Celiotomy—Current Status

David E. Freeman, MVB, PhD*, Anje G. Bauck, DVM, PhD

KEYWORDS

- Colic • Surgery • Repeat celiotomy • Complications • Postoperative reflux

KEY POINTS

- Repeat celiotomy is a life-saving procedure in horses that have developed a surgically treatable postoperative obstruction; however, identifying the cause of obstruction can be difficult, before and during the second surgery.
- Timing of repeat celiotomy is critical because a delay in the decision process can worsen the prognosis and put the total cost of treatment out of reach for the owner.
- Complications of repeat celiotomy can be life threatening, including incisional complications and adhesions; however, repeat celiotomy does not seem to exacerbate postoperative ileus, despite the additional surgical manipulation required.
- An important benefit of repeat celiotomy is termination of hopeless cases, thereby reducing cost and suffering.
- Although postoperative ileus is a recognized cause of postoperative reflux, overemphasis of its role in postoperative reflux can delay the decision for a necessary repeat celiotomy.

INTRODUCTION

Horses that require a repeat celiotomy during the same hospitalization period as the first surgery (defined as early repeat celiotomy) can constitute 5% to 15% of all surgical colic cases, mostly in horses treated for small intestinal diseases.[1–13] In this article, the emphasis will be on early repeat celiotomy after small intestinal surgery, although large intestinal diseases will be addressed briefly.

Surgeons can experience a considerable mental block to repeat celiotomy, largely because of the possible perception of a surgical error,[2] and such errors can account for 33% to 57% of early repeat celiotomies.[4,9] The decision for repeat celiotomy relies on many of the same diagnostic approaches as for the first surgery but with the additional possible finding of a deviation from the expected response to that surgery.[1] This applies to signs of postoperative colic (POC), which should usually be eliminated by the first surgery. Postoperative reflux (POR) and systemic inflammatory response syndrome (endotoxemia) should also be resolved by the first surgery but their persistence

University of Florida, College of Veterinary Medicine, Gainesville, FL, USA
* Corresponding author.
E-mail address: freemand@ufl.edu

Vet Clin Equine 39 (2023) 325–337
https://doi.org/10.1016/j.cveq.2023.03.012
0749-0739/23/© 2023 Elsevier Inc. All rights reserved.
vetequine.theclinics.com

can be erroneously accepted as a typical response to small intestinal surgery.[10] Recognition of risk factors for repeat celiotomy could also guide the decision, such as jejunocecostomy at the first surgery.[9,11–13]

INDICATIONS FOR REPEAT CELIOTOMY

The most common reasons for repeat celiotomy are POR and POC.[1,6,9] Although POC can be managed by nasogastric decompression and analgesic drugs, severe signs can demand a more aggressive approach.[1,4,7] Suspicion of a postoperative bleeder is a tempting reason for repeat celiotomy but identification of the responsible vessel can be difficult.[14] Although POR is regarded largely as postoperative ileus (POI), a dysmotility induced by surgical manipulation, it is more likely a multifactorial response with possible causes that require surgical treatment.[1,10] However, this presents a unique challenge because the clinical manifestation of POR is the same, regardless of a functional or physical cause.[2] A favorable response to medical treatment is possible in most horses with POR[15] but this response neither confirms POI nor rules out a minor technical problem or physical obstruction that resolves with time.[5] The degree of pain in horses with POR varies and contributes little to the distinction between POI and a physical obstruction.[2,16] Some horses with POR can initially display mild-to-moderate signs of colic that seem to resolve after gastric decompression.

Difficulty in maintaining either a packed cell volume (PCV) less than 50% after 24 hours of fluid therapy or an increasing PCV and decreasing total plasma protein concentration could support the decision for a repeat celiotomy.[2,17] Although increasing heart rate could indicate the need for repeat celiotomy,[17,18] this can be misleading. Attempts have been made to identify clinical features of POR that would distinguish between POI and a physical obstruction but the efficacy of these has not been tested.[18] The volume and duration of reflux can be similar in a horse with a surgical reason for POR as in horses with a presumptive medical reason.[15] Postoperative fever was associated with finding a surgical cause of POR in one study but a cause and effect relationship between these complications could not be determined.[15] However, in a potential candidate for repeat celiotomy, a persistent fever could be another contributor to the decision process.[15]

Transabdominal sonographic examination can fail to distinguish between physical obstruction and POI because both cause small intestinal distention, static hypomotile loops of normal wall thickness, and sedimentation of contents. Sonographic examination can be used to assess the linea alba closure if it is considered the problem,[6] as related to disruption, adhesions, and entrapment or inclusion of intestine in it. Sonographic examination and abdominocentesis can be used to diagnose postoperative hemorrhage or peritonitis. Abdominal palpation per rectum is of limited value compared with sonographic examination and could stress the abdominal closure.[19] Diagnostic findings per rectum might include cecal impaction,[20] small intestinal distention, or a tight mesenteric band.[9] Abdominocentesis is helpful if the horse has severe septic peritonitis but increased peritoneal fluid neutrophils and total protein can be expected within the first week of the initial surgery.[21] A repeat celiotomy should be regarded as an important diagnostic procedure, in the same way as the first surgery was considered.

TIMING OF REPEAT CELIOTOMY

Early repeat celiotomy is usually related in time to the first surgery,[6] although the duration of signs is probably a more critical issue.[1] The time element is important because prolonged medical treatment can put a repeat celiotomy beyond the owner's financial reach, create complications from protracted treatment, including those related to fluid therapy and delayed feeding, and favor adhesion formation. A tendency to overemphasize the role of POI in pathogenesis of POR can evoke the need for protracted medical therapy and thereby delay the need for a repeat celiotomy. However, underestimating the importance of POI could prompt an unnecessary repeat celiotomy.[15] The authors' approach for POR that persists for the first 24 hours after it starts is to discuss the possible need for repeat celiotomy with the owner. If POR decreases in volume during the first 24 to 48 hours, continued medical treatment is justified; however, persistence to 48 hours and beyond should invoke a stronger consideration for repeat celiotomy. Signs of POC, especially if difficult to control, can force an earlier decision than POR.

TEAMWORK FOR REPEAT CELIOTOMY

Even experienced surgeons have limited experience with repeat celiotomy, and many lesions that necessitate a second surgery can be subtle and different to what is typically encountered in colic surgery. Ideally, an experienced surgeon should be involved in the repeat celiotomy.[2] An experienced surgeon can guide the decision to reoperate and can expedite the surgery so that the horse's chances of survival are improved.

APPROACH AND EXPLORATION

The high incisional infection rate in the original midline incision if reused[1] could justify a paramedian approach[22] (**Fig. 1**). If the paramedian and original ventral midline

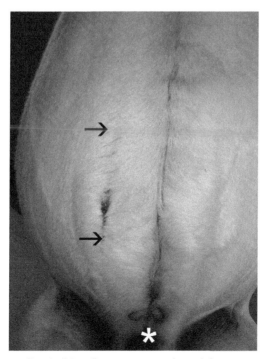

Fig. 1. Healed paramedian incision (between *arrows*) used for repeat celiotomy because midline incision was infected. Although the paramedian incision became infected, both incisions healed without forming hernias. Prepuce is indicated (*asterisk*).

incisions both become infected,[6] the abdominal wall can be weakened. However, full recovery and return to expected use is still possible (**Fig. 2**).

If the original incision is used, the ventral abdomen is scrubbed and draped as for any celiotomy, the adhesive skin drape is incised along the original incision, and skin sutures are removed. Instruments used to that point are discarded and gloves are changed.[17] The exposed subcutaneous tissues can be rinsed with sterile physiologic saline and wiped gently to remove the excess solution and blood clots.[17] The subcutaneous and linea alba sutures are removed by cutting each strand below the knots. Granulation tissue and draining tracts can be debrided as part of the surgical approach or immediately before closure. An alternative approach is to remove the skin sutures during the preliminary scrub, so that the linea alba edges can be scrubbed. This approach might be preferred by some surgeons but could be irritating to raw tissue edges.

In most cases, peritoneal surfaces are not inflamed and peritoneal fluid is sparse and serosanguinous. The degree of small intestinal distention can be less than expected, possibly because of effective preoperative decompression through a nasogastric tube. The anastomosis or previously strangulated segment should be sought by tracing from the ileocecal fold orally. The anastomosis should be exteriorized with care to void damage to it and should be checked for a kink or excess tension caused by an error in placement or orientation.[17] A jejunocecal anastomosis can be difficult to exteriorize, especially if it's most aboral part was placed high on the cecal body. Access can be improved with careful traction on the cecum and possibly exteriorization of the large colon. Some fibrin might be evident on the anastomosis and surrounding tissues (**Fig. 3**) but this can resolve in time. Serositis close to or on an anastomosis or enterotomy is not unusual and possibly not clinically important unless associated with another finding. Peritonitis is usually evident as excess serosanguinous peritoneal fluid with numerous fibrin tags (**Fig. 4**). If accompanied by an odor, then intestinal leakage from an anastomosis, enterotomy, or ruptured viscus should be suspected.

TYPICAL FINDINGS

Potential causes of postoperative obstruction that indicate a need for early repeat celiotomy can be categorized as failure to correct the original lesion, development

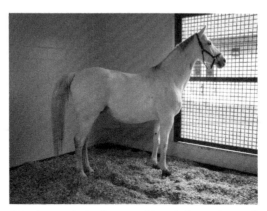

Fig. 2. Horse in **Fig. 1** to demonstrate absence of hernia formation and satisfactory abdominal contour, despite infection in midline and paramedian incisions after repeat celiotomy 6 years previously.

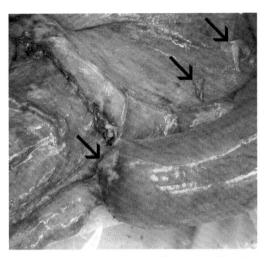

Fig. 3. Impacted jejunojejunostomy that caused reflux in less than 12 hours after the first surgery (before feeding) and necessitated a repeat celiotomy 38 hours postoperatively. Note fibrin tags on intestine and mesentery (*arrows*).

of a new lesion, recurrence of the primary lesion, or surgery-related complication. The most common pathologic or obstructive findings are stenosis or impaction at an anastomosis (see **Fig. 3**), distended small intestine (as the sole finding or secondary to an obstruction), adhesions, torsion/volvulus, flexion, intussusception, and intestinal

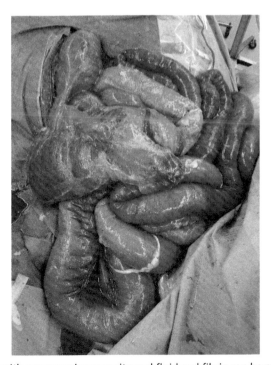

Fig. 4. Peritonitis with serosanguinous peritoneal fluid and fibrin can be managed in milder cases if the cause can be eliminated.

ischemia or necrosis.[1,2,4,8,9,12,16,23–25] Although focal adhesions usually cause obstruction after hospital discharge, they can cause POR and POC during hospitalization,[24] even within 5 days after surgery.[9] Although anastomotic impaction is regarded as a risk of early feeding, it usually develops before feed is offered, probably with dry matter already in the stomach.[1,2,9,25] Consequently, this common cause of postoperative obstruction should not be ruled out because of an early onset of signs, and can develop in all anastomoses, including jejunocecostomy (**Fig. 5**), with a possible greater risk with jejunoileostomy. Jejunoileostomy was associated with more repeat celiotomies in one study than with other small intestinal anastomoses,[26] which can be related to anastomotic impaction in the author's experience.[9]

Vascular complications can develop from failure to ligate a mesenteric vessel during resection, failure to accurately identify nonviable intestine, progression of vascular changes from the primary disease, continued ileal necrosis, coagulopathy, and venous thrombosis in one or more sites.[1,24–28] Mucosal ischemia extending orally or aborally from an anastomosis might not be apparent on inspection of the serosal surface.[1] Less common lesions revealed at repeat celiotomy include anastomotic leakage, mesenteric hematoma, blind-loop syndrome, mesenteric abscess, gastric impaction.[1–3,5,9,26]

TREATMENTS AT REPEAT CELIOTOMY

Treatment of the obstruction revealed at repeat celiotomy should include the prevention of recurrence whenever possible. For example, manual disruption or softening of an impacted jejunojejunostomy by water infusion by any means could risk reimpaction because of stenosis or a possible functional defect that interrupts transit. Consequently, resection and revision of an impacted anastomosis are recommended. Conversion to jejunocecostomy is recommended for an impacted jejunoileostomy. An impacted jejunocecostomy is difficult to revise because opportunities for the replacement on the cecum are limited. Instead, lavage through a jejunal enterotomy followed by the extension of the oral end of the anastomosis should be effective[29] (**Fig. 6**).

Adhesions to the anastomosis or nearby intestine usually require adhesiolysis and even resection of the involved intestine and anastomosis.[8] Extensive and mature adhesions are usually beyond treatment. Anastomotic leakage is a very rare complication in small intestine, and it can be treated by resection of the affected anastomosis.

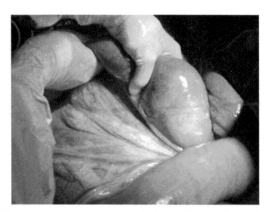

Fig. 5. Impacted jejunocecostomy at repeat celiotomy. Manual breakdown of such impactions can be traumatic (see text).

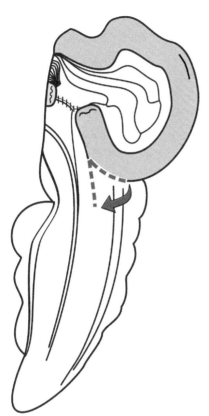

Fig. 6. Incisions required in jejunum and cecum (*red broken lines*) to extend a stoma considered too small in a horse diagnosed with impacted jejunocecostomy at repeat celiotomy. The edges thus created are apposed from jejunum to cecum to end at the red arrow. The impaction is resolved beforehand (see text) through an enterotomy in jejunum about 1 m from the anastomosis, indicated by the short black line.

Abdominal lavage might be required if obvious septic peritonitis has developed. A focal leak in a jejunocecostomy could be repaired with interrupted sutures without resection if the margins are viable[17] and the lumen can be preserved because revision and relocation to another site on the cecum is difficult.

If a jejunocecostomy needs revision at early repeat celiotomy, the jejunum is detached from the cecum and resected as needed and the remaining opening in the cecum can be used for the revised handsewn side-to-side or end-to-side anastomosis. Any excess in the cecal opening is closed separately to meet the new anastomosis. Placing the new anastomosis further distally or laterally on the cecum (between the dorsal and lateral cecal bands) or even bypass of the cecum with a jejunocolostomy might be considered in some cases.

In horses that have had a small intestinal strangulation, the large colon can acquire a "vacuum-packed" appearance (**Fig. 7**), presumably the consequence of correcting systemic dehydration by intense water absorption from the large intestine.[30] Response to colotomy for the removal of dehydrated contents can be favorable, even when this is the only procedure performed at repeat celiotomy following a primary small intestinal disease.[1] This response can be explained by the observation

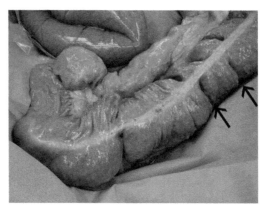

Fig. 7. Vacuum-packed ventral colon at repeat celiotomy with deep crenellations (*arrows* on examples) caused by dehydration and contraction of contents. Removal of such contents by colotomy could contribute to resolution of reflux.

that such impactions can be slow to resolve, which could delay cecal emptying and thereby cause downstream resistance to small intestinal transit.

EXPECTED RESPONSE TO REPEAT CELIOTOMY

In most cases, early repeat celiotomy saves horses that might otherwise die but it can also terminate a hopeless case at a reasonable cost and with reduced suffering.[1] Most horses should demonstrate an immediate favorable response to a repeat celiotomy, evident as improved attitude and interest in food shortly after recovery from anesthesia. After a repeat celiotomy, horses can be fed according to a typical postoperative schedule,[9] thereby deriving full benefits from early postoperative feeding. Early feeding and voluntary water consumption can be beneficial through reducing IV fluid therapy and hospital stay.

Finding "nothing abnormal" at the second surgery and only decompressing distended small intestine might lead to a favorable outcome. It might also indicate that a lesion was missed. This could be attributed to the rarity of some complications and their subtle manifestation, such as an anastomosis that does not function normally despite normal physical appearance. The intestine is usually distended proximal to the anastomosis in such cases. Repeat celiotomy would seem counterintuitive as a treatment of POR because of the risk of exacerbating POI through intestinal manipulation.[31] However, one study on small intestinal strangulation reported that manual decompression resolved POR in 3 of 4 horses,[8] possibly by eliminating some of the adverse effects of persistent intestinal distention.[32,33] In a more recent study on strangulating diseases in the jejunum, repeat celiotomy (1 or 2) completely eliminated POR in 81% of horses with this complication and eliminated POC in all horses[1] (**Fig. 8**). Apparently, tissue handling associated with the second surgery, possibly as much or more than at the first surgery, does not increase the risk of POR[1] (see **Fig. 8**).

COMPLICATIONS AND SURVIVAL RATES

Short-term postoperative complications following repeat celiotomy include incisional complications and adhesions. If the original ventral midline incision is reused, the risk of postoperative incisional infection and hernia formation is approximately 4-fold higher compared with a single celiotomy in the same hospitals.[1,4,6,9,34] This suggests

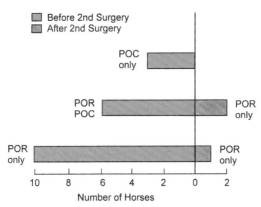

Fig. 8. Response to repeat celiotomy in 19 horses recovered from surgery to treat POR only, POR and POC, and POC only. Repeat surgery resolved POC in all horses, and 1 or 2 repeated surgeries resolved POR in all but 3 with this complication. (*Data from* Ref.[1])

a deep infection with profound adverse effects on wound healing.[6] The high rate of incisional complications after repeat celiotomy can reduce client satisfaction and return to athletic activity, and increase cost of treatment. Consequently, this risk must be included in the decision process, balanced against the life-saving benefits.

Repeat celiotomy has earned a negative reputation, largely based on highly variable short-term survival rates compared with a single surgery (27% to 86% survival for repeat celiotomy).[1–4,6–9,23,26,27,35] Long-term studies suggest a decline in survival rates,[3,4,6–9,27] possibly because of a greater risk of adhesion formation than after a single surgery.[2,4,36] Horses that had multiple celiotomies in one study were almost 3 times less likely to start a race compared with horses that had only one colic surgery.[37] However, some horses can survive to the ends of their expected life spans after repeat celiotomy.[1,38]

Intraoperative euthanasia has been identified as the most common cause of death for horses that had a repeat celiotomy[2–4,35] at 21% to 30%, probably because of financial constraints, irreparable lesions,[7] and a poor prognosis.[35] Findings that lead to euthanasia during repeat celiotomy include severe peritonitis with extensive fibrin deposition and adhesions (**Fig. 4**), intestinal rupture or necrosis, or uncontrollable intra-abdominal bleeding.[2] Reasons for euthanasia after repeat celiotomy are peritonitis, ischemic intestinal necrosis, ruptured viscus, anastomotic leakage, obstructive adhesions, POR, POC, severe endotoxemic shock, and colitis.[3,4,39]

A favorable prognosis for survival[7] and a positive response to a second surgery have been associated with POC as the clinical indicator for repeat celiotomy[1] (see **Fig. 8**). Possibly uncontrollable pain pushes the surgeon and owner to a repeat surgery promptly, whereas other complications, including POR and peritonitis, can have a more insidious course and induce a lower sense of urgency. A favorable outcome could also be expected in a horse with distended small intestine at the second surgery,[1,7] possibly because this finding is associated with a lesion that is amenable to correction. Increased PCV at 24 hours after the first surgery, peritonitis as the reason for repeat celiotomy, and adhesions as the major findings at the second surgery yield a poor prognosis for recovery.[7]

WHEN TO STOP

Horses can undergo repeat celiotomy 2 or more times during the same hospitalization, and survive to hospital discharge.[1,3–5,9,24] If repeat celiotomy reveals an untreatable problem, such as extensive adhesions, peritonitis from a nontreatable source (see **Fig. 4**), and hemorrhage from an inaccessible vessel, euthanasia spares the horse from further suffering and the owner from the expense of protracted and ineffective medical treatment.

SUMMARY—SMALL INTESTINAL SURGERY

- No single guideline should be interpreted in isolation as an indicator of repeat celiotomy, with the possible exception of uncontrollable POC.
- Delays in repeat celiotomy consume the owner's finances to the point that a repeat celiotomy is beyond his/her financial reach and might adversely affect the outcome.
- Owners should be informed of the need for a second surgery shortly after the relevant complications develop.
- Overemphasis on POI and its treatment can delay the decision process for a repeat celiotomy.
- If in doubt about an anastomosis at repeat celiotomy, it should be resected, especially if it was impacted.
- Future studies should focus on ways to reduce incisional complications after repeat celiotomy.
- A critical goal of repeat celiotomy is to learn why the first surgery failed and then to take that information to subsequent cases.

LARGE INTESTINE

The prevalence of POR is low after surgery for large colon diseases, and hence, a repeat celiotomy is rarely indicated after this surgery. However, large colon displacements are common causes of colic in horses and many of them, especially right dorsal displacement of the colon, nephrosplenic entrapment (NSE), and large colon volvulus (LCV) can recur.[40] However, recurrence of these diseases is usually, but not always, later in the postoperative course, within weeks to months after hospital discharge. Consequently, when these horses are presented with a recurrent episode, their abdominal incision has healed and they are in favorable systemic and cardiovascular states. However, a preventive procedure might need to be considered by owner and surgeon for these cases, such as colopexy or colon resection, or, in the case of NSE, nephrosplenic space ablation.

Horses treated for impaction of the small colon at the first surgery could be at some risk of reimpaction, especially in a small equid or foal. However, this is rare. A pelvic flexure enterotomy can be performed at the first surgery to remove colon bulk and thereby decrease this risk. A rare indication for repeat celiotomy in the large colon is severe melena caused by a bleeding vessel in a colotomy.[41] Recurrence of a cecal impaction is always a concern after the first surgical treatment of this disease,[20,42] especially if a jejunocolostomy is not performed or if a predisposing orthopedic disease persists.[20,42] Recurrent cecal impaction can be late in the postoperative period but can also develop within a few days after the first surgery. Colon resection can cause POC but this is usually managed medically rather than by repeat celiotomy, and usually resolves within 24 hours after onset. Repeat celiotomy because of poor postoperative progress after large colon resection is usually unsuccessful, presumably because of the greater bacterial and endotoxin loads from the colon and limited access for further resection. A repeat celiotomy after correction of an LCV, without resection, is rarely successful, even if the colon is resected at the second surgery. Examples of large intestinal diseases that can be missed at the first surgery and cause persistent POC are small colon strangulation by lipoma,[4] a small colon enterolith,[43] or impaction in the cecal cupola.[44]

DISCLOSURE

The authors have no relationship with a commercial company that has a direct financial interest in subject matter or materials discussed in this article. The authors did not receive any financial support for any part of this study.

REFERENCES

1. Bauck AJ, Easley JT, Cleary OB, et al. Response to early repeat celiotomy in horses after a first surgery for jejunal strangulation. Vet Surg 2016;46:843–50.
2. Huskamp B, Bonfig H. Relaparotomy as a therapeutic principle in postoperative complications of horses with colic. Proc Equine Colic Res Symp 1985;2:317–21.
3. Parker JE, Fubini SL, Todhunter RJ. Retrospective evaluation of repeat celiotomy in 53 horses with acute gastrointestinal disease. Vet Surg 1989;18:424–31.
4. Mair TS, Smith LJ. Survival and complication rates in 300 horses undergoing surgical treatment of colic. Part 4: early (acute) relaparotomy. Equine Vet J 2005;37:315–8.
5. Gorvy DA, Edwards GB, Proudman CJ. Intra-abdominal adhesions in horses: a retrospective evaluation of repeat laparotomy in 99 horses with acute gastrointestinal disease. Vet J 2008;175:194–201.
6. Dunkel B, Mair TS, Marr CM, et al. Indications, complications, and outcome of horses undergoing repeated celiotomy within 14 days after the first colic surgery: 95 cases (2005-2013). J Am Vet Med Assoc 2015;246:540–6.
7. Findley JA, Burgess R, Salem S, et al. Factors associated with survival of horses following relaparotomy. Equine Vet J 2016. https://doi.org/10.1111/evj.12635.
8. Vachon AM, Fischer AT. Small intestinal herniation through the epiploic foramen: 53 cases (1987-1993). Equine Vet J 1995;27:373–80.
9. Freeman DE, Hammock P, Baker GJ, et al. Short- and long-term survival and prevalence of postoperative ileus after small intestinal surgery in the horse. Equine Vet J Suppl 2000;32:42–51.
10. Freeman D. Post-operative reflux – a surgeon's perspective. Equine Vet Educ 2018;30:671–80.
11. Pankowski RL. Small intestinal surgery in the horse: A review of ileo and jejunocecostomy. J Am Vet Med Assoc 1987;190:1608.
12. Holcombe SJ, Rodriguez KM, Haupt JL, et al. Prevalence of and risk factors for postoperative ileus after small intestinal surgery in two hundred and thirty-three horses. Vet Surg 2009;38:368.
13. Espinosa P, Le Jeune SS, Cenani A, et al. Investigation of perioperative and anesthetic variables affecting short-term survival of horses with small intestinal strangulating lesions. Vet Surg 2017;46:345–53.
14. Gray SN, Dechant JE, LeJeune SS, et al. Identification, management and outcome of postoperative hemoperitoneum in 23 horses after emergency exploratory celiotomy for gastrointestinal disease. Vet Surg 2015;44:379–85.
15. Jacobs CC, Stefanovski D, Southwood LL. Use of perioperative variables to determine the requirement for repeat celiotomy in horses with postoperative reflux after small intestinal surgery. Vet Surg 2019;48:1204–10.
16. Hunt JM, Edwards GB, Clarke KW. Incidence, diagnosis and treatment of postoperative complications in colic cases. Equine Vet J 1986;18:264–70.

17. Ducharme NG. Repeat laparotomy. In: Mair T, Divers T, Ducharme N, editors. Manual of equine Gastroenterology. London: W.B. Saunders Co.; 2000. p. 184–7.

18. Merritt AM, Blikslager AT. Postoperative ileus: to be or not to be? Equine Vet J 2008;40:295–6.

19. Kirker-Head CA, Kerwin PJ, Steckel RR, et al. The in vivo biodynamic properties of the intact equine linea alba. Equine Vet J Suppl 1989;7:97–106.

20. Smith LCR, Payne RJ, Boys Smith SJ, et al. Outcome and long-term follow-up of 20 horses undergoing surgery for caecal impaction: A retrospective study (2000–2008). Equine Vet J 2010;42:388–92.

21. Santschi EM, Grindem CB, Tate LP, et al. Peritoneal fluid analysis in ponies after abdominal surgery. Vet Surg 1988;17:6–9.

22. Anderson SL, Vacek JR, Macharg MA, et al. Occurrence of incisional complications and associated risk factors using a right ventral paramedian celiotomy incision in 159 horses. Vet Surg 2011;40:82–9.

23. Mezerova J, Zert Z, Kabes R, et al. Analysis of therapeutic results and complications after colic surgery in 434 horses. Vet Med 2008;53:12–28.

24. MacDonald MH, Pascoe JR, Stover SM, et al. Survival after small intestine resection and anastomosis in horses. Vet Surg 1989;18:415–23.

25. Freeman DE, Schaeffer DJ. Clinical comparison between a continuous Lembert pattern wrapped in a carboxymethylcellulose and hyaluronate membrane with an interrupted Lembert pattern for one-layer jejunojejunostomy in horses. Equine Vet J 2011;43:708–13.

26. Stewart S, Southwood LL, Aceto HW. Comparison of short- and long-term complications and survival following jejunojejunostomy, jejunoileostomy and jejunocaecostomy in 112 horses: 2005-2010. Equine Vet J 2014;46:333–8.

27. van den Boom R, van der Velden MA. Short- and long-term evaluation of surgical treatment of strangulating obstructions of the small intestine in horses: a review of 224 cases. Vet Quart 2001;23:109–15.

28. Martin-Cuervo M, Gracia LA, Vieitez V, et al. Postsurgical segmental mesenteric ischemic thrombosis in a horse. Can Vet J 2013;54:83–5.

29. Bauck AG and Freeman DE. Review of repeat celiotomy following small intestinal strangulation: decision guidelines, intraoperative findings, and outcomes. Proceedings of the 64th Annual Meeting of American Association of Equine Practitioners. San Francisco, California. pp. 401-406, 2018.

30. Lester GD, Merritt AM, Kuck HV, et al. Systemic, renal, and colonic effects of intravenous and enteral rehydration in horses. J Vet Intern Med 2013;27:554–66.

31. Bauer AJ, Boeckxstaens GE. Mechanisms of postoperative ileus. Neuro Gastroenterol Motil 2004;16(Suppl 2):54–60.

32. Dabareiner RM, Sullins KE, White NA, et al. Serosal injury in the equine jejunum and ascending colon after ischemia-reperfusion or intraluminal distention and decompression. Vet Surg 2001;30:114.

33. Dabareiner RM, White NA, Donaldson LL. Effects of intraluminal distention and decompression on microvascular permeability and hemodynamics of the equine jejunum. Am J Vet Res 2001;62:225–36.

34. Gibson KT, Curtis CR, Turner AS, et al. Incisional hernias in the horse incidence and predisposing factors. Vet Surg 1989;18:360–6.

35. Morton AJ, Blikslager AT. Surgical and postoperative factors influencing short-term survival of horses following small intestinal resection: 92 cases (1994-2001). Equine Vet J 2002;34:450–4.

36. Mair TS, Smith LJ. Survival and complication rates in 300 horses undergoing surgical treatment of colic. Part 3: Long-term complications. Equine Vet J 2005;37: 310–4.
37. Santschi EM, Slone DE, Embertson RM, et al. Colic surgery in 206 juvenile Thoroughbreds: Survival and racing results. Equine Vet J Suppl 2000;32:32–6.
38. Freeman DE, Schaeffer DJ. A comparison of handsewn versus stapled jejunocecostomy in horses - complications and long-term survival: 32 cases (1994-2005). J Am Vet Med Assoc 2010;237:1060–7 [Erratum appears in J Am Vet Med Assoc 2011;238:65].
39. French NB, Edwards GB, Smith JE, et al. Long term survival of equine colic cases. Part 3: Risk factors for postoperative complications. Equine Vet J 2002; 34:443–9.
40. Smith LJ, Mair TS. Are horses that undergo an exploratory laparotomy for correction of a right dorsal displacement of the large colon predisposed to postoperative colic, compared to other forms of large colon displacement? Equine Vet J 2010;42:44–6.
41. Doyle AJ, Freeman DE, Rapp H, et al. Life-threatening hemorrhage from enterotomies and anastomoses in 7 horses. Vet Surg 2003;32:553–8.
42. Aitken MR, Southwood LL, Ross BM, et al. Outcome of Surgical and Medical Management of Cecal Impaction in 150 Horses (1991–2011). Vet Surg 2015; 44:540–6.
43. Blikslager AT, Bowman KF, Levine JF, et al. Evaluation of factors associated with postoperative ileus in horses: 31 cases (1990-1992). J Am Vet Med Assoc 1994; 205:1748–52.
44. Sherlock CE, Eggleston RB. Clinical signs, treatment, and prognosis for horses with impaction of the cranial aspect of the base of the cecum: 7 cases (2000-2010). J Am Vet Med Assoc 2013;243:1596–601.

Role of Laparoscopy in Diagnosis and Management of Equine Colic

Ann Martens, DVM, PhD, Dip. ECVS*, Hanna Haardt, DVM

KEYWORDS

- Laparoscopy • Horse • Colic • Diagnosis • Treatment • Nephrosplenic • Adhesion

KEY POINTS

- Laparoscopy is most commonly used for diagnosis and treatment of chronic recurrent colic in horses.
- Laparoscopy can be performed in standing and recumbent horses depending on the area of interest.
- Preventative measures such as closure of anatomic spaces, as well as treatment of some acute causes of colic, and taking biopsies for further diagnostic testing can be performed.

INTRODUCTION

Laparoscopy in horses was first described in 1970 in mares for characterization of reproductive events.[1,2] The first description of laparoscopy on horses with abdominal abnormalities was published in 1986 by Fischer and colleagues.[3] Since then laparoscopy has become a frequently used diagnostic and surgical tool in equine medicine.[4] Presently, equine laparoscopy is most commonly used for the diagnosis and treatment of disorders of the urogenital tract, with the two most common procedures being laparoscopic ovariectomy and cryptorchidectomy. Nevertheless, laparoscopy has also found its place in the broad field of diagnosis, treatment, and prevention of several gastrointestinal disorders causing colic in horses.

Horses with acute abdominal pain are generally poor patients for laparoscopic exploration and treatment, as they are often too painful to be restrained in stocks for standing laparoscopy. Moreover, horses with acute abdominal pain typically have distended intestines, which preclude good visualization of the abdomen and increase the chance of inadvertent intestinal puncture when introducing a trocar. Therefore, laparoscopy is most commonly performed in horses with chronic recurrent colic to establish a diagnosis, take biopsies, or if possible, perform a treatment. Globally,

Department of Large Animal Surgery, Anaesthesia and Orthopaedics, Faculty of Veterinary Medicine, Ghent University, Salisburylaan 133, 9820 Merelbeke, Belgium
* Corresponding author.
E-mail address: ann.martens@ugent.be

Vet Clin Equine 39 (2023) 339–349
https://doi.org/10.1016/j.cveq.2023.03.003
0749-0739/23/© 2023 Elsevier Inc. All rights reserved.

the diagnostic sensitivity of laparoscopy for recurrent colic and or weight loss was 63% to 66%, whereas the diagnostic specificity was low (17%–25%), meaning that the cause of colic or weight loss can often be missed.[5,6]

SYSTEMATIC LAPAROSCOPIC VISUALIZATION OF THE EQUINE ABDOMEN

Laparoscopy can be performed in the standing or recumbent horse. The left flank and right flank approaches in the standing horse as well as the ventral approach in the dorsally recumbent horse have different indications and offer a different view and approach to the abdominal structures. For either procedure, it is strongly advised to withhold feed for at least 12 hours before surgery to facilitate safe access to the abdomen and maximize visualization of the abdominal organs.[5] The authors prefer a fasting period of 24 to 36 hours in which horses are also walked to encourage defecation. Water should not be withheld.

Standing Laparoscopy

Laparoscopy is most frequently performed in the standing, sedated horse with infiltration of the flank region with local anesthetic. This approach has the advantage of avoiding the risks of general anesthesia and providing a good view and access to several abdominal organs that can be involved in pathology causing colic (eg, nephrosplenic space, epiploic foramen (EF), inguinal rings, and diaphragm). Moreover, standing laparoscopy is also more suitable for horses in which general anesthesia seems undesirable due to old age, weakness due to chronic diseases, or severe lameness.

Depending on the region of interest and procedure planned, the left or right flank is approached by making a stab incision through the skin just dorsal to the crus of the internal abdominal oblique muscle, halfway between the tuber coxae and the last rib.[5] In general, it is considered safer to make this portal on the left side of the abdomen due to the risk of inadvertently puncturing the cecum on the right side.[7] Palpation per rectum can be used to check for cecal distention before making a portal on the right side. Overall, the authors consider the risks of intestinal damage minimal if the correct technique and appropriate instrumentation are used for a first portal on the right side. A cannula with conical obturator is introduced through the abdominal muscles aiming toward the opposite coxofemoral joint. After removal of the trocar, air is allowed to spontaneously enter the abdomen by introducing a slim instrument into the outer opening of the cannula. Then, a laparoscope is introduced into the cannula, and the abdomen is insufflated with carbon dioxide to a pressure of approximately 15 mm Hg. Instrument portals are made under direct vision in the locations needed for the planned procedure. Typically, one portal is made between the 17th and 18th rib and the laparoscope is switched to that portal to allow free instrument manipulation through several flank portals.

The anatomy visible on laparoscopy has been thoroughly described. From the left flank, parts of the diaphragm, liver, stomach, spleen, left kidney and segments of jejunum, descending and ascending colon as well as the urinary bladder, rectum, ovary, and uterus in mares and vaginal ring in males are visible. From the right flank parts of the liver including its caudate process, the stomach including the pylorus, the EF and omental bursa, the duodenum, the base of the cecum, the right dorsal colon, segments of the jejunum, descending, and ascending colon, urinary bladder and right reproductive organs as well as the rectum can be evaluated.[7]

Recumbent Laparoscopy

As mentioned above, standing laparoscopy is unsuitable for acute colic in most cases. The need for the horse to remain still and standing is alleviated during recumbent laparoscopy. However, many clinicians prefer an open approach to the abdomen for easier manipulation of the intestines. Colic-related interventions described using a recumbent laparoscopic approach include adhesiolysis and colopexy,[6] but this approach could also be used to obtain intestinal biopsies.

In the dorsally recumbent horse, the ventral part of the abdomen can be inspected laparoscopically. For access to the abdomen, a ventral portal is made at the caudal extend of the umbilical depression.[6] A cannula with a blunt obturator is introduced into the abdomen. Care must be taken to avoid penetration of the intestines and lifting the abdominal wall using Backhaus towel clamps placed on the linea alba close to the stab incision can help to prevent this. Alternatively, a teat cannula can be used for safe abdominal access. The following steps are identical to the approach for standing laparoscopy including introduction of the laparoscope and insufflation of the abdominal cavity. Further portals are created as needed for the respective procedure. In the cranial region of the abdomen, the following structures can be found: ventral surface of the diaphragm, falciform ligament and round ligaments of the liver, ventral portion of the liver, spleen, right and left ventral colons, sternal flexure of the ascending colon, apex of the cecum, and stomach.[8] Good visualization of the caudal region of the abdomen is facilitated by positioning the horse in Trendelenburg position (elevation of the caudal portion of the body up to 30°, ensuring that the horse is fixed to the table well). Structures that can be observed in the caudal abdomen are the urinary bladder, mesorchium and ductus deferens (left and right), vaginal ring (left and right), insertion of the prepubic tendon, various segments of jejunum and descending colon, pelvic flexure of the ascending colon, body of the cecum, and cecocolic fold.

INTESTINAL BIOPSY AND TREATMENT OF SMALL INTESTINAL LESIONS

As mentioned, laparoscopy is often used for the minimally invasive diagnosis of causes of chronic weight loss and recurrent colic. Inflammatory bowel disease, grass sickness, and neoplasia are common causes and can be diagnosed by taking biopsies of the small intestine with the aid of laparoscopy. To identify the appropriate section for sampling, the small intestine must be evaluated in its entirety. To achieve the maximum visibility, a right flank approach should be used. According to Schambourg and Marcoux, this allows for 15 to 20 cm of the duodenum and about 40 cm more of the ileum to be viewed compared with a standard ventral midline laparotomy.[9] The exploration of the small intestine starts at the level of the duodenum. Its short mesentery keeps it in place, and minimal manipulation is necessary. The long mesentery of the jejunum, however, makes running of the small intestine imperative. This is readily performed using two atraumatic clamps to pass the intestine from the one to the other (**Fig. 1**, Video 1). Schambourg and Marcoux state that Babcock clamps provide inadequate purchase and recommend the use of Kelly or atraumatic intestinal forceps.[9]

Once the appropriate segment of the small intestine for biopsy is identified, the surgeon can chose between two different techniques: one involves intracorporeal suturing or stapling and the other one relies on exteriorization of the small intestinal segment of which the biopsies are taken. The latter technique is the most straightforward to perform in the authors' experience.

The intracorporeal technique comes with two options. Schambourg and Marcoux describe a two-step biopsy procedure during which first only serosa and muscularis are removed with laparoscopic scissors. The incision is then partially closed with a Lembert pattern, ensuring that the submucosa and mucosa are everted through the non-sutured part of the incision. Kelly clamps are used to keep traction on the submucosa and mucosa, which are then resected using scissors before closing the incision

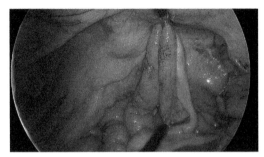

Fig. 1. Running the small intestine: a section of jejunum is held with Babcock forceps, whereas another atraumatic intestinal forceps is used to grasp a more aboral section. There is light serosal hemorrhage due to manipulation of the small intestine.

with the last suture.[9] Bracamonte and colleagues describe the use of a 45-mm endoscopic articulating linear stapler (ELS) with a 440-mm shaft: The ELS is applied to the small intestine at a 10-degree angle to the antimesenteric border. The ELS is then reapplied crossing the first cut in a 120-degree angle. This created a V-shaped segment that is safely removed. Bracamonte and colleagues then compared the ELS-technique to a double-layer hand-sewn technique via a laparotomy approach. They found that the segments closed with the ELS had a higher bursting strength and a smaller reduction in luminal diameter than the double-layer hand sewn segments.[10]

For the extracorporeal biopsy technique, the abdomen is first examined laparoscopically. Then, a 10-cm grid flank laparotomy incision is made through which the small intestine can be exteriorized. In order to choose the appropriate segment, the length of the accessible intestine can either be manipulated intra-abdominally with the aid of two atraumatic laparoscopic forceps or be exteriorized and repositioned with hand assistance through the grid incision. The flank incision can be protected with a plastic sleeve (**Fig. 2**A, B, Video 2) to facilitate the atraumatic exteriorization of the intestinal loop and to decrease the risk of incisional infection.[11] A routine biopsy can then be taking using conventional techniques.

Acute small intestinal lesions are typically treated via a ventral midline laparotomy, should medical treatment not be sufficient. However, Klohnen describes the laparoscopic removal of a lipoma in a standing horse.[12] The small intestine had not been compromised in this case. Similarly, Klohnen describes the laparoscopic removal of a lipoma obstructing the small colon.[12] Coomer and colleagues describe the use of laparoscopy for a small intestinal resection by exteriorizing the affected part of the small intestine as described in the previous paragraph. However, the resection only comprised a small section of the small intestine including a small adenocarcinoma.[13]

NEPHROSPLENIC ENTRAPMENT OF THE ASCENDING COLON AND CLOSURE OF THE NEPHROSPLENIC SPACE

Nephrosplenic entrapment of the large colon is a common cause of colic in horses with an incidence rate of 2.5% to 11%.[14] Although acute cases are most commonly treated either conservatively or surgically via a midline laparotomy, Munoz described the laparoscopic treatment of a left dorsal displacement: in a case series of 12 horses the displacement was first corrected in the standing horse using a modified grid laparotomy, after which the nephrosplenic space was closed laparoscopically. The authors first introduced a laparoscope through a 4 to 5 cm long flank incision to

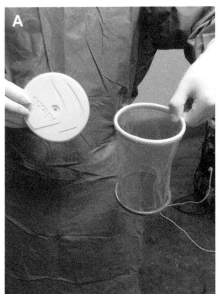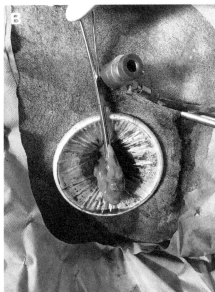

Fig. 2. Use of a plastic sleeve (Alexis O Wound Protector-Retractor, Applied Medical Resources Corporation, Rancho Santa Margarita, USA) for extracorporeal biopsy technique: (*A*) Alexis O protector-retractor with two rings that are connected by a plastic sleeve and a cap to avoid the loss of insufflation of the abdomen when using the ring as a portal and (*B*) the blue ring is placed intra-abdominally, whereas the white retraction ring remains on the skin. The white ring is gently grasped at 10 and 2 o'clock and pulled up until the green ring sits tightly against the peritoneal layer. It is then flipped inward or outward until the desired retraction is achieved. A piece of jejunum has been exteriorized and a biopsy has been taken.

explore the abdomen. After creation of a second portal between the 17th and 18th intercostal space, the first incision was enlarged to exteriorize the colon and allow for decompression and later manual replacement into the ventral abdomen, as well as repositioning of the spleen dorsally to close the nephrosplenic space. The closure of the nephrosplenic space was performed laparoscopically without manual assistance. Eight horses developed minor complications after surgery, 10 horses returned to their intended purpose, whereas the other two were retired or euthanized due to unrelated problems.[15]

Closure of the nephrosplenic space to prevent recurrence of a nephrosplenic entrapment of the large colon is reported in literature. Many different techniques and materials are described to close the space: these include simple suture material, barbed sutures and various implants.[14,16,17] A standard left laparoscopic approach allows for visualization of the nephrosplenic space. A large diameter (25–30 mm) cannula is introduced through the most dorsal left flank portal to allow for direct vision of the nephrosplenic space and to facilitate suturing. Suture material is used as per the surgeon's preference, however, a needle size that just fits through the large diameter cannula while fixed on the needle holder is recommended, as it avoids the challenges of intracorporeal needle repositioning. Barbed suture makes an extracorporeal starting knot redundant and obviates the need to keep the suture tight in between the bites, as the suture cannot glide back through the tissue. The space is closed from cranial to caudal, suturing the perirenal fascia to the splenic capsule (**Fig. 3**A, B, Video 3).

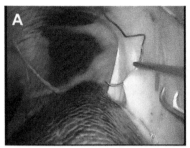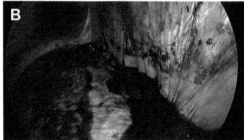

Fig. 3. Closure of the nephrosplenic space, the laparoscope is placed through a portal in the last intercostal space on the left side. A 25 to 30 mm diameter cannula is used for insertion of the needle holder and fixed needle. At this point, there is no gas insufflation of the abdomen. (*A*) The first bite is taken through the renal fascia and splenic capsule. (*B*) Appearance after closure of the nephrosplenic space.

A trocar with incorporated light emitting diode (LED) light (eg, Trocar Large Animal GR®, GR Vet Innovation, Saint Saturnin, 72, France) allows for direct visualization of the nephrosplenic space, making a laparoscope redundant.[18] Yet, when laparoscopic instruments are available, this device does not offer additional benefit.

Alternatively, a polypropylene mesh can be applied to the nephrosplenic space. The mesh needs to be 2 to 4 cm wider than the distance between the perirenal fascia and the spleen. It is draped over the dorsolateral edge of the spleen making sure that the space is sufficiently covered and the mesh lays cranial to the caudal border of the spleen to avoid intestinal adhesions. It is first attached to the renal fascia and then to the splenic capsule using laparoscopic staples or tacking devices.[16,19] Gialletti and colleagues compared the use of mesh and barbed suture for nephrosplenic space ablation and concluded that the suture was faster, more cost-efficient and caused fewer complications.[16] Spagnolo and colleagues described the use of homologous pericardium implants harvested from horses euthanized for orthopedic disease. The study included six Arabian horses without previous related abdominal disease. The complete closure of the nephrosplenic space was achieved in all horses without signs of colic for the 36-month follow-up period.[14]

The reported recurrence rates of nephrosplenic entrapment in horses after laparoscopic closure of the nephrosplenic space are low: Röcken and Nelson reported 0% to 3% recurrence after closure versus 21% to 23% in the control groups.[17,20] Rodriguez described a recurrence of colic of unspecified cause in 19% of horses undergoing closure versus 42% in the control group.[21] In the study by Burke and Parente, none of the horses treated by mesh obliteration showed recurrence of nephrosplenic entrapment. However, 38% of them showed signs of colic within a year after mesh obliteration. This included 15% of horses that had a surgically confirmed diagnosis of nephrosplenic entrapment versus 50% of horses in which the diagnosis was made based on palpation per rectum only. This difference was attributed to the possibility of additional causes of colic that were unrecognized at the time of treatment or an incorrect diagnosis made at presentation.[19] Reasons for recurrence of colic are most commonly other types of displacements or volvulus of the large colon as well as other causes of mild colic or displacement of the colon between the spleen and the body wall.[17,21] In the authors' experience, true nephrosplenic entrapment of the large colon after ablation of the nephrosplenic space only occurs after failure of the mesh or suture.

EPIPLOIC FORAMEN ENTRAPMENT AND PREVENTIVE CLOSURE OF THE FORAMEN

Just like the nephrosplenic space, the EF can be closed to prevent colic associated with intestinal EF entrapment (EFE). Recent work has demonstrated the funnel-like shape of the omental vestibule with two openings: a smaller one on the right side of the median plane, which is the EF, and a large one on the left side, which is the opening from the omental vestibule to the caudal recess of the omental bursa.[22,23] It has been suggested that the funnel-like shape of the equine omental vestibule, as it tapers toward the EF, acts as a trap that allows intestines to enter the wide opening of the omental vestibule, and then move through it from the left to the right toward the smaller EF, where intestines become entrapped.[24] Main risk factors are crib-biting and wind-sucking as well as height and a previous history of colic.[25] Compared with other strangulating small intestinal lesions, EFE has been identified as having a worse prognosis for long-term survival.[26] Recurrence of EFE has been described in 2% to 14% of cases.[23] To prevent entrapment, the EF can be closed laparoscopically through a standing right flank approach. A long (58 cm) 30° laparoscope is advanced cranially between the caudate process of the liver and the duodenum until the EF can be visualized between the base of the caudate process and the hepatoduodenal ligament. The first described technique uses titanium helical coils to staple the gastropancreatic fold to the right lobe of the liver.[27] This resulted in complete closure of the EF in five of the six horses on which this procedure was performed, albeit with a relatively thin fold. The technique described by van Bergen and colleagues uses a self-folded diabolo-shaped polypropylene implant (**Fig. 4**) which is introduced through a stainless steel applicator tube into the EF. The implant is self-retaining and positioned with its smallest part at the level of the portal vein (Video 4). In their study, van Bergen and colleagues successfully closed all EFs of the six horses enrolled.[28] In a further study evaluating this laparoscopic procedure, including 34 horses that had colic surgery due to EFE, the EF had closed spontaneously in 32% of cases, most likely caused by the local inflammation after entrapment of the intestines. In the remaining 23 horses, the EF was obliterated using the diabolo-mesh technique without major complications.[29]

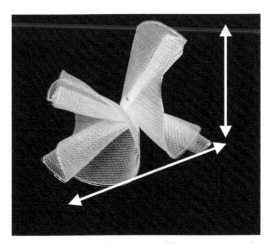

Fig. 4. Diabolo-shaped expandable mesh construct (diameter: 10 cm, length: 10 cm) used in horses for laparoscopic closure of the epiploic foramen. It is made of two preformed knitted polypropylene meshes (3DMax Mesh, BD, Franklin Lakes, New Jersey, USA) used for inguinal hernia repair in men.

ADHESIOLYSIS

Adhesions are one of the most common postoperative complications after laparotomy in the horse with a reported occurrence rate of 8% to 28%. In their study, Röcken and colleagues describe adhesions in 20 horses with chronic recurrent colic signs. Most of these adhesions (65%) involved abdominal reproductive organs and 17/20 could be successfully resolved laparsocopically.[30] In general, the adhesions that can be treated laparoscopically are clearly demarcated and a definite differentiation between adhesion and hollow organs is possible (**Fig. 5**). The use of sharp dissection, vessel sealing devices (Ligasure, Medtronic, Dublin, Ireland, Enseal, Johnson & Johnson, New Brunswick, New Jersey, USA), laser surgery, and high-frequency electrosurgery are described.[30] Furthermore, a stapling devise can be used to create a safe dissection; two lines of staples are placed on the transition of the adhesion to its origin. The staple line at the base of the adhesion closes the hollow organ or cavity, allowing the surgeon to cut between the two lines of staples without inadvertently opening any hollow structure.[30,31] In the authors' experience, converting to a hand-assisted laparoscopy is essential in those cases where a sharp delineation of the hollow organ and the adhesion is not possible. Hereby, one portal is enlarged to allow the surgeon's hand to enter the abdomen. This allows for tactile feedback as well as easier manipulation. Despite the encouraging success rates in the literature, extensive adhesions can seldomly be treated laparoscopically (Video 5).

SUTURE OF MESENTERIC RENTS

Some causes of acute colic can be treated with laparoscopy after the initial lesion has been corrected via a standard ventral midline laparotomy. One of those conditions is the laparoscopic closure of mesenteric rents or tears with or without entrapment of intestine through the opening. Even though the entrapment is usually not resolved laparoscopically, this technique provides surgical access to the most dorsal aspects of the mesentery, which are not accessible via ventral midline laparotomy. In all reports at hand, the acute colic was treated via laparotomy, during which the entrapment of the intestines was corrected, and further intraoperative interventions were effectuated as necessary. Laparoscopic closure of the mesenteric defect was then performed 24 hours to 18 days after laparotomy. In all cases, it had been impossible to close the tear during the celiotomy due to its dorsal extend. All authors used the standard laparoscopic approach to the abdominal cavity in standing horses described above.[32-35] In the authors' opinion, converting the standard laparoscopic approach to a hand-assisted procedure greatly facilitates both the visualization and the

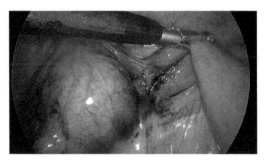

Fig. 5. Adhesions between a mass at the dorsal body wall and the duodenum seen from a portal in the 17th intercostal space on the right side.

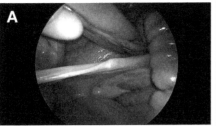 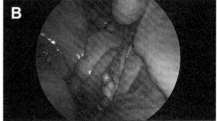

Fig. 6. Closure of a mesenteric rent: (*A*) depicting the hand-assisted approach to the large mesenteric rent and (*B*) showing the result after suturing the rent with barbed suture (Courtesy T. de Beauregard).

manipulations needed to identify and close of the defect (**Fig. 6**A, B). Mesenteric rents can be closed either with barbed suture, hemostatic staples or regular suture material. In the reports available, all horses recovered without complications.[32–35]

DIAPHRAGMATIC HERNIA

Another, arguably less common, cause of colic is diaphragmatic hernias. In their case report, Röcken and colleagues treated a horse with severe acute colic due to a diaphragmatic hernia with laparoscopic closure of the hernia 12 days after a standard ventral midline laparotomy. The horse presented with acute severe colic due to small intestinal strangulation. The diaphragmatic hernia was located dorsally to the nephrosplenic space, which had rendered a repair during the ventral midline laparotomy impossible. Laparoscopy was performed using standard left flank portals in the standing horse, revealing the defect in the tendinous part of the diaphragm. The defect was covered by the spleen and was deemed impossible to repair using flank portals. The repair was then finally performed a week later via thoracoscopy.[36] Klohnen also describes the laparoscopic closure of diaphragmatic hernias and mentions the use of a mesh if a tear in the muscular part cannot be fully closed.[12]

CLINICS CARE POINTS

- Feed should be withheld for at least 12 hours before laparoscopy to improve visualization and to avoid inadvertent puncture of the intestine when introducing a trocar.
- For standing laparoscopy, the horse has to be able to remain standing for the procedure which excludes most cases of acute colic.
- Transrectal palpation before the laparoscopy is advisable to identify distended intestines to avoid inadvertent puncture of the large intestine.
- Although laparoscopic visualization of the abdominal organs is typically good, manipulation is restricted. Conversion to a hand-assisted procedure can facilitate interventions.
- Intestinal biopsies are easiest to obtain using a laparoscopy-assisted extra-corporeal approach.

DISCLOSURE

The authors have no relevant financial or non-financial interests to disclose.

SUPPLEMENTARY DATA

Supplementary data related to this article can be found online at https://doi.org/10.1016/j.cveq.2023.03.003.

REFERENCES

1. Witherspoon DM, Talbot RB. Nocturnal ovulation in the equine animal. Vet record 1970;87:302–4.
2. Witherspoon DM, Talbot RB. Ovulation site in the mare. J Am Vet Med Assoc 1970;157:1452–9.
3. Fischer AT Jr, Lloyd KC, Carlson GP, et al. Diagnostic laparoscopy in the horse. J Am Vet Med Assoc 1986;189:289–92.
4. Hendrickson DA. Diagnostic Techniques. In: Advances in equine laparoscopy. Hoboken, U.S.: Wiley; 2012. p. 83–91.
5. Graham S, Freeman D. Standing diagnostic and therapeutic equine abdominal surgery. Vet clin North America Equine practice 2014;30:143–68.
6. Walmsley JP. Review of equine laparoscopy and an analysis of 158 laparoscopies in the horse. Equine Vet J 1999;31:456–64.
7. Galuppo LD, Snyder JR, Pascoe JR. Laparoscopic anatomy of the equine abdomen. Am J Vet Res 1995;56:7–28.
8. Galuppo LD, Snyder JR, Pascoe JR, et al. Laparoscopic anatomy of the abdomen in dorsally recumbent horses. Am J Vet Res 1996;57:923–31.
9. Schambourg MM, Marcoux M. Laparoscopic intestinal exploration and full-thickness intestinal biopsy in standing horses: a pilot study. Vet Surg 2006;35:689–96.
10. Bracamonte JL, Boure LP, Geor RJ, et al. Evaluation of a laparoscopic technique for collection of serial full-thickness small intestinal biopsy specimens in standing sedated horses. Am J Vet Res 2008;69:431–9.
11. Wilderjans H, Advances in standing laparoscopy, European veterinary conference voorjaarsdagen, meeting held The Hague, Netherlands on 05 July 2017.
12. Klohnen A. Evaluation of horses with signs of acute and chronic abdominal pain, In: Ragle C.A. In: *Advances in equine laparoscopy.* Ames, IA: Wiley-Blackwell; 2012. p. 93–118.
13. Coomer R, McKane S, Roberts V, et al. Small intestinal biopsy and resection in standing sedated horses. Equine Vet Educ 2016;28:636–40.
14. Spagnolo JD, Castro LM, Correa RR, et al. Nephrosplenic Space Ablation in Horses After Homologous Pericardium Implant Using a Laparoscopic Stapler. J Equine Vet Sci 2020;95.
15. Munoz J, Bussy C. Standing Hand-Assisted Laparoscopic Treatment of Left Dorsal Displacement of the Large Colon and Closure of the Nephrosplenic Space. Vet Surg 2013;42:595–9.
16. Gialletti R, Nannarone S, Gandini M, et al. Comparison of Mesh and Barbed Suture for Laparoscopic Nephrosplenic Space Ablation in Horses. Animals : an open access. Journal from MDPI 2021;11.
17. Rocken M, Schubert C, Mosel G, et al. Indications, surgical technique, and long-term experience with laparoscopic closure of the nephrosplenic space in standing horses. Vet Surg 2005;34:637–41.
18. Bussy C, Benredouane K, Munoz J, et al. Closure of the Equine Nephrosplenic Space Using a Single LED Powered Trocar via Standing Mini-Laparotomy. Open J Vet Med 2019;11–20.

19. Burke MJ, Parente EJ. Prosthetic Mesh for Obliteration of the Nephrosplenic Space in Horses: 26 Clinical Cases. Vet Surg 2016;45:201–7.
20. Nelson BB, Ruple-Czerniak AA, Hendrickson DA, et al. Laparoscopic Closure of the Nephrosplenic Space in Horses with Nephrosplenic Colonic Entrapment: Factors Associated with Survival and Colic Recurrence. Vet Surg 2016;45:O60–9.
21. Rodriguez JMA, Grulke S, Salciccia A, et al. Nephrosplenic space closure significantly decreases recurrent colic in horses: a retrospective analysis. Vet Rec 2019;185.
22. van Bergen T, Doom M, van den Broeck W, et al. A topographic anatomical study of the equine epiploic foramen and comparison with laparoscopic visualisation. Equine Vet J 2015;47:313–8.
23. van Bergen T, Wiemer P, Martens A. Equine colic associated with small intestinal epiploic foramen entrapment. Vet J 2021;269.
24. Freeman DE, Pearn AR. Anatomy of the vestibule of the omental bursa and epiploic foramen in the horse. Equine Vet J 2015;47:83–90.
25. Archer DC, Pinchbeck GK, French NP, et al. Risk factors for epiploic foramen entrapment colic: an international study. Equine Vet J 2008;40:224–30.
26. Proudman CJ, Smith JE, Edwards GB, et al. Long-term survival of equine surgical colic cases. Part 1: Patterns of mortality and morbidity. Equine Vet J 2002;34:432–7.
27. Munsterman AS, Hanson RR, Cattley RC, et al. Surgical Technique and Short-Term Outcome for Experimental Laparoscopic Closure of the Epiploic Foramen in 6 Horses. Vet Surg 2014;43:105–13.
28. van Bergen T, Wiemer P, Bosseler L, et al. Development of a new laparoscopic Foramen Epiploicum Mesh Closure (FEMC) technique in 6 horses. Equine Vet J 2016;48:331–7.
29. van Bergen T, Martens A. Epiploic foramen entrapment colic in horses. Equine Vet Educ 2021;33:181–3.
30. Rocken M, Scharner D, Gerlach K, et al. Laparoskopischer Nachweis und Verteilungsmuster intraabdominaler Adhäsionen beim chronisch rezidivierenden, nicht voroperierten Koliker. PFERDEHEILKUNDE 2006;18:574–8.
31. Bartmann CP, Schiemann V, Bubeck K. Laparoskopische Adhäsiolyse am Urogenitaltrakt des Pferdes. PFERDEHEILKUNDE 2006;22:153–9.
32. Sutter WW, Hardy J. Laparoscopic repair of a small intestinal mesenteric rent in a broodmare. Vet Surg 2004;33:92–5.
33. O'Neill HD. Hand-assisted laparoscopic reattachment of a mesoduodenojejunal defect in a broodmare. Equine Vet Educ 2020;32:E184–8.
34. Cypher EE, Blackford J, Snowden RT, et al. Surgical correction of entrapment of the large colon and caecum through a mesoduodenal rent with standing laparoscopic repair in a mare. Equine Vet Educ 2020;32:185–8.
35. Witte TH, Wilke M, Stahl C, et al. Use of a hand-assisted laparoscopic surgical technique for closure of an extensive mesojejunal rent in a horse. Javma-J Am Vet Med A 2013;243:1166–9.
36. Rocken M, Mosel G, Barske K, et al. Thoracoscopic diaphragmatic hernia repair in a warmblood mare. Vet Surg 2013;42:591–4.

Neonates and Periparturient Mares

Tips and Tricks for Diagnosis and Management

Nathan Slovis, DVM, CHT*, Leci Irvin, DVM

KEYWORDS

- Foal • Peripartum mare • Meconium • Congenital • Colic • Uroperitoneum • Hernia
- Hemorrhage

KEY POINTS

- Distinguishing between medical and surgical colic can be difficult in foals because abdominal palpation per rectum is not feasible; however, ultrasonography can replace palpation per rectum with a high sensitivity yet low specificity.
- In addition to fetal loss through abortions, life-threatening situations for the mare may develop in late gestation such as ventral body wall ruptures, peripartum hemorrhage, uterine torsion, and hydrops of the fetal membranes.
- For foals and mares with acute colic, the ability to differentiate between surgical and medical lesions early in the course of the disease will affect the prognosis.

INTRODUCTION

Abdominal pain in the foal can be a frustrating diagnostic challenge as the differential diagnoses are extensive (**Box 1**). Abdominal pain can progress rapidly leading to septicemia or even death. The approach to a neonate with a painful or distended abdomen includes history, type and dose of analgesics administered, and whether there are any other animals affected with diarrhea. Surgical versus medical treatment may be determined with a proper history and physical examination. Mild colic signs (eg, meconium impactions or Rotavirus) may include restlessness, attempts to defecate, tail swishing, straining to urinate/urinating frequently, walking around the stall, and not nursing. Severe colic signs should not be ignored and may include bloating, lying down and rolling, abdominal distention, and diffuse sweating. Immediate placement of a stomach tube should be performed in any foal which presents with chronic mild colic signs or acute onset of violent colic signs. Distinguishing between medical and surgical colic can be difficult in foals because abdominal palpation per rectum is

Hagyard Equine Medical Institute, McGee Medical Center, 4250 Ironworks Pike, Lexington, KY 40511, USA
* Corresponding author.
E-mail address: nslovis@hagyard.com

Vet Clin Equine 39 (2023) 351–379
https://doi.org/10.1016/j.cveq.2023.03.013   vetequine.theclinics.com

---

Box 1
Differential diagnosis of colic in foals by age group

0 - 7 days
  Congenital conditions
  • Atresia ani/ atresia coli
  • Lethal white
  Meconium impaction
  Prematurity/dysmaturity (Dysmotility)
  Ruptured bladder syndrome
  Thoracic or abdominal trauma following rib fractures
  Infectious enteritis/colitis
  Gastric/duodenal ulceration
  Physiological ileus (electrolyte disturbances)
  Peritonitis
  Chyloabdomen
  Surgical lesions
  • Complicated hernias—inguinal, scrotal, or umbilical
  • Intestinal volvulus or displacement
  • Intussusception

1–6 weeks
  Congenital conditions
  Ruptured bladder syndrome
  Thoracic or abdominal trauma following rib fractures
  Infectious enteritis/colitis
  Non-infectious diarrhea, eg, lactose intolerance, antibiotic-induced diarrhea.
  Gastric /duodenal ulceration
  Duodenal stricture
  Strangulating obstructions
  Non-strangulating obstructions (ascarid or feed-related impactions, intussusceptions foreign bodies)
  Complicated hernias

Other less common causes of colic:
  • Adhesions(post-surgery or following severe enteritis)
  • Fecaliths in miniature horses
  • White muscle disease

6–10 weeks
  Intrabdominal abscess secondary to *Rhodococcus equi*
  Infectious enteritis/colitis

---

not feasible; however, ultrasonography can replace palpation per rectum with a high sensitivity yet low specificity. A "monitor and wait" approach has as much risk as exploratory surgery in foals. In foals presenting with acute pain, a period of somnolence can be noted and mistaken for a positive response to the medical treatments, when, in fact, this type of medical state could indicate marked deterioration likely caused by severe septic shock.

The age of the animal is also important in determining the risk associated with different pathologic conditions. During the first 6 to 24 hours of age, congenital atresia of the colon, rectum, or anus as well as meconium impactions are the most frequent causes of colic. Primarily white Paint horse foals whose dam and sire are overo are at risk for ileocolonic aganglionosis (lethal white foal syndrome, LWFS). Older foals, 2 to 5 days of age, are more likely to suffer from intussusceptions, rupture bladder, enteritis, gastroduodenal ulceration, inguinal hernias, and small intestinal volvulus. Ultrasonography can be used to help diagnose conditions that cause colic signs. For example, distended (>2.5 cm diameter), amotile small intestine, and the absence of gastric distention is suggestive of a small intestinal volvulus whereas a large volume of peritoneal fluid with a history of infrequent urination is suggestive of a ruptured bladder. Notably, severe abdominal pain is not pathognomonic for a surgical lesion. Tachycardia in excess of 120 beats per minute that is non-responsive to pain medication and in the absence of fever is suggestive of a surgical lesion. This article provides an overview of the differential diagnoses for foal colic with general guidelines for therapy.

NEONATES
Congenital

Intestinal atresia (atresia coli and atresia ani)

Atresia of the large, transverse, and small colon as well as the rectum and anus, termed atresia coli and atresia ani, respectively, have been documented in foals. In human medicine, congenital atresias are currently thought to be associated with vascular accidents, involving a segment of intestine during fetal development, which results in atrophy and potentially complete disappearance of the affected portion of the bowel.[1] Affected foals may seem normal for the first 24 hours of life. Feces and gas accumulate orad to the intraluminal membrane or blind-ended portion of the gastrointestinal tract causing an obstruction which results in progressive abdominal distension along with increasing severity of colic signs. Affected foals nurse well initially and then become anorexic as pain progresses. Both atresia coli and atresia ani are uncommon congenital abnormalities. Atresia coli, although still rare, is the most common type of intestinal atresia noted in foals.[2] It is associated with more severe and earlier onset of signs than atresia ani. In cases of atresi coli and subsequent secondary gastrointestinal rupture, transient periods of improvement are often noted followed by rapid clinical deterioration associated with fulminant septic peritonitis. Via a similar mechanism, fillies with atresia ani can develop rectovaginal fistulas secondary to persistent straining and increased intraluminal pressure. Rectovaginal fistulation may coincide with decreased severity of colic signs depending on the amount of feces and gas that can be passed. The perineum should be examined for evidence of a normal anus. In some cases of atresia ani, the anus is absent whereas in others, an external anus is visible yet not patent. If feces is present in or around the vulva, vaginal examination for a rectovaginal fistula should be performed.[3] Diagnosis of atresia ani is achieved by visual inspection, digital palpation, and proctoscopy if needed. Diagnosis of atresia coli is more difficult than that of atresia ani because the lesion is not evident grossly. Meconium impaction is often suspected initially based on a history of no fecal passage since birth and progressive abdominal distension. Foals with atresia coli will only have mucus evident on a glove following digital rectal palpation whereas foals with a meconium impaction will have a small amount of feces-colored mucus on the glove following digital rectal palpation (**Fig. 1**). Confirmation of a suspected diagnosis of atresia coli can be accomplished in some cases with proctoscopy/colonoscopy. Contrast radiography following the administration of a barium enema can confirm a gastrointestinal obstruction but cannot differentiate between intestinal atresia and other types of gastrointestinal obstructions.[4] Exploratory celiotomy may be required for definitive diagnosis of intestinal atresia. Atresia coli should be regarded as a fatal condition. Intestinal motility issues or failure of the anastomosis have resulted in cases where surgical correction of atresia coli was attempted. On the other hand, in some cases, surgical correction of atresia ani has been successful; a more favorable prognosis accompanies cases in which the anal sphincter is normal and intestinal obstruction is caused by only a thin layer of tissue. Following successful surgical correction of atresia ani, while

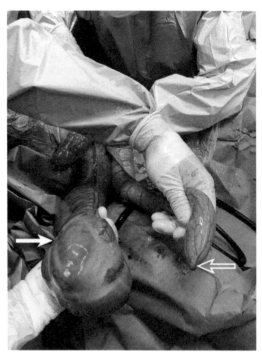

Fig. 1. Atresia in a 30-hour-old Thoroughbred colt. The agenesis was located between the ventral and dorsal colons. Dark arrow: Ventral colon and open arrow: dorsal colon.

not proven, some veterinarians recommend that horses should not be bred due to a potential underlying genetic basis of this condition.

Lethal white foal syndrome

LWFS, also known as ileocolonic aganglionosis, is an inherited, congenital condition resulting in aberrant development of the enteric nervous system that affects white American Paint horse foals born from overo-overo breeding. It has also been reported in one foal with a solid-colored Quarter horse parent.[5] It occurs when foals are homozygous for the lethal white gene, a mutated endothelin B receptor gene, resulting in abnormal migration and colonization of neural crest cell progenitors during gastrointestinal development. The latter results in the absence of enteric neurons that make up the myenteric plexus. The endothelin B receptor is also involved in the development of neural crest cells, which are committed to differentiate into melanocytes hence the association between intestinal aganglionosis and coat color phenotypes.[6] Hirschsprung disease, or aganglionic megacolon in humans, is similar in pathogenesis to LWFS.[7] Heterozygotes usually have the overo color pattern, which is most common in American Paint horses and may also be found in Quarter horses, Pintos, and Saddlebreds. White foals born to other breeds are not affected. Most foals with LWFS are entirely white with blue or white irises but some may have small areas of pigmentation on the forelock and tail. They may also be deaf.[8] Within 24 hours of life, abdominal distention and colic signs develop due to ileus resulting from aganglionosis of the distal small intestine and large intestine. The affected foals pass minimal or no feces. The abdominal radiographs reveal gas-distended gastrointestinal viscera and transabdominal sonographic evaluation shows distended, hypomotile to amotile intestine and colon. In summary, a white foal born to an overo-overo mating with progressive abdominal distention and minimal fecal production is highly suggestive of LWFS. This history and the aforementioned progression of clinical signs are used to make a diagnosis. This is a fatal condition, therefore, the affected foals should be humanely euthanized.

Umbilical hernia

Umbilical hernias are common congenital defects of the body wall with an overall estimated incidence of 0.5% to 2%.[9] Congenital umbilical hernias are more likely to occur in females than males. In addition, Quarter horses and Thoroughbreds have been shown to be at greater risk when compared with Standardbreds, Arabians, and ponies.[10] Congenital umbilical hernia is usually uncomplicated, defined as a hernia that does not contain intestine or only contains non-incarcerated intestine. The affected foals, therefore, often present with no clinical abnormalities except for a visually apparent hernia that is reducible on palpation. It is important to differentiate an umbilical hernia from a hematoma or seroma in the same location and, most commonly in older foals, an enlarged or abscessed external umbilical remnant. Although less likely, umbilical hernias can also be complicated, containing incarcerated or strangulated intestine, which corresponds with an increase in hernia size, firmness, edema, and pain on palpation.[11] The palpation and presence of intestine within the hernia is not necessarily a concern unless the hernia is irreducible. Colic signs are often, yet not always, observed when strangulation has occurred and will develop as intestinal distention and vascular compromises progress. Sonographic evaluation of the hernia and ventral abdomen is helpful in determining the contents of the hernia in addition to whether or not it is complicated by entrapped intestine. Sonography can also help differentiate non-reducible hernias from umbilical remnant abscesses. Surgical correction of complicated umbilical hernias involving entrapped intestine with or without ischemic injury is straightforward and associated with an excellent prognosis for survival. Early recognition and surgical correction is critical for success.

Inguinal-scrotal hernia

Inguinal-scrotal hernias are typically soft tissue swellings on one side of the scrotal area and are rarely bilateral. Most inguinal-scrotal hernias are indirect, that is, the intestine passes through the vaginal ring into the vaginal tunic (**Figs. 2** and **3**). Initial

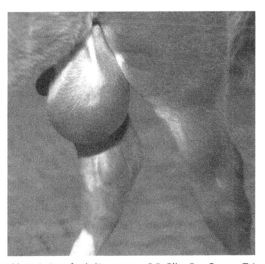

Fig. 2. Indirect scrotal hernia in a foal. (Bartmann C-P, Glitz F, v. Oppen T, Lorber K J, Bubeck K, Klug E, Deegen E: Diagnosis and surgical management of colic in the foal. Pferdeheilkunde 17:676-680, 2001.)

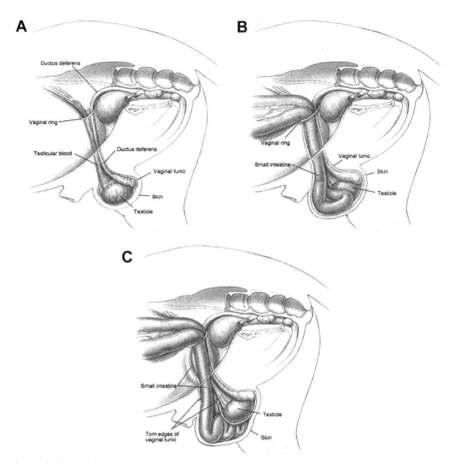

Fig. 3. (A) Normal inguinal structures (B) Indirect inguinal hernia (C) Direct inguinal hernia. (Bartmann CP, Freeman DE, Glitz F, et al. Diagnosis and surgical management of colic in the foal: Literature review and a retrospective study. Clinical Techniques in Equine Practice. 2002;1(3):125-142. https://doi.org/10.1053/ctep.2002.35574.)

management is directed at repeated manual reduction of the scrotal contents or application of a truss bandage. A hernia truss bandage consists of gauze/rolled cotton followed by elastic adhesive bandaging applied in a figure-of-eight pattern to help reduce the hernia. Successful manual reduction is typically achieved in the first month.[12,13] Foals with an irreducible, direct inguinal hernia will present with signs of colic several hours after birth (4–48 hours). This is caused by rupture of the common vaginal tunic, such that the jejunum migrates into the subcutaneous space associated with the scrotum and prepuce. Direct inguinal-scrotal hernias can also cause severe scrotal and preputial swelling and edema. Immediate surgical intervention is recommended **(Fig. 4)**.[14]

Stomach

Gastric distention/perforation
Gastric rupture is a fatal consequence of neonatal colic that results from loss of tissue integrity associated with severe gastric ulceration and subsequent gastric perforation

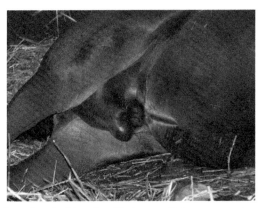

Fig. 4. Irreducible direct inguinal hernia with loops of jejunum noted under the scrotal skin with marked scrotal and preputial swelling.

or marked distention of the stomach wall.[15] Gastric distention and perforation may be primary or secondary in nature. Primary gastric perforation results from excessive intake or, more likely, decreased outflow due to a physical or functional obstruction such as congenital pyloric stenosis or acquired pyloric stenosis and/or duodenal stricture secondary to severe gastric and duodenal ulceration. Secondary gastric perforation is associated with a physical or functional intestinal obstruction aboral to the stomach. It is, therefore, a complication of a primary intestinal lesion, most commonly small intestinal in origin. Occasionally gastric perforation is caused by a large intestinal obstruction.[14] There have been several documented cases of idiopathic gastric rupture in foals.[16] It is presumed these cases result from marked gastric dilation based on the overall configuration of the rupture with a suspected underlying structural, and more likely, functional defect predisposing affected horses to gastric rupture. Investigations into human neonatal idiopathic gastric perforation have noted an association with reduced gastrointestinal pacemaker cells and gastric motility disorders.[17] Foals, before gastric perforation, whether it be primary or secondary, initially display nonspecific colic signs such as anorexia, ptyalism, and increased time in lateral or dorsal recumbency. If not detected early, the stomach could perforate resulting in fulminant diffuse septic peritonitis and ultimately generalized signs of sepsis and cardiovascular collapse characterized by tachycardia, tachypnea, weak peripheral pulses, varying degrees of abdominal discomfort, and death within hours. Diagnosis of gastric perforation may be difficult and often cannot be based on gastroscopic assessment alone due to the sometimes-benign surface appearance of perforating gastric ulcers. For this reason, transabdominal sonography, which may reveal increased or abnormal echogenicity of peritoneal fluid, followed by abdominocentesis are important in confirming gastric perforation or rupture. Identification of plant material on peritoneal fluid analysis is pathognomonic for gastrointestinal perforation. The identification of intracellular and/or extracellular enteric bacteria is highly suggestive of gastrointestinal leakage. Humane euthanasia is indicated once gastric perforation is confirmed.

Gastric ulceration
Gastroduodenal ulcer disease (GDUD) is common in foals, usually suckling and weanling-aged foals, especially those which are systemically stressed or compromised. Foals with a history of ill-thrift, recent or ongoing disease, hospitalization, non-steroidal anti-inflammatory therapy, transport, early weaning or management

changes as well as orphaned foals are at higher risk of developing gastric ulcers.[18] Unlike the typical squamous mucosal ulcers seen in adult horses, foals often have ulceration of the glandular mucosa and/or duodenum.[19] The pathogenesis of gastroduodenal ulcers in foals is unknown. It is assumed, however, to be similar to that in other species where gastric epithelial injury occurs when noxious irritants including gastric acid, bile acids, pepsin, and other enzymes overcome the protective factors which maintain healthy gastric and duodenal mucosa.[20] Gastric acid production is highly variable in neonatal foals leading to an often alkaline environment. Ulceration, therefore, likely arises from the suppression of protective factors including production of mucus, bicarbonate, prostaglandin E2, and epithelial growth factor rather than from an excess of acid production.[21] GDUD is divided into four syndromes, which include (1) subclinical or silent ulcers, (2) clinical or active ulcers, (3) perforating ulcers, and (4) ulcers associated with functional and/or physical gastric or duodenal obstruction. Functional disorders are associated with gastroduodenal inflammation, which can impair the myoelectric activity of the gastrointestinal tract leading to delayed gastric emptying.[17] Physical obstructive disorders would include pyloric stenosis or duodenal stricture formation, both of which can occur secondary to severe gastroduodenal ulceration (**Fig. 5**). Pyloric stenosis can also be a congenital condition. Foals with GDUD most commonly present with intermittent colic signs. In addition, they may display more specific signs including ptyalism, bruxism, and lying on their back for prolonged periods. Diarrhea has also been reported. In cases of pyloric stenosis or duodenal stricture formation, marked gastric distention with associated ileus and reflux may be seen. Even in these cases, signs of colic are variable but tend to become more severe with gastric distention and reflux. The reflux could be a large volume of 500 mL or more every 2 to 4 hours, despite the restriction of oral fluids. Some foals with endoscopically evident gastric and/or duodenal ulceration do not show any of the above clinical signs and, therefore, are deemed to have subclinical disease. Gastroscopy is required for a definitive diagnosis of GDUD as well as the sequelae of GDUD specifically, acquired pyloric stenosis or duodenum stricture formation. In some foals with duodenal ulceration, thickening of the duodenal wall is sonographically evident. Bleeding ulcers are uncommon in foals and, even if considerable gastrointestinal bleeding occurs secondary to gastric or duodenal ulceration, fecal occult blood is undetected. Severe gastric and/or duodenal ulceration can lead to gastrointestinal perforation resulting in fulminant septic peritonitis.

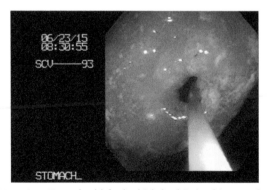

Fig. 5. Pyloric stricture in a 3-week-old foal which had 3-day history of colic and anorexia. On arrival, the foal had 1 L of reflux. Gastroscopy illustrating the biopsy instrument going through the pyloric sphincter that had a 4 mm patency.

Treatment of GDUD predominantly consists of anti-ulcer therapy specifically sucralfate and proton pump inhibitors such as omeprazole. With moderate to severe ulceration, a minimum of 3 to 4 weeks of anti-ulcer therapy should be recommended as the initial treatment course ideally followed by a recheck gastroscopy. As an aside, routine anti-ulcer treatment of hospitalized, high-risk, or systemically ill foals, is controversial due to the possibility that gastric acid suppression could predispose neonates to infectious diarrhea.[20]

As discussed above, pyloric stenosis and duodenal stricture formation are uncommon but serious sequelae of GDUD. Medical management involves anit-ulcer therapy and increasing gastric emptying via prokinetics such as metoclopramide (0.1–0.2 mg/kg IV TID-QID or 0.1–0.25 mg/kg PO QID) or bethanechol (0.02 mg/kg SQ TID-QID). Supportive therapy in the form of intravenous fluids and parenteral nutrition is often indicated. Surgical intervention via a gastrojejunostomy or gastroduodenostomy may be required in severe cases although reports documenting survival to racing age and normal growth rates in these foals are limited. In general, if there is no prompt improvement of severe GDUD with medical management, prognosis is guarded.[17]

Small Intestine

Small intestine volvulus

Small intestinal volvulus (SIV) is defined as a rotation of a segment of jejunum or ileum greater than 180° about its mesentery.[22] SIV has been reported as the most common indication for intestinal surgery in foals where pain may seem to fluctuate but quickly becomes severe and the affected foal's abdomen becomes markedly distended.[21,23] SIV may occur as a secondary complication in foals treated for a primary disease process such as neonatal septicemia or enteritis. This is believed to occur because of the potential for segmental ileus associated with excessive recumbency or changes in feeding regimen. Initial clinical signs are consistent with acute onset of severe abdominal pain. As the intestinal distention increases so does the abdominal distention. The pain associated with this strangulating lesion can initially be severe and then decline because of intestinal ischemia and subsequent necrosis. Ileus secondary to an enteritis may have clinical signs similar to an SIV; however, many of these foals present with fevers, unlike foals with an SIV.[24] Clinical signs alone cannot be used to differentiate between ileus and SIV. Diagnostic imaging techniques such as transabdominal sonography can be used to help correctly differentiate these conditions. Sonographic visualization of markedly distended (>2.5 cm diameter), poorly motile segments of the small intestine with ventral sedimentation of particulate material is strongly suggestive of a small intestinal strangulating lesion such as an SIV. Peritoneal fluid analysis can be performed, however, the use of lactate peritoneal fluid assessment versus peripheral lactate levels, in the author's experience (NMS), is dissimilar to that of adults. The author has noted that foals which have enterocolitis can have elevated lactate levels in the peritoneal fluid, and therefore, does not use peritoneal lactate levels to determine if surgical intervention is required. Serosanguineous abdominal fluid would prompt immediate surgical intervention. Prompt surgical management of a foal with an SIV, ideally before intestinal resection becomes necessary, is critical for a favorable outcome. A multi-institutional study evaluating outcomes of foals with small intestinal strangulating obstruction (SISO) revealed 24 of 25 (96.0%) foals and 66 of 75 (88.0%) adults which were recovered from surgery for small intestinal strangulating obstruction survived to hospital discharge. These findings provide a more optimistic outlook on prognosis following surgical correction of SISO in foals.[25]

Mesodiverticular band

The mesodiverticular band (MDB) is an embryologic remnant of the vitelline circulation, which provides arterial blood to the Meckel's diverticulum. In the event of an error of involution, a patent or nonpatent arterial band persists and extends from the mesentery to the apex of the antimesenteric diverticulum. This creates a snare-like opening through which bowel loops may herniate and become obstructed. Foals which present with a small intestinal obstruction due to an MDB are usually in severe pain and are difficult to differentiate from those with an SIV. **Fig. 6**.

Ascarid impactions

Ascarid impactions usually occur in foals which are 3 to 5 months of age. Most of these cases occur in foals, 54% of which had a history of being dewormed 6 days before the onset of clinical signs.[24] Ascarid impactions have a poorer prognosis for long-term survival when compared with other colic surgeries. The reason for the poor prognosis is not exactly known but is thought to be related to damage to the intestinal wall from the toxins/allergens that are released by the ascarids leading to prolonged ileus. For this reason, prevention of *Parascaris equorum* infection or minimizing a foal's ascarid burden through environmental management as well as regular monitoring and deworming of both mares and foals is essential. A tentative diagnosis of ascarid impaction can be made based on clinical signs of colic in a young horse with a poor deworming history and the presence of larval or mature ascarids in the feces or nasogastric reflux. Transabdominal sonography can also be used to detect the presence of ascarids in dilated loops of the small intestine. As many ascarid impactions are caused by immature worms, there might be no ascarid eggs in the feces, and therefore, the foal may have a negative fecal egg count although it is important to remember that fecal egg count is not a reliable indicator of overall worm burden.[26] Treatment consists of gastric decompression, pain management, fluid replacement, and the use of anthelmintics. The use of mineral oil (4-8 ml/kg via nasogastric tube [NGT]) before the use and after the use of anthelmintics has been proposed to help treat the current ascarid impaction and prevent another impaction post anthelmintics. The use of fenbendazole (10 mg/kg PO SID for 5 consecutive days) is the preferred anthelmintic because ivermectin and moxidectin are less effective because of resistance. The recommendation of a lower dose of an anthelmintic to help prevent complications (ie, another impaction) is debatable. Currently, there is no data which illustrates that reducing the

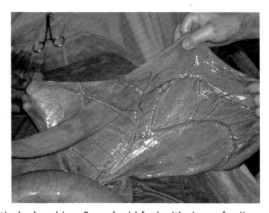

Fig. 6. Mesodiverticular band in a 2-week-old foal with signs of colic and marked small intestine distention with ileus.

dose of an anthelminthic reduces the effect or subsequently reduces the risk of adverse reactions such as another impaction.

Enterocolitis

Enterocolitis is one the most common causes of neonatal foal mortality and subsequently results in economic losses worldwide.[27] One retrospective study looking at 137 foals less than 30 days of age noted that colic-associated enterocolitis was the most common diagnosis for foal colic, representing 27% of all cases.[28] Until 6 months of life, up to 20% of foals have been reported to have diarrhea caused by infectious agents.[25] The etiology of diarrhea in neonatal foals is complex and involves infectious agents, management, and facilities, as well as nutritional, environmental, and physiologic conditions.[25,27,29] Infectious causes of enteritis in neonates include *Rotavirus*, Coronavirus, *Salmonella*, *Clostridium perfringens A* and *C*, *Clostridium difficile*, *Campylobacter*, *Enterococcus durans*, *Bacteroides fragilis*, and *Rhodococcus equi*.

Clinical signs in foals range from low-grade diarrhea to fulminate colitis with ileus. Foals can become very painful which can mimic a surgical gastrointestinal lesion; however, foals with enterocolitis tend to be pyrexic while foals with gastrointestinal surgical lesions are typically normothermic. In addition to diarrhea, foals become tachypneic, which may be secondary to discomfort associated with enterocolitis, pyrexia, metabolic acidosis, and/or the anxiety of being treated. Diagnostic sonography usually reveals marked fluid distention of the small intestine, large colon, or both. Foals with severe ileus will also have fluid distention of the stomach, which may necessitate the passage of a nasogastric tube to prevent gastric perforation. Foals with severe enterocolitis become anorexic and dehydrated; therefore, therapy is aimed at maintaining hydration and electrolyte balance. Foals less than 30 days of age with diarrhea were documented to have a high prevalence of bacteremia (50%) and, therefore, the use of broad-spectrum antimicrobials such as ampicillin and amikacin or ceftiofur (if azotemia is noted) should be made with these differences in mind.[30–32] In adult horses, antibiotic therapy is targeted at the specific pathogen causing enterocolitis. In young foals with enterocolitis, due to the higher prevalence of bacteremia, broad-spectrum antimicrobial therapy should be initiated regardless of the cause.

Intussusception

Foals with an intussusception (jejunal, ileocecal, cecocolic) can have signs that are initially intermittent and indicates low-grade pain. Colic signs may then progress to those characteristic of violent pain. Small intestinal intussusception has been regarded as a common cause of colic in foals; however, in three retrospective studies, only 1 case was identified out of 227 foals which presented for colic.[26,33,34] Intussusceptions on occasion can cause acute colic signs and, therefore, can be difficult to distinguish from an SIV. Subacute cases have been documented in young foals which have diarrhea or have recently recovered from diarrhea. Enteritis may be a predisposing factor. In older foals, tapeworm infestation may also be a risk factor. One of the authors (NMS), has diagnosed foals with jejunal intussusceptions that are transient, and therefore, corrected on their own, while the foal was medically managed with maintenance intravenous fluids, non-steroidal anti-inflammatory drugs, and feed restriction. If the foal is not showing severe colic signs, it is recommended to serially monitor the intussusception via transabdominal sonography for edema. If edema is noted and colic signs persist or worsen, surgical exploration should be pursued. Transabdominal sonography will reveal a "bull's eye" lesion caused by telescoping of the intussusceptum (inner part) into the intussuscipiens (outer part)[35] **(Fig. 7)**. The

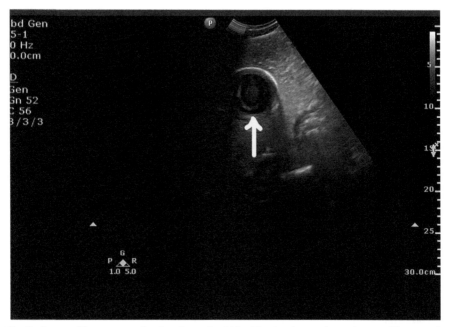

Fig. 7. Ileocecal intussusception in a 3-week-old foal having intermittent bouts of low-grade abdominal pain. Image was taken from the right flank. Yellow Arrow: Ileum intucception in the cecum.

small intestine proximal to the intussusception can be dilated, especially if the intussusception is chronic.

Large Colon

Meconium impaction

Meconium retention or impaction is one of the most common causes of neonatal colic, exceeded only by enterocolitis, and is the leading cause of intestinal obstruction which occurs in foals ranging from less than 1 day to approximately 2 days of age.[26] Meconium is a mucilaginous mixture of bile, mucus, amniotic fluid, and epithelial cellular debris which is normally passed within the first hours after birth.[36] Complete retention or incomplete passage of meconium can result in progressive intestinal and subsequent abdominal distention due to accumulation of gastrointestinal fluid and gas orad to the obstruction. Meconium may be impacted anywhere from the large colon to the rectum. Colts are more commonly affected as they have a narrower pelvis than fillies.[37] Signs of abdominal pain, including dorsal recumbency, flank watching, rolling, tail swishing, tail flagging, anorexia, and, specifically, tenesmus, are common. These signs often occur after nursing; between colic episodes, the foal is often bright and alert. Foals with a complete obstruction caused by a meconium impaction show colic signs within the first few hours of life. These foals will also have signs of tenesmus, (kyphotic body position with a hunched back classic of foals straining to defecate), and even signs similar to stranguria during bouts of abdominal pain. This can cause confusion as some clinicians who identify a patient with stranguria may focus on the urinary bladder when in fact the foal is having issues related to a meconium impaction. History of minimal or no passage of meconium, clinical signs, and age will assist with reaching a tentative diagnosis. A history of passing a small volume of meconium does not rule out a meconium impaction. Digital examination of the rectum may, yet not always, allow palpation of meconium. Identification of a mass of meconium may be possible on manual palpation of the abdominal wall of a relaxed, recumbent foal; transabdominal sonography and/or abdominal radiography provide more sensitive and specific information when attempting to diagnose meconium obstructions. Sonography can be used to identify meconium, which appears as a mottled intraluminal mass with an echogenicity similar to that of fat or the liver (**Fig. 8**). Although sonography may not consistently confirm an impaction if present, it is useful to rule out other causes of neonatal colic. In some cases, retrograde contrast via barium enemas or proctoscopy can be useful to identify impactions that are not easily visualized with abdominal radiography or ultrasound examination.

In mild cases, a single enema (mild soap and water) may resolve the meconium impaction. Concurrent administration of N- butylscopolammonium bromide (Buscopan) may decrease colonic spasm and aid in the passage of meconium. Repeated administration of commercial enemas should be avoided due to the risk of phosphate toxicosis. If there is a poor response to a single routine enema, an acetylcysteine enema (250 mL 4% acetylcysteine) should be administered and may be repeated if non-productive. During the administration of an acetylcysteine enema, the foal is sedated with 0.1 to 0.3 mg/kg diazepam IV with or without 1 mg of butorphanol tartrate IV per 50 kg. If nursing is restricted, intravenous fluid therapy and parenteral nutrition are indicated. Conservative over-hydration with intravenous fluids may also be useful in cases that are refractory to the immediate aforementioned therapy. On rare occasions, surgical intervention is required due to increasing severity of colic signs related to bloating and poor response to medical management.

Large colon volvulus
Large colon displacement and subsequent volvulus occur much less often in foals compared with mature horses.[26,38] Small intestinal or small colon lesions are much more commonly identified than large colon lesions in foals, including neonates,

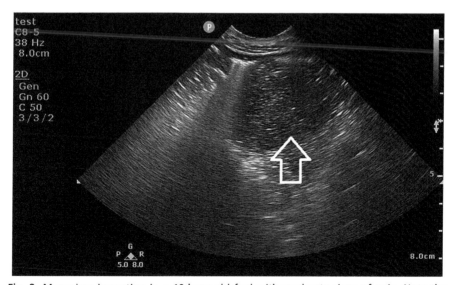

Fig. 8. Meconium impaction in a 10-hour-old foal with moderate signs of pain. Note the meconium in the large colon (*arrow*).

presenting for colic requiring surgical intervention.[37] The lower incidence of large colon-related colic in foals compared with adults may be associated with the limited large intestinal fermentation and gas production that occur in foals and, therefore, decreased risk of gaseous distention and subsequent colonic displacement.[39] Possible predisposing factors for large colon volvulus in neonates include perinatal hypoxic damage to the colon or colitis which would both contribute to ileus/dysmotility and subsequent gaseous distention of the colon. Congenital anatomic malformations of the colon and/or mesenteric attachments could also predispose a neonate to large colon displacement and volvulus. In horses, the density of neurons and ganglions, comprising the myenteric plexus, is greatest in the pelvic flexure and left dorsal colon pacemaker regions; therefore, theoretically, congenital abnormalities in neural function affecting these regions as seen with colonic myenteric hypoganglionosis and ileocolonic aganglionosis could predispose a neonate to large colon volvulus.[40–42] Foals with large colon volvulus present with progressive and marked abdominal distention accompanied by severe colic signs. These foals are often tachycardic, consistent with the degree of gastrointestinal pain, toxemia, and hypovolemia. Vascular compromise can develop rapidly and, as this occurs, the mucous membrane color will deteriorate and other signs of cardiovascular compromise such as weak peripheral pulses and cool extremities may be observed. Affected foals can progress from mild to uncontrollable pain rapidly. Reaching a definitive diagnosis of large colon volvulus in a foal is difficult without surgical exploration. Abdominal sonography and radiography will reveal intestinal distention. Colonic edema may be present depending on the duration and degree of vascular compromise as well as colonic distention. In foals less than 2 days of age, it is important to determine if the foal has ever defecated to rule out congenital intestinal atresia or a severe meconium impaction, which would also result in gastrointestinal distention followed by marked abdominal distention and severe colic signs. Rapid surgical exploration is required. At surgery, the viability of the colon can be assessed.

Colitis/necrotizing enterocolitis

Necrotizing enterocolitis (NEC) is one of the most serious human infant gastrointestinal emergencies and often requires surgical intervention due to the presence of necrotic bowel.[43] Perinatal asphyxia syndrome produces hypoxic-ischemic encephalopathy resulting in neurologic deficits ranging from hypotonia to grand mal seizures. Foals affected with perinatal asphyxia also experience gastrointestinal disturbances ranging from mild ileus and delayed gastric emptying to severe, bloody diarrhea, and NEC (**Fig. 9**). It has been postulated that when a preterm infant is stressed by periods of hypoxia or hypotension, blood flow is redistributed, via input from the adrenergic system, away from the splanchnic bed. Subsequent reperfusion of the gastrointestinal system results in the production of oxygen-free radicals and tissue damage characteristic of reperfusion injury. If the hypoxic event is severe, NEC can occur resulting in bloody diarrhea, pneumatosis intestinalis, ascites, and/or intestinal perforation. This type of gastrointestinal injury in neonates is believed to predispose them to bacterial invasion and translocation.[29,41] A diagnosis of hypoxic-ischemic ileus is presumptive when the patient has a history of peripartum asphyxia (placentitis, premature placental separation), negative fecal diagnostics for infectious diseases, and distended small intestine with decreased motility noted on transabdominal sonography. Treatment of foals with NEC includes supportive care and restricted nursing. Foals are usually administered broad-spectrum antimicrobials, maintenance fluids, and total parenteral nutrition to allow the mucosa of the injured bowel to start healing.

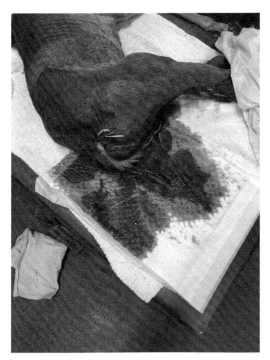

Fig. 9. Necrotizing enterocolitis in a 30-hour-old Thoroughbred colt. Foal was a dystocia and had severe perinatal asphyxia syndrome. Hemorrhagic diarrhea with blood clots noted in the manure. The foal did make a full recovery after 10 days of supportive therapy including TPN nutrition and no oral intake of milk.

Urinary Tract

Uroperitoneum

Uroperitoneum, or urine in the peritoneal cavity, is a common problem in neonatal foals.[44,45] It is a sign of perforation of some portion of the urinary tract. The urinary bladder is the most common site of rupture, but renal, ureteral, and urethral perforations or injuries can also occur and result in leakage of urine into the peritoneal cavity.[42,43,46] Uroperitoneum, arising from bladder rupture, may be associated with a congenital bladder abnormality or directly result from traumatic injury to the urinary tract sustained during parturition. Bladder perforation can also result from septic foci and subsequent necrosis from septicemia in foals greater than 5 to 7 days of age. Traditionally, bladder rupture has been more frequently documented in colts. In the author's (NMS) experience, however, the frequency at which systemically ill or recumbent foals, of either sex, are affected is approximately equal.

Hospitalized foals may not void urine voluntarily and, therefore, can develop ruptured bladders after a period of hospitalization, during which time they have been receiving intravenous crystalloid fluids as supportive therapy. In these foals, the classic electrolyte imbalances may be absent or reduced in severity. Azotemia is almost always noted. Clinical signs, in otherwise healthy neonates which develop ruptured bladders, include repeated posturing to urinate or stranguria during the first 2 days of life. When visualized, the urine stream is typically weaker and more sporadic than that seen with a normal neonate. If there is a large volume of urine in the peritoneal cavity due to a large rent in the bladder wall, urine communicates freely between the peritoneal cavity and bladder lumen, although some voiding of urine via the urethra continues. Therefore, observation of the foal voiding urine should not rule out the possibility of a ruptured bladder. Stranguria can easily be misinterpreted as tenesmus making the initial diagnosis difficult. Urine progressively accumulates in the abdomen resulting in a dull demeanor and progressive abdominal distension over 2 to 4 days. As the condition progresses, these foals develop hyponatremia, hypochloremia, hyperkalemia, and azotemia. Depending on the timing of presentation, the metabolic derangements that develop can result in other signs: hyponatremia can result in neurologic disturbances including seizures, and progressive hyperkalemia can result in cardiac dysrhythmias. Lethargy, dull demeanor, and a loss of interest in nursing develops as the foal's metabolic status deteriorates. Diagnosis with transabdominal sonography is useful and can quickly reveal increased anechoic-to-hypoechoic-free fluid in the peritoneal cavity such that bowel loops and other viscera appear suspended within the peritoneal fluid (**Fig. 10**). The rent in the bladder, whether congenital (rare) or acquired, is nearly always located in the dorsal bladder wall. Importantly, uroperitoneum is a metabolic rather than a surgical emergency in foals, and detection of voluminous anechoic-to-hypoechoic peritoneal fluid is supportive of a presumptive diagnosis in the field. If sonography is unavailable, a fluid sample may be obtained via abdominocentesis and assayed for creatinine concentration. If the creatinine concentration in the peritoneal fluid is twice or greater than twice that of the serum creatinine concentration, a diagnosis of uroperitoneum is made. It is important to note that serum electrolyte and creatinine concentrations may be normal in the early stages of the disorder and should not be used as a means of ruling out the condition. In foals, the prognosis for full recovery following surgical repair is very good barring complications.[42–44] Foals tend to present to the clinic with severe hyponatremia (<120 mmol/ L or mEq/L) and need to be stabilized before surgery. Although acute hyponatremia

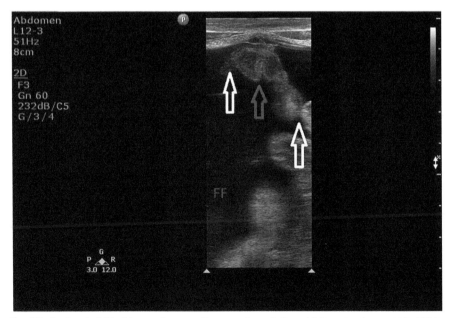

Fig. 10. Perforated bladder and uroperitoneum in a 4-day-old Quarter horse colt. White arrows: Umbilical arteries. Red arrow is the collapsed bladder. FF, Free fluid: Uroperitoneum.

(<48 hours duration) can be corrected relatively quickly, fast correction of chronic hyponatremia carries a risk of osmotic demyelination. Unfortunately, information about the duration of the condition is difficult to accurately establish in clinical cases, even in human patients. Due to this uncertainty, current recommendations are to treat chronic and acute hyponatremia equally conservatively if Na^+ concentrations are less than 120 mmol/L. In symptomatic cases, an increase of 4 to 8 mmol/L (approximately 5% increase in Na^+ concentration) over the first 6 hours of therapy often alleviates clinical signs and further increases should not exceed a total of 10 mmol/L/day[8,15] In cases with no neurologic symptoms, a gradual increase of 10% per day should be targeted. The author (NMS) will send cases to surgery once the Na^+ concentrations are greater than 123 mmol/L and the patient is showing no signs of neurologic dysfunction. Drainage of the abdomen may also be necessary to help remove the low Na^+ and high K+ concentrations of the urine which can further exacerbate the systemic electrolyte abnormalities. Patients who are hyperkalemic can be treated with the use of fluids that contain either dextrose or sodium bicarbonate to reduce the K+ concentration to less than (5.0 mmol/L or mEq/L). Occasionally, uroperitoneum may recur after surgery as a result of ongoing necrosis and leakage. When this occurs, and the volume of free fluid in the peritoneal cavity related to direct communication between the bladder and abdominal cavity is small, it often can be managed conservatively by the placement of an indwelling urinary catheter for 3 to 5 days. A second celiotomy may be required in other cases.

Pregnant Mares

In addition to fetal loss through abortions, life-threatening situations for the mare may develop in late gestation such as ventral body wall ruptures, uterine torsion, and hydrops of the fetal membranes. Accurate diagnosis and timely intervention may not only save the life of the mare but may also result in the birth of a viable foal in cases of ventral body wall ruptures and uterine torsions. The following reviews some of these late gestation complications.

Uterine torsion

Torsion of the uterus is uncommon, constituting between 5% and 10% of all serious obstetric problems.[47] It can affect mares of any age or parity and most frequently has an acute onset in the last 60 days of gestation. It can also occur earlier in gestation, although it is less likely. Although uterine torsions usually present acutely, there have been reports of chronic torsions with clinical signs noted for up to 2 months before diagnosis.[48,49] They can also present as dystocias in term mares, although this is rare and most torsions occur before parturition. Falling or rolling, the presence of a large fetus and relatively small volume of fetal fluids, and/or increased fetal movement are events that may increase the risk of gravid horn rotation. In most cases, no precipitating events or factors are confirmed. Several studies have described higher survival rates for both mare and fetus when the torsion occurs and corrected prior to 320 days of gestation.[50] The affected mares often present with a quiet or dull demeanor and signs of colic that are mild to moderate in severity but tend to be poorly responsive to analgesics. The degree of discomfort has been likened to a horse with a large colon impaction, although colic signs are much more severe if the gastrointestinal tract is incorporated into the torsion such as with concurrent incarceration of the small intestine or small colon.[51] In one retrospective study involving 19 mares, 50% of the mares had concurrent gastrointestinal disease including inflammatory bowel disease, large colon impaction, large colon volvulus, right dorsal displacement of the large colon, or gastric rupture.[52] Therefore, it is important to evaluate both the gastrointestinal and reproductive tracts when presented with a pregnant mare showing colic signs. The severity of clinical signs is also related to the degree of uterine rotation and subsequently the degree of uterine vascular compromise. Uterine torsions that are greater than 360° create clinically relevant tension on the vascular structures in the broad ligament resulting in impaired placental perfusion and decreased fetal oxygen delivery. Rupture of the uterus can occur with prolonged torsion or marked vascular compromise and will result in fulminant peritonitis and signs of sepsis.

Examination per rectum is usually necessary for the diagnosis of uterine torsion. Torsion of the uterus can occur clockwise, to the right: the left broad ligament is stretched horizontally over the top of the uterus and the right broad ligament courses tightly ventrally or vertically under the uterus toward the opposite side. The uterus may also rotate in a counter-clockwise direction, to the left: the right broad ligament is palpable as a dorsal sheet of tissue going to the left side and the left broad ligament is pulled ventrally, toward the midline. Rotation can range from 180° to 360°. Unlike cattle, in the mare, the cervix and cranial vagina are usually not involved unless the degree of rotation is severe or fibrous tissue has formed. It is therefore imperative, in all pregnant mares which develop colic, to perform an examination per rectum, given that a vaginal examination can be unrewarding as well as potentially contraindicated.[45] Transrectal and transabdominal sonography can aid in the assessment of uterine compromise by enabling the determination of uterine wall thickness as well as evaluation of placental integrity, vascular distension, fetal viability, and condition of the fetal fluid.[45] If there is concern about intestinal involvement, abdominocentesis may be performed to aid in determining the appropriate mode of replacement and/or overall prognosis.

There are various non-surgical and surgical techniques implemented to correct uterine torsions; the technique chosen depends on the stage of gestation of the mare, the condition as well as the value of the mare and fetus, and the duration of clinical signs. Non-surgical options include manual de-rotation of the uterus in a term mare facilitated by grasping the fetus through the dilated cervix and using momentum to rotate the fetus and the uterus back into an anatomically normal position as well as rolling a preterm mare using the pressure of planks to stabilize the uterus during rotation. Cited disadvantages to these techniques include potentially making the condition worse if the direction of torsion is misdiagnosed, the potential to displace the colon, and a high incidence of placental detachment. Surgical intervention via a standing flank laparotomy can be more difficult in term mares with large fetuses or in cases in which the fetus is dead but carries less anesthetic risks than a ventral midline celiotomy. The ventral midline celiotomy is recommended in cases where gastrointestinal involvement or uterine compromise is suspected to avoid uterine rupture or gastrointestinal damage. The prognosis for the fetus depends on the degree of vascular compromise which in turn depends on the severity of uterine torsion and speed of correction. Mare and foal survival is significantly greater when uterine torsion occurs at less than 320 days of gestation.[53] However, in many cases, correction is not timely enough and frequently uterine torsion results in abortion or, in term mares, delivery of a dead foal. When fetal life is confirmed following correction of uterine torsion in a term mare, preparations should be made for resuscitation and aggressive medical management following birth due to the increased risk of neonatal encephalopathy secondary to in utero hypoxic-ischemic damage. In preterm mares, administration of progestins to suppress myometrial activity is recommended following successful re-rotation of the uterus and confirmation of fetal life.

Diaphragmatic hernia

Diaphragmatic hernias are an uncommon cause of colic in pregnant mares.[54] In mature horses, diaphragmatic rent formation and subsequent gastrointestinal herniation are thought to be primarily associated with a traumatic event, such as impact injury during racing/pasture accident or instances of markedly increased intraabdominal pressure such as those experienced during foaling.[55] One of the authors (NMS) has also noted diaphragmatic hernias in older mares with pituitary pars intermedia dysfunction (PPID) due to an overall decrease in muscle mass and presumptive muscle atrophy.[56] The location of acquired rent formation varies, but it has been most commonly documented in the left hemiabdomen at the level of the musculotendinous junction.[52] In foals, diaphragmatic hernias are more likely associated with congenital diaphragmatic rents or difficult foaling events that result in rib fractures and subsequent laceration of the diaphragm. In cases where the rent is formed via a traumatic event, there can be a long interval between the trauma and onset of clinical signs as severe and persistent abdominal pain is associated with migration and secondary incarceration of gastrointestinal contents and not with the formation of the diaphragmatic rent. The severity of colic signs can range from mild to severe and often correspond with the degree of vascular compromise of the herniated contents. Colic is the most common clinical sign and is caused by a simple or strangulating obstruction of the herniated bowel as well as tension on the mesentery. Signs of respiratory distress including tachypnea and shallow breathing have also been documented.[57] Signs of respiratory distress depend on the amount and type of herniated contents, with larger gastrointestinal viscera resulting in a proportional reduction in pulmonary functional capacity and ventilation-perfusion mismatching. The small intestine or large colon is most commonly involved and herniation of liver, stomach, and spleen has been documented.[58] Absence or asymmetry of bronchovesicular lung sounds associated with one hemithorax may suggest the presence of a diaphragmatic hernia, especially in conjunction with auscultation of loud borborygmi in the thorax and absent borborygmi in the abdominal cavity. Sonographic evaluation is a useful tool in the diagnosis of diaphragmatic hernias involving the small intestine by identifying fluid- or gas-filled tubular structures within the thorax as well as those involving the large colon, which appears as a thick-walled, sacculated, fluid-filled structure within the thorax.[59] Depending on the location of the diaphragmatic rent, the rent itself may not be visible on ultrasonographic evaluation. Thoracic radiographs are helpful in confirming a suspected diagnosis of diaphragmatic hernia in which gastrointestinal viscera are not sonographically seen in the thoracic cavity. Confirmation is based on the identification of intrathoracic large colon, which appears as a large, sacculated fluid- and gas-filled structure. Contrast radiography can also help highlight small intestinal loops within the thoracic cavity.[60]

Pre-partum hemorrhage

Hemorrhage from the middle uterine, external iliac, utero-ovarian, and vaginal arteries has been described in late pregnancy and after parturition. Periparturient hemorrhage (PPH) is an important cause of colic and fatality in broodmares with an estimated incidence of 2% to 3% in the broodmare population.[61] In a retrospective study investigating causes of death in the immediate postpartum period, 41% of the 98 mares involved in the study died of uterine arterial rupture and subsequent internal hemorrhage.[62] Although most cases occur in older, multiparous mares, it is becoming more of a problem in younger, primiparous mares from 5 to 24 (median, 14) years of age.[63] Hemorrhage most commonly occurs within the first 48 hours following foaling.

Pre-partum hemorrhage has also been seen. Therefore, peripartum hemorrhage should be considered as a differential when middle or late gestation mares as well as 24- to 72-hour post-parturient mares present for colic. In some instances, mares are simply found dead because of acute arterial hemorrhage. More often, however, mares develop signs within 24 hours of parturition, and most are associated with a rupture of the right uterine artery. Although the etiology of uterine artery rupture has not been definitively ascertained, three hypotheses have been proposed: (1) arterial rupture usually occurs on the right side of the mare's uterus, possibly as a result of the cecum displacing the uterus and increasing tension on the right uterine artery in addition to direct pressure on the artery by the cecum; (2) normal age-related vascular degeneration; and (3) copper deficiency interfering with the elasticity of the vessels.[64]

Hemorrhage usually originates from the uterine artery, resulting in hematoma formation if blood exclusively dissects within the planes of the broad ligament, between the myometrium and the serosa of the uterus, or a hemoabdomen if the hemorrhage is uncontrolled and escapes from the confines of the broad ligament. Clinical signs associated with PPH can be non-specific and depend on the extent of hemorrhage as well as if it is controlled or uncontrolled. If hemorrhage is contained within the broad ligament, affected mares usually present with acute onset of colic signs, likely associated with stretching of the broad ligament and its dorsal attachments. Colic signs can range from mild to severe, including flank watching and rolling as well as intermittent flehmen response. Flehmen is thought of as characteristic of pain localized to the broad ligament in periparturient mares.[59] If hemorrhage overwhelms the confines of the broad ligament or if the broad ligament ruptures, both resulting in uncontrolled bleeding into the peritoneal cavity, signs of cardiovascular shock specifically tachycardia, agitation, dull demeanor, muscle fasciculations, sweating, vocalizing and weakness will often predominate signs of abdominal discomfort. At this time, mucous membranes appear pale. It is not unusual to initially identify pink mucous membranes in mares with an acute bleed (<3–4 hours) due to splenic contraction and the release of pooled red blood cells. The absence of previous colic signs should not eliminate PPH as a differential diagnosis in this scenario. Since mares with PPH can present with relatively non-specific clinical signs, diagnosis can be difficult although, signalment and clinical signs specifically, a peripartum mare presenting with signs of colic and/or hemorrhagic shock should lead to uterine artery rupture being high on the differential diagnosis list. Transabdominal sonography, abdominocentesis, and bloodwork are useful to confirm the diagnosis of hemorrhage. When evaluating the hemogram, in the peracute phase of hemorrhage, hematocrit and protein values are normal because the relative proportion of red blood cells to plasma is unaltered until hemodilution occurs with the movement of interstitial fluid into the intravascular space in an attempt to preserve total circulating blood volume and pressure. Splenic contraction is stimulated by the sympathetic-mediated response to hemorrhage resulting in an increased circulating erythrocyte mass which can elevate hematocrit such that serial blood monitoring will reveal a decrease in total protein before a decrease in hematocrit. Assuming hemorrhage ceases, the lowest values for hematocrit and protein are usually seen at about 48 hours following the onset of hemorrhage. Blood lactate concentration can also be used as a helpful marker of circulatory perfusion and is high (>4 mmol/L) in mares with hemorrhage. Transabdominal sonography is the most efficient diagnostic tool to support a diagnosis of hemoperitoneum based on the unique swirling sonographic appearance of free peritoneal blood. Careful transrectal sonography can also be useful when hemorrhage is confined to the broad ligament. If the arterial rupture is confined to the broad ligament, a hematoma can often be palpated in the broad ligament and seromuscular surface of the uterus per rectum.

Some clinicians warn against performing examinations per rectum in mares suspected of having PPH due to the risk of precipitating an episode of uncontrolled hemorrhage because of the increased stress and agitation associated with the procedure. Abdominocentesis is indicated when other differential diagnoses such as uterine rupture or gastrointestinal disease are suspected.

Treatment is aimed at restoring perfusion, enhancing coagulation, providing antimicrobial prophylaxis, controlling pain with analgesia and sedation, and reducing the effects of endotoxemia. Mares with PPH can be successfully managed with antifibrinolytic drugs (aminocaproic acid 40 mg/kg in 1 L of 0.9% saline loading dose and then 20 mg/kg QID or tranexamic acid 20 mg/kg IV BID diluted on 1 L of 0.9% saline). Blood transfusions may be indicated based on clinical signs (HR > 80 BPM), abdominal ultrasound findings, and bloodwork(red blood cell count, total protein, and albumin). In a study, one of the authors (NMS) found that mares with PPH have an 84% survival rate. Mares in this study with pre-partum bleeds had a survival rate of 60% while mares with post-partum hemorrhage had a survival rate of 87.3%.[60] We attribute the successful treatment of these mares to early recognition of the disease and aggressive medical management.

Prepubic tendon and abdominal wall rupture

The prepubic tendon serves as the pelvic attachment of the linea alba and therefore acts as the ventral abdominal sling in the pregnant mare. It consists of the tendons and aponeuroses associated with the muscles that define the ventral and lateral body walls, which include the rectus abdominus, transverse abdominus, and oblique muscles.[65] Rupture of the muscles comprising the ventrolateral body wall is much more common than complete prepubic tendon rupture.[59] Most prepubic tendon ruptures and body wall defects occur within the last 2 months of gestation. Both of these conditions are emergencies due to the increased risk of evisceration that accompanies the loss of the ventral abdominal support. Older and Draft breed mares are predisposed to prepubic tendon rupture.[59] Other reported predisposing factors are hydrops allantois, hydrops amnion, trauma, and twins.[66] One of the authors (NMS), has also noted this to occur in older mares with PPID due to a decrease in muscle mass and presumptive muscle atrophy.[53] Body wall ruptures are usually preceded by the development of marked ventral edema (**Fig. 11**). On initial presentation, clinical signs commonly

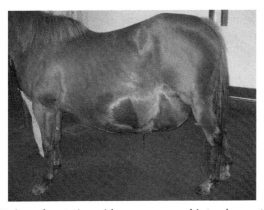

Fig. 11. Mare at 300 days of gestation with a severe prepubic tendon rupture secondary to a hydroallantois. She was euthanized due to severe extra abdominal hemorrhage from her torn muscles resulting in pain.

associated with ventral body wall defects include ventral pitting edema that is painful on palpation, easily depressible abdominal wall tissue, ventral displacement of the abdominal wall, hemorrhagic mammary secretions indicative of regional tissue trauma, and reluctance to walk forward. Progressive enlargement of the abdomen secondary to the body wall defect may result in tachycardia as well as colic signs. It can also lead to the incarceration of a segment of the intestine and, therefore, a more acute onset of severe colic signs. Complete prepubic tendon rupture classically results in tilting of the pelvis which leads to a subsequent elevation of the tail head and ischial tuberosities; lordosis occurs and the mare typically adopts a "sawhorse stance."[63] Cranial and ventral displacement of the mammary gland also occurs due to the loss of its caudal attachment to the pelvis.[67] Definitive diagnosis can be difficult as ventral edema may arise from many other conditions such as the typical development of ventral edema in late gestation following decreased venous and lymphatic drainage secondary to the compressive weight of the gravid uterus, large hematoma formation secondary to external trauma, hydrops allantois/hydrops amnion, or twin pregnancy. It is especially important to differentiate prepubic tendon rupture from hydrops as ventral abdominal wall ruptures can also be sequelae of these conditions. Monitoring creatinine kinase and aspartate transferase as markers of muscle damage can be helpful in determining the severity of the condition with increases in these enzymes indicating further compromise to the ventral body wall musculature directly related to the compressive weight of the gravid uterus.[63] Clinical suspicion of ventral body wall defects can be confirmed with transabdominal sonography via identification of increased intramuscular edema and increased echogenicity consistent with hemorrhage.

Conservative management is recommended as the treatment of choice for mares with body wall defects when possible. However, not all mares can be comfortably controlled in this way when the tear is too severe or is rapidly enlarging, or where pain cannot be controlled, will necessitate intervention (Cesarean if appropriate) and/or euthanasia. Conservative management would consist of analgesia, stall rest, and an abdominal support wrap (https://www.cmequine-products.com/) that is tightened daily. Any mare with a history of a ruptured prepubic tendon should be retired from breeding due to the high level of risk for both mare and foal in subsequent gestations.

Large colon volvulus

Strangulating displacement of the large colon is most commonly, yet not exclusively, seen in broodmares and accounts for 10% to 20% of all surgical colic cases.[68] Recent parturition is an established risk factor, specifically within the first 100 days following parturition. Large colon volvulus has, however, also been reported in the last trimester of pregnancy. Other proposed risk factors include a recent increase in dietary concentrates as well as exposure to lush pasture.[69] Thoroughbred broodmares are overrepresented in the population of horses which develop large colon volvulus. Recent studies involving Thoroughbred mares located in Kentucky suggested a potential heritable basis and, therefore, genetic predilection for the development of a large colon volvulus, based on the shared use of sires among affected progeny.[70] The markedly increased incidence of this condition in recently postpartum mares is likely multifactorial. Affected mares usually reside in rich pastures during the spring and consume increased amounts of high-energy concentrates to support lactation and pregnancy, both of which could contribute to changes in the cecal and colonic microbiome. It is also historically thought that there is more room within the abdomen of a recently postpartum mare, which could facilitate displacement and subsequent volvulus. However, large colon volvulus also occurs in pre-partum mares and non-pregnant horses. The hallmark presentation of this condition involves the acute onset of violent colic signs and progressive abdominal distention. Less commonly, these mares may present with a history of intermittent mild colic signs and subsequent acute onset of severe and intractable pain that occurs with complete strangulation of the colon. Physical examination in the early stages of the disease may be relatively unremarkable but within a short period, increasing severity of colic signs, tachycardia, increasing abdominal distention, signs of hypovolemia as well as shock become apparent. Transabdominal sonography often reveals dilation of colonic mesenteric vessels as well as edematous thickening of the large intestinal wall, as a result of venous and lymphatic engorgement secondary to strangulation. Dilated colonic vessels are best visualized in the right abdomen between intercostal spaces 12 and 15. On palpation per rectum, marked gas distention of the large colon is noted. With marked colonic gas distention, increased pressure is placed on the diaphragm, which impairs the diaphragm's ability to engage in effective ventilatory excursions, therefore tachypnea and dyspnea can occur. In summary, large colon volvulus should be suspected in a periparturient mare displaying severe colic signs and progressive abdominal distention. The presence of abdominal distention can help differentiate this condition from the aforementioned causes of colic in the periparturient mare. Mares have a good prognosis with early surgical treatment. In a recent study, Thoroughbred broodmares had successful breeding careers following surgical correction of ≥360° LCV that compared favorably with previous reports of Thoroughbred broodmare career longevity and productivity; 81.7% of the mares which were bred after surgery produced live foals. These foaling rates are similar to live foaling rates reported for other populations of well-managed Thoroughbred mares.[71]

Hydrops allantois/hydrops amnion

Hydrops conditions of the placenta in the mare are uncommon, with hydrops allantois being reported more frequently than hydrops amnion.[72] The condition in the mare usually develops during the last trimester of pregnancy and is characterized by the excessive accumulation of allantoic (hydrops allantois) or amnionic fluid (hydrops amnion). The sequelae of unnoticed or untreated hydrops allantois/amnion can be substantial, including abdominal wall hernias, prepubic tendon rupture, and even cardiovascular shock associated with unattended foaling and dystocia.[73–75] This condition is often detected by the horse owner/caregiver due to a sudden onset of abdominal enlargement (over a period of a few weeks), ventral edema, varying degrees of colic, lethargy, anorexia, tachycardia, and, on occasion, dyspnea associated with intra-abdominal hypertension. Differential diagnoses include twins, other causes of colic as well as other causes of ventral edema.

Definitive diagnosis requires a transrectal examination of the reproductive tract and transabdominal sonographic examination to detect abnormally abundant fetal fluids. The allantoic fluid volume in mares with hydrops allantois can range from 110 to 230 L, while a normal volume at term ranges from 8 to 18 L.[76] Examination per rectum will reveal a large fluid-filled uterus of varying tightness with the dorsal wall potentially protruding above the level of the pubis and absence of fetal ballottment.[60] Examination per rectum for hydrops amnion is similar to that of hydrops allantois except the uterus will not be protruding above the level of the pubis.[60] Transabdominal sonography for hydrops allantois will reveal excessive allantoic fluid, with a depth greater than 18 cm being highly suggestive of hydrops allantois. The normal amount of allantoic fluid depth is 4.7 to 22.1 cm with a mean maximal depth of 13.4 ± 4.4 cm (**Fig. 12**).[64,77] Imaging of the non-pregnant horn also usually reveals an abnormal amount of allantoic fluid.

Treatment of choice for hydrops allantois or amnion is early termination of pregnancy via drainage of the allantoic or amniotic fluid using a sterile technique under

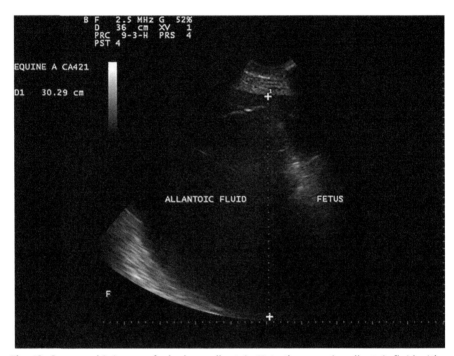

B F   2.5 MHZ G   52%
D   36 cm XV   1
PRC 9-3-H PRS   4
PST 4

EQUINE A CA421

D1   30.29 cm

ALLANTOIC FLUID   FETUS

F

Fig. 12. Sonographic image of a hydrops allantois. Note the excessive allantoic fluid with a depth of 30.29 cm (normal allantoic depth: 4.7–22.1 cm).

standing sedation.[71] The prognosis for a viable foal from a mare that has hydrops allantois is poor. One of the authors (NMS) as well as other veterinarians have successfully managed a mare with hydrops amnion. The mare was close to her expected date of parturition (2 weeks) and therefore the pregnancy was maintained and the mare had a viable foal. If early termination of the preganacy is warranted then prostaglandin E[a] or N-butylscopolammoniumbromide[b] gel is gently massaged onto the cervix if cervical dilation is desired. A PGE_1 gel can be made by crushing 200 µg misoprostol[c] tablets, resuspending in 1.5–2 mL of saline and further mixing with 1.5–2 mL of sterile lubricant. After 5 minutes, the cervix can be gently dilated manually. The veterinarian should be careful not to excessively dilate the cervix because they will not be able to control the rate of drainage of the fluid. Vaginal-assisted delivery is recommended, however, care should be taken not to traumatize the cervix. Retention of fetal membranes should be expected and treatment of removal in the form of uterine lavages as well as prophylactic metritis care should be implemented. Placement of an intravenous catheter before transcervical gradual fluid drainage of the allantoic or amniotic fluid is important to allow for intravenous fluid support during the procedure and avoid hypotensive shock. The prognosis for survival and future fertility of hydrops mares is good; 90% of mares surviving to hospital discharge with 95% of those mares successfully delivering future foals, provided the hydrops is diagnosed and treated

---

[a] Prepidil, Pharmacia & Upjohn, Kalamazoo, MI 49001.

[b] N-butylscopolammonium bromide 5 mg/mL gel, Hagyard Pharmacy, Lexington KY 40511.

[c] Misprostol Tablets 200mcg, ANI Pharmaceuticals, Inc. Baudette, MN 56623.

appropriately with transcervical gradual fluid drainage and no damage to the reproductive tract or abdominal wall occurs.[78]

SUMMARY

Distinguishing between medical and surgical colic can be very difficult in foals because palpation per rectum is not feasible. Sonography can replace palpation per rectum with a high sensitivity but low specificity. A "monitor and wait" approach has as much risk as exploratory surgery in foals. These patients present different considerations than in older foals and adults. The clinician must consider these differences in the evaluation when making a diagnosis, a decision for surgery, and formulating a prognosis for the owner.

Diagnosis of colic in the pregnant mare also presents some peculiar challenges. The presence of a gravid uterus may prevent adequate examination of the intestinal tract *per rectum.*

It may also be difficult or impossible to obtain peritoneal fluid in heavily pregnant mares, in which the uterus overlies the ventral abdominal wall. It may be difficult to distinguish between gastrointestinal and reproductive causes of abdominal pain, although, with the exception of uterine torsion, the gravid uterus is rarely the source of moderate to severe abdominal pain in pregnant mares.

CLINICS CARE POINTS

- The most common causes of neonatal colic are enterocolitis and meconium impactions.
- A "monitor and wait" approach has as much risk as exploratory surgery in foals.
- Abdominal ultrasound is a vital diagnostic tool when assessing neonates that present with colic signs since abdominal palpation per rectum is not feasible.
- Abdominal ultrasound in pregnant mares with colic is also beneficial to distinguish between gastrointestinal and reproductive causes of abdominal pain.
- Deciding the best course of treatment for a pregnant mare with colic can be further complicated by concerns regarding fetal viability.
- Accurate diagnosis and timely intervention may not only save the life of the mare but may also result in the birth of a viable foal especially in cases such as uterine torsions and ventral body wall ruptures. Transabdominal ultrasound of the fetus should be performed and can provide information regarding fetal distress or death

REFERENCES

1. Aggerwal N, Sugandhi N, Kour H, et al. Total Intestinal Atresia: Revisiting the Pathogenesis of Congenital Atresias. J Indian Assoc Pediatr Surg 2019;24(4): 303–6.
2. Young RL, Linford RL, Olander HJ. Atresia coli in the foal: a review of six cases. Equine Vet J 1992;24(1):60–2.
3. Nappert G, Laverty S, Drolet R, et al. Atresia coli in 7 foals (1964–1990). Equine Vet J 2010;24:57–60.
4. Hunter B, Belgrave RL. Atresia coli in a foal: Diagnosis made with colonoscopy aided by N-butylscopolammonium bromide. Equine Vet Edu 2010;22:429–33.
5. Lightbody T. Foal with Overo lethal white syndrome born to a registered quarter horse mare. Can Vet J 2002;43(9):715–7.
6. Giancola F, Gentilini F, Romagnoli N, et al. Extrinsic innervation of ileum and pelvic flexure of foals with ileocolonic aganglionosis. Cell Tissue Res 2016;366(1):13–22.

7. McCabe L, Griffin LD, Kinzer A, et al. Overo lethal white foal syndrome: equine model of aganglionic megacolon (Hirschsprung disease). Am J Med Genet 1990;36(3):336–40.

8. Magdesian KG, Williams DC, Aleman M, et al. Evaluation of deafness in American Paint Horses by phenotype, brainstem auditory-evoked responses, and endothelin receptor B genotype. J Am Vet Med Assoc 2009;235(10):1204–11.

9. Stick JA. Abdominal hernias. In: Auer JA, Stick JA, editors. Equine surgery. 3rd edition. Sydney (Australia): W.B Saunders; 2006. p. 491–9.

10. Freeman DE, Spencer PA. Evaluation of age, breed, and gender as risk factors for umbilical hernia in horses of a hospital population. Am J Vet Res 1991; 52(4):637–9.

11. Bodaan CJ, Panizzi L, Stewart AJ, et al. Extensive umbilical herniation of the large colon in a foal. Equine Vet Educ 2014;26:341–4.

12. Adams R, Koterba AM, Brown MP, et al. Exploratory celiotomy for gastrointestinal disease in neonatal foals: a review of 20 cases. Equine Vet J 1988;20(1):9–12.

13. Bartmann CP, Freeman DE, Glitz F, et al. Diagnosis and surgical management of colic in the foal: Literature review and a retrospective study. Clin Tech Equine Pract 2002;1(3):125–42.

14. Ryan CA, Sanchez LC. Nondiarrheal disorders of the gastrointestinal tract in neonatal foals. Vet Clin North Am Equine Pract. 2005;21(2):313–32.

15. Winfield LS, Dechant JE. Primary gastric rupture in 47 horses (1995-2011). Can Vet J 2015;56(9):953–8.

16. Borst GH, van der Weij PJ, Vos JH. [Idiopathic gastric rupture in a Friesian foal]. Tijdschr Diergeneeskd 2004;129(8):270–1.

17. Ohshiro K, Yamataka A, Kobayashi H, et al. Idiopathic gastric perforation in neonates and abnormal distribution of intestinal pacemaker cells. J Pediatr Surg 2000;35(5):673–6.

18. Coleman MC, Slovis NM, Hunt RJ. Long-term prognosis of gastrojejunostomy in foals with gastric outflow obstruction: 16 cases (2001–2006). Equine Vet J 2009; 41(7):653–7.

19. Andrews FM, Nadeau JA. Clinical syndromes of gastric ulceration in foals and mature horses. Equine Vet J Suppl 1999;(29):30–3.

20. Isenberg JI, Hogan DL, Koss MA, et al. Human duodenal mucosal bicarbonate secretion. Evidence for basal secretion and stimulation by hydrochloric acid and a synthetic prostaglandin E1 analogue. Gastroenterology 1986;91(2):370–8.

21. Sanchez LC, Lester GD, Merritt AM. Intragastric pH in critically ill neonatal foals and the effect of ranitidine. J Am Vet Med Assoc 2001;218(6):907–11.

22. Freeman DE: Small intestine, in JA Auer, JA Stick (eds): Equine Surgery (ed 2). Philadelphia, PA, Saunders, 1999, pp 232– 257. White NA: Epidemiology and etiology of colic, in NA White (ed): The Equine Acute Abdomen. Philadelphia, PA, Lea and Febiger, 1990, pp 49– 65.

23. Orsini JA. Abdominal surgery in foals. Vet Clin North Am Equine Pract 1997;13(2): 393–413.

24. Stephen JO, Corley KT, Johnston JK, et al. Small intestinal volvulus in 115 horses: 1988-2000. Vet Surg 2004;33(4):333–9.

25. Erwin SJ, Clark ME, Dechant JE, et al. Multi-Institutional Retrospective Case-Control Study Evaluating Clinical Outcomes of Foals with Small Intestinal Strangulating Obstruction: 2000-2020. Animals (Basel) 2022;12(11).

26. Reinemeyer CR, Nielsen MK. Parasitism and colic. Vet Clin Equine Pract 2009; 25(2):233–45.

27. Frederick J, Giguère S, Sanchez LC. Infectious Agents Detected in the Feces of Diarrheic Foals: A Retrospective Study of 233 Cases (2003–2008). J Vet Int Med 2009;23(6):1254–60.
28. Mackinnon MC, Southwood LL, Burke MJ, et al. Colic in equine neonates: 137 cases (2000-2010). J Am Vet Med Assoc 2013;243(11):1586–95.
29. Magdesian KG. Neonatal foal diarrhea. Vet Clin N Am Equine Pract 2005;21(2): 295–312.
30. Radostits OM, Gay C, Hinchcliff KW, et al. Veterinary Medicine E-Book: a textbook of the diseases of cattle, horses, sheep, pigs and goats. St. Louis (MO): Elsevier Health Sciences; 2006. p. 274–7.
31. Theelen MJP, Wilson WD, Byrne BA, et al. Initial antimicrobial treatment of foals with sepsis: Do our choices make a difference? Vet J 2019;243:74–6.
32. Hollis AR, Wilkins PA, Palmer JE, et al. Bacteremia in equine neonatal diarrhea: a retrospective study (1990-2007). J Vet Intern Med 2008;22(5):1203–9.
33. Bernard WV, Reef VB, Reimer JM, et al. Ultrasonographic diagnosis of small-intestinal intussusception in three foals. J Am Vet Med Assoc 1989;194(3):395–7.
34. Vatistas NJ, Snyder JR, Wilson WD, et al. Surgical treatment for colic in the foal (67 cases): 1980-1992. Equine Vet J 1996;28(2):139–45.
35. Sanchez LC, Giguère S, Lester GD. Factors associated with survival of neonatal foals with bacteremia and racing performance of surviving Thoroughbreds: 423 cases (1982-2007). J Am Vet Med Assoc 2008;233(9):1446–52.
36. Pusterla N, Magdesian KG, Maleski K, et al. Retrospective evaluation of the use of acetylcysteine enemas in the treatment of meconium retention in foals: 44 cases (1987–2002). Equine Vet Educ 2004;16(3):133–6.
37. McCue P. Meconium impaction in newborn foals. J Equine Vet Sci 2006;26:152–5.
38. Cable CS, Fubini SL, Erb HN, et al. Abdominal surgery in foals: a review of 119 cases (1977-1994). Equine Vet J 1997;29(4):257–61.
39. Hennessy SE, Fraser BS. Right dorsal displacement of the large colon as a cause of surgical colic in three foals in New Zealand. N Z Vet J 2012;60(6):360–4.
40. Schusser GE, White NA. Morphologic and quantitative evaluation of the myenteric plexuses and neurons in the large colon of horses. J Am Vet Med Assoc 1997;210(7):928–34.
41. Murray MJ, Parker GA, White NA. Megacolon with myenteric hypoganglionosis in a foal. J Am Vet Med Assoc 1988;192(7):917–9.
42. Santschi EM, Purdy AK, Valberg SJ, et al. Endothelin receptor B polymorphism associated with lethal white foal syndrome in horses. Mamm Genome 1998; 9(4):306–9.
43. Noerr B. Current controversies in the understanding of necrotizing enterocolitis. Part 1. Adv Neonatal Care 2003;3(3):107–20.
44. Kablack KA, Embertson RM, Bernard WV, et al. Uroperitoneum in the hospitalised equine neonate: retrospective study of 31 cases, 1988-1997. Equine Vet J 2000; 32(6):505–8.
45. Divers TJ, Perkins G. Urinary and hepatic disorders in neonatal foals. Clin Tech Equine Pract 2003;2(1):67–78.
46. Castagnetti C, Mariella J, Pirrone A, et al. Urethral and bladder rupture in a neonatal colt with uroperitoneum. Equine Vet Edu 2010;22(3):132–8.
47. Lefevre L, Nollet H, Vlaminck L, et al. Uterine torsion in the mare: a review and three case reports. Vlaams Diergeneeskundig Tijdschrift 2008;77:397–405.
48. Doyle AJ, Freeman DE, Sauberli DS, et al. Clinical signs and treatment of chronic uterine torsion in two mares. J Am Vet Med Assoc 2002;220(3):349–53, 323.

49. Taylor EL, Blanchard T, Varner D. Management of dystocia in mares: uterine torsion and cesarean section. Compend Contin Educ Pract Vet 1989;11:1265–72.

50. Spoormakers TJ, Graat EA, ter Braake F, et al. Mare and foal survival and subsequent fertility of mares treated for uterine torsion. Equine Vet J 2016;48(2):172–5.

51. Barber SM. Torsion of the uterus–a cause of colic in the mare. Can Vet J 1979; 20(6):165–7.

52. Jung C, Hospes R, Bostedt H, et al. Surgical treatment of uterine torsion using a ventral midline laparotomy in 19 mares. Aust Vet J 2008;86(7):272–6.

53. Chaney KP, Holcombe SJ, LeBlanc MM, et al. The effect of uterine torsion on mare and foal survival: a retrospective study, 1985–2005. Equine Vet J 2007; 39(1):33–6.

54. Auer DE, Wilson RG, Groenendyk S, et al. Diaphragmatic rupture in a mare at parturition. Equine Vet J 1985;17(4):331–3.

55. Kelmer G, Kramer J, Wilson DA, editors. Diaphragmatic hernia: etiology clinical presentation, and diagnosis, Comp Cont 2008;3:28–35.

56. Pleasure DE, Walsh GO, Engel WK. Atrophy of skeletal muscle in patients with Cushing's syndrome. Arch Neurol 1970;22(2):118–25.

57. Romero AE, Rodgerson DH. Diaphragmatic herniation in the horse: 31 cases from 2001-2006. Can Vet J 2010;51(11):1247–50.

58. Edwards GB. Diaphragmatic hernia - a diagnostic and surgical challenge. Equine Vet Educ 1993;5(5):267–9.

59. Everett KA, Chaffin MK, Brinsko SP. Diaphragmatic herniation as a cause of lethargy and exercise intolerance in a mare. Cornell Vet 1992;82 3:217–23.

60. Mair TS, Pearson H, Waterman AE, et al. Chylothorax associated with a congenital diaphragmatic defect in a foal. Equine Vet J 1988;20(4):304–6.

61. Arnold CE, Payne M, Thompson JA, et al. Periparturient hemorrhage in mares: 73 cases (1998-2005). J Am Vet Med Assoc 2008;232(9):1345–51.

62. Lu KG, Sprayberry KA. Managing Reproduction Emergencies in the Field: Part 2: Parturient and Periparturient Conditions. Vet Clin North America: Equine Practice 2021;37(2):367–405.

63. McAuliffe SB, Slovis NM. The Pregnant Mare. In: McAuliffe S, Slovis N, editors. Color atlas of diseases and disorders of the foal. Philadelphila, PA: Saunders/ Elsevier; 2008. p. 25–30.

64. Reef VB, Vaala WE, Worth LT, et al. Ultrasonographic evaluation of the fetus and intrauterine environment in healthy mares during late gestation. Vet Radiol Ultrasound 1995;36:533–41.

65. Habel RE, Budras KD. Anatomy of the prepubic tendon in the horse, cow, sheep, goat, and dog. Am J Vet Res 1992;53(11):2183–95.

66. Ross J, Palmer JE, Wilkins PA. Body wall tears during late pregnancy in mares: 13 cases (1995-2006). J Am Vet Med Assoc 2008;232(2):257–61.

67. Hanson RR, Todhunter RJ. Herniation of the abdominal wall in pregnant mares. J Am Vet Med Assoc 1986;189(7):790–3.

68. Proudman CJ, Smith JE, Edwards GB, et al. Long-term survival of equine surgical colic cases. Part 1: patterns of mortality and morbidity. Equine Vet J 2002;34(5): 432–7.

69. Suthers JM, Pinchbeck GL, Proudman CJ, et al. Survival of horses following strangulating large colon volvulus. Equine Vet J 2013;45(2):219–23.

70. Petersen JL, Lewis RM, Embertson R, et al. Preliminary heritability of complete rotation large colon volvulus in Thoroughbred broodmares. Vet Rec 2019; 185(9):269.

71. Leahy ER, Holcombe SJ, Hackett ES, et al. Reproductive careers of Thorough-bred broodmares before and after surgical correction of ≥360 degree large colon volvulus. Equine Vet J 2018;50(2):208–12.
72. Sertich PL, Reef VB, Oristaglio-Turner RM, et al. Hydrops amnii in a mare. J Am Vet Med Assoc 1994;204(9):1481–2.
73. Sertich PL. Periparturient emergencies. Vet Clin North Am Equine Pract 1994;10(1):19–36.
74. Slovis NM, Lu KG, Wolfsdorf KE, et al. How to manage hydrops allantois/hydrops amnion in a mare. Proc Annu Conv Am Assoc Equine Pract 2013;34–9.
75. Blanchard T, Varner D, Buonanno A, et al. Hydrallantois in two mares. J Equine Vet Sc 1987;7(4):222–5.
76. Frazer GS. Chapter 59 Dystocia and Fetotomy. Current Therapy in Equine Repro-duction 2006;417.
77. Reef VB, Vaala WE, Worth LT, et al. Ultrasonographic assessment of fetal well-being during late gestation: development of an equine biophysical profile. Equine Vet J 1996;28(3):200–8.
78. Lemonnier LC, Wolfsdorf KE, Kreutzfeldt N, et al. Factors Affecting Survival and Future Foaling Rates in Thoroughbred Mares with Hydrops. J Equine Vet Sci 2022;113:103941.

What Is the Microbiota and What Is Its Role in Colic?

Carolyn E. Arnold, DVM, PhD, DACVS[a],*, Rachel Pilla, DVM, PhD[b]

KEYWORDS

• Equine • Colic • Microbiome • Gastrointestinal bacteria

KEY POINTS

- The gastrointestinal microbiome plays an important role in the health of the horse.
- Horses with colic and diarrhea exhibit dysbiosis of the gastrointestinal microbiome compared with healthy horses.
- Antimicrobial drugs disrupt the healthy microbiota.
- Although we are continuing to learn more about the equine gastrointestinal microbiome in health and disease, more studies are need using consistent methodology for sample processing and analysis to interpret results published to date.
- Ultimately, the goal is to better understand the role of the microbiome in horses with colic potentially leading to methods to optimize the microbial populations of the gastrointestinal tract to prevent disease.

INTRODUCTION TO THE MICROBIOME

Colic is the principal cause of equine deaths worldwide[1] as well as a source of economic and emotional loss to owners. Historically, researchers have implicated factors such as modern management practices (diet,[2–5] exercise,[3,6] and stabling/access to pasture[5,7]), hindgut fermentation resulting in the production of gas,[8] and anatomic features of the gastrointestinal (GI) tract itself[9] (intralumenal narrowing that predisposes to obstruction, ischemic lesions created by entrapment of portions of bowel with a long mesenteric attachment) as the contributing factors to GI disease causing signs of colic. Although great strides have been made in the treatment of individual horses with colic, the prevalence of colic in the equine population remains high and unchanged over the last 25 years.[10–12] These statistics indicate that the *underlying cause of GI disease remains unknown* and poses an important, yet unanswered, clinical question.

[a] School of Veterinary Medicine, Texas Tech University, 7671 Evans Street, Amarillo, Texas 79106, USA; [b] Gastrointestinal Laboratory, Department of Small Animal Clinical Sciences, School of Veterinary Medicine, Texas A&M University, College Station, TX, USA
* Corresponsing author. School of Veterinary Medicine, Texas Tech University, 7671 Evans Street, Amarillo, Texas 79106.
E-mail address: Carolyn.Arnold@ttu.edu

Vet Clin Equine 39 (2023) 381–397
https://doi.org/10.1016/j.cveq.2023.03.004
0749-0739/23/© 2023 Elsevier Inc. All rights reserved.

Recent research into human GI disease has brought to light the importance of the microorganisms residing within the gut. Known as the microbiome, this collection of bacteria, bacteriophages, fungi, protozoa, and viruses has coevolved over thousands of years to form a symbiotic relationship with its host.[13,14] For the purposes of this discussion, the term microbiome will refer only to bacteria as they have been more thoroughly investigated. The commensal bacteria of the GI tract serve important metabolic functions such as nutrient breakdown and absorption, the production of short-chain fatty acids (SCFAs), the conversion of primary to secondary bile acids, the biosynthesis of vitamins and amino acids, the regulation of the inflammatory environment of the gut, and the modulation of the immune system in response to pathogens.[15] Changes in the normal bacterial populations result in alterations in these metabolic functions. Oftentimes, these metabolic responses result in inflammatory changes that are associated with disease. The term *dysbiosis* has been used to describe the alterations in the bacterial community composition and subsequent functional changes in metabolism associated with disease states.[15,16] In humans, the identification of the microbiome and its role in various GI diseases has enabled advances in the understanding, diagnosis, and treatment of ulcerative colitis, Crohn's disease, obesity, and metabolic disease.[17] Similar progress has been made in companion animals suffering from acute and chronic enteropathies.[18–20] Owing to the success of these efforts, equine researchers have begun to investigate the gut microbiota in healthy horses and those with GI disease.

Characterization of the Gastrointestinal Microbiota

Until recently, the culture-based methods were used to identify bacteria. This limited the number of identifiable species to only cultivable bacteria, an estimated 10% of the total number of known species.[21] With the advent of next-generation sequencing (NGS), over 1000 species of bacteria previously unrecognized by microbial culture can now been identified.[21,22] Two methods of NGS have been used to discover GI microbiome composition: 16S rRNA gene sequencing and whole genome or shotgun sequencing. With each method, DNA is purified from a sample and its nucleic acid sequence is defined. With 16S rRNA or short-read sequencing, primers target and amplify a marker gene (the 16S ribosomal subunit) with conserved regions common to all bacteria flanking variable regions unique to each species. This short sequence of DNA (about 450 bp) is subsequently assigned to an operational taxonomic unit (OTU) or amplicon sequence variant (ASV) depending on the pipeline used, and the OTUs/ASVs will be compared with a library of bacterial sequences for identification. In contrast, whole genome or shotgun sequencing identifies the entire genome of a sample which is later assembled and compared with a database. Because it includes areas of the genome beyond the 16S rRNA gene, it allows for investigation beyond taxonomic classification, identifying functional genes such as virulence factors, antimicrobial resistance genes, and genes associated with bacterial metabolism. It is also not limited to bacteria (which possess a 16S ribosomal subunit) but includes sequences from other kingdoms such as viruses, fungi, archaea, and the host itself.

Data provided by both types of NGS include a taxonomic description of the bacteria at the level of phylum, class, order, family, genus, and species as well as their abundance. Although 16S rRNA sequencing is cheaper, faster, and more commonly used than shotgun sequencing, it does not provide the resolution needed to identify bacteria to the species level.[23] It also does not include any functional genes, limiting itself to answering "who is there?" but skipping the more pressing question of "what are they doing?"

How to Interpret Microbiome Data

Microbiome data are typically analyzed and reported as alpha diversity, beta diversity, and taxonomy. Alpha diversity is used to summarize the diversity within a sample and is reported as a single metric. This term can take into account either the number of different species present in a sample (richness) and also their distribution among each species (evenness).[24] Frequently reported metrics of alpha diversity may report just richness (number of unique taxa) or evenness (distribution among each taxa) or a combination of both. Alpha diversity can include the OTUs or ASVs (richness), Chao1 (richness), Shannon (richness and evenness), or Simpson's (richness and evenness) indices.[25] In **Fig. 1**, five healthy horses were administered metronidazole after sample collection on Day 0 which was discontinued on Day 3 due to adverse effects. However, fecal samples were collected on Days 7 and 14 (post-antibiotic administration). There is a significant loss in the number of species found in feces on Day 3 compared with Day 0 and followed by a recovery period by Day 14.

Beta diversity examines the composition of the bacterial community between samples, attributing a number to quantifiy similarity or differences between groups of samples. It is commonly reported as the Bray–Curtis index (composition), Jaccard index (presence or absence of species without abundance), and UniFrac distances (phylogenic relatedness with or without abundance).[25] Beta diversity is displayed using a 2- or 3-dimensional principal coordinate analysis (PCoA) or principal component (PCA) plots. Each individual animal is represented on the plot, with samples that are spatially clustered together on the plot having similar bacterial composition than samples that are distant from each other. In **Fig. 2**, Ericsson and colleagues demonstrated how samples from each compartment of the GI tract clustered on a PCoA plot. The

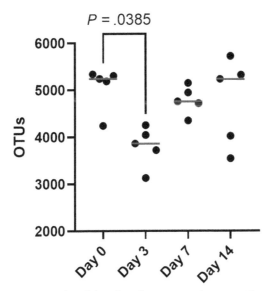

Fig. 1. A plot demonstrating the alpha diversity measured as operational taxonomic units (OTUs) for five horses treated with metronidazole. The red bar indicates the median for each Day. There is a reduction in the number of species found in fecal samples between Day 0 (pre-metronidazole administration) and Day 3 (post-metronidazole administration). Although the Day 14 median OTUs was similar to Day 0, there was more variability in the OTUs between horses.

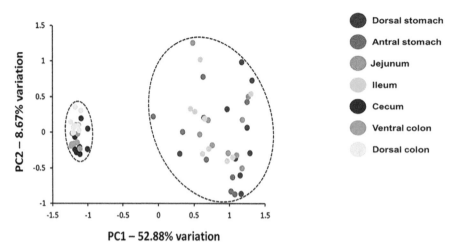

Fig. 2. Principal component analysis (PCA) of luminal gut microbial populations of samples from the dorsal stomach, antral stomach, jejunum, ileum, cecum, ventral colon, and dorsal colon of nine healthy adult horses. Of note is that the samples from the proximal GI tract (dorsal stomach to ileum) cluster distinctly from samples of the distal GI tract (cecum to dorsal colon). This indicates significant differences in bacterial populations. (*Adapted from* Ericsson AC, Johnson PJ, Lopes MA, et al. A Microbiological Map of the Healthy Equine Gastrointestinal Tract. *PLoS One* 2016 with permission.)

microbiome of the proximal GI tract (stomach to the ileum represented by brown, orange, and yellow spheres) clustered separately from the distal GI tract (cecum, ventral, and dorsal colons in shades of blue). This indicates different microbial community composition.

Finally, the abundance of bacterial taxa (phylum, class, order, family, genus, and species) in each sample is reported. Standard statistical methods are used to determine significant differences between groups of samples for each individual bacterial taxa, such as healthy horses versus those with GI disease, and methods to adjust for multiple comparisons must be used to prevent false discoveries. Histograms of the fecal microbiome at the phylum level for horses on five different diets are presented in **Fig. 3**.

It is important to note that methods for microbiome sequencing are not standardized and different DNA extraction methods, primer sets for 16S rRNA sequencing, databases for taxa identification, and pipelines for data analysis are often used in different combinations. In addition, high inter-individual variation is another known factor which means that studies with small sample sizes often have highly variable taxa abundance. Any one of these factors can introduce bias to the results, favoring the identification of certain taxa in detriment of others. Therefore, when looking at the literature it is important to focus not on the individual percentages themselves, but rather the main trends that are common across studies.

The Microbiome of Equine Gastrointestinal Tract

The fecal microbiome is thought to be representative of the distal (aboral) GI tract. Fecal samples are also readily available and obtained using minimally invasive methods of collection. In humans and companion animals,[26–28] the resident bacterial populations of each GI compartment are reflective of the anatomic and functional components of that segment as well as the substrate that reaches it.[29] These distinct

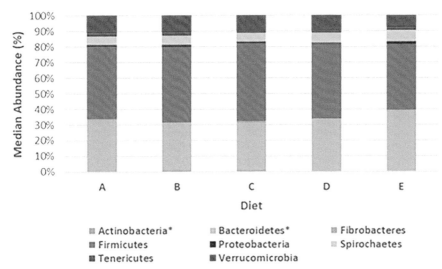

Fig. 3. Histograms representing the abundance of each phyla from healthy horses on different diets: Diet A: horses fed forage only (hay and/or pasture); Diet B: horses fed forage plus low fiber concentrate (5%–7%) at ≤0.5% of body weight in kg/d; Diet C: forage plus medium fiber concentrate (10%–15%) fed at ≤0.5% of body weight in kg/d; Diet D: forage plus high fiber concentrate (18%–33%) fed at ≤0.5% of body weight in kg/d; Diet E: forage plus medium fiber concentrate (10%–15%) fed at 1% to 2% of body weight in kg/d. Asterisks represent significant differences between bacterial phyla. Actinobacteria is significantly more abundant in Diet E compared with Diet B–D, whereas Bacteroidetes is more abundant in Diet E compared with B. (*From* Arnold, CE, Pilla, R, Chaffin, MK, et al. The effects of signalment, diet, geographic location, season, and colitis associated with antimicrobial use or Salmonella infection on the fecal microbiome of horses. J Vet Intern Med. 2021; 35(5): 2437–2448. https://doi.org/10.1111/jvim.16206.)

anatomical regions have specific pH ranges, enzymes, oxygen tensions, and microbiome compositions. Studies on the bacteria of the equine GI tract have found similar results. There seems to be distinct differences in the bacterial community composition, between the proximal (oral, stomach, and small intestine) and distal (aboral, cecum, and large colon) GI tract in horses (see **Fig. 2**).[29–32] These studies have confirmed that feces are an adequate proxy for the hindgut of the horse,[30,31] allowing for minimally invasive sampling from a portion of the gastrointestinal tract (GIT) frequently affected by GI disease.

Is There a Core Microbiome in the Hindgut of the Horse?

Researchers have attempted to define the "core microbiome" of the horse by identifying bacterial populations consistently present among healthy individuals. These taxa likely perform critical metabolic functions that are altered in dysbiosis or disease states.[33] As hindgut fermenters, the equine large colon contains fibrolytic bacteria that break down non-soluble plant material and convert it into SCFAs that supply the majority of the horse's energy needs.[34] Multiple studies in healthy horses have identified 17 to 20 phyla with varying abundances in equine feces.[30,31,35–39] The major phyla that seem consistently present across studies include Firmicutes, Bacteroidetes, and Verrucomicrobia.

At this point in time, the functional role of these bacteria has not been definitely characterized, and there is likely redundancy of function among taxa. Firmicutes, the most abundant phyla in the equine fecal microbiome, has an important role in the degradation of complex plant material.[40] Firmicutes includes many commensal groups belonging to the class Clostridia, which has previously been associated with pathogenic species. However, taxa within this class such as Lachnospiraceae (which produce butyrate, the main nutrient for colonic enterocytes) and Ruminococcaceae (production of acetate, propionate, and butyrate) perform important metabolic functions that are altered by GI disease. Bacteroidetes and Verrucomicrobia are often cited as the second or third most abundant phyla.[30,37,38,41–43] Bacteroidetes also contributes to the production of SCFA from fiber breakdown. Verrucomicrobia uses mucin in the GI tract as a nutrient and plays a pivotal role in maintaining the mucosal barrier at the epithelial surface. Depletion of Verrucomicrobia has been associated with the loss of barrier function in GI diseases such as colitis.[44,45] Other phyla that are present in lower abundance include Spirochaetes, Tenericutes, Fibrobacteres, Proteobacteria, and Actinobacteria.[30,38,43,46]

Factors Affecting the Healthy Horse Microbiome

The healthy equine fecal microbiome is affected by a number of factors that have been previously implicated as risk factors for colic by epidemiological studies. Studies using culture-based and non-culture-based methods have found inherent factors such as breed,[35,37,47] age,[42,48] and pregnancy status[49] in addition to external factors such as geographic location,[35] transport,[50] exercise intensity[51–53] fasting,[54,55] and season[56] seem to have some influence on the fecal microbiome. Dietary variables such as exposure to pasture,[35,57] abrupt feed change,[57–59] and feeding concentrate versus forage[60] can alter the microbiome to some degree, whereas the feeding of high-starch concentrates can not only alter the colonic environment but also induce laminitis.[42,61] These studies are commendable in their effort to characterize the response of the healthy equine fecal microbiome to external factors; however, the magnitude of the effect that these factors have on the microbiome with regard to changes in alpha diversity, beta diversity, and taxonomy is unclear, particularly if these changes are not associated with states of dysbiosis. Furthermore, it is often hard to compare studies because of their small sample size, the use of university teaching herds, or horses housed at single locations.[62,63] Finally, early studies often used culture-based or early NGS sequencing methodologies (ie, terminal-restriction fragment length polymorphism,[60] Illumina, 454-pyrosequencing),[37,42,61] as well as a variety of methods for sample collection, storage, and DNA extraction, which makes comparison across studies unreliable.

In a study using the largest number of healthy horses to date, the fecal bacterial microbiota of 80 adult horses from diverse geographical areas of the United States was examined by 16S rRNA sequencing.[43] Diet, a known driver of microbiome composition, individual animal factors such as breed, sex, age, state of residence, and season were evaluated. Individual animal factors had only minor influences on either alpha or beta diversity. Diet was stratified by forages and concentrates of varying fiber content. Only the most extreme diet (feeding concentrate at 1%–2% of body weight) influenced microbial community composition (beta diversity) and increased in the abundance of Actinobacteria. A PCoA plot of healthy horses stratified by diet is compared, as presented in **Fig. 4**.

Although the high-concentrate diet had a clear impact on microbiome composition, it is important to quantify that impact and differentiate whether it reflects an adaptation to the diet or a true dysbiosis (ie, changes in microbiome function associated with disease). For that, a comparison with samples from horses with colitis (due to antimicrobial usage or *Salmonella* infection) was compared with the healthy horse population

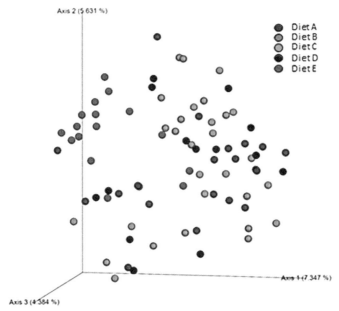

Fig. 4. A three-dimensional principle component analysis (PCA) showing the effect of diet on the fecal bacterial microbiota. Diet A: horses fed forage only (hay and/or pasture), purple. Diet B: horses fed forage plus low fiber concentrate (5%–7%) at ≤ 0.5% of body weight in kg/d, green. Diet C: forage plus medium fiber concentrate (10%–15%) fed at ≤ 0.5% of body weight in kg/d, orange. Diet D: forage plus high fiber concentrate (18%–33%) fed at ≤ 0.5% of body weight in kg/d blue. Diet E: forage plus medium fiber concentrate (10%–15%) fed at 1% to 2% of body weight in kg/d, red. Of note is that horses fed Diet E (high concentrate) clustered together and were spatially separated from horses fed Diets A to D. (*From* Arnold, CE, Pilla, R, Chaffin, MK, et al. The effects of signalment, diet, geographic location, season, and colitis associated with antimicrobial use or Salmonella infection on the fecal microbiome of horses. J Vet Intern Med. 2021; 35(5): 2437–2448. https://doi.org/10.1111/jvim.16206.)

(**Fig. 5**). Although samples from horses on diet E (high-concentrate) cluster together from healthy horses on the other diets, they remain well within the main group of healthy horses, suggesting that the size effect of an extreme diet is smaller than that of a true disease-associated dysbiosis.

Microbiome Studies of Horses with Gastrointestinal Disease

Colic

Although there is evidence that dysbiosis plays a role in equine colic, there are relatively few studies that have evaluated the fecal microbiome in horses with colic. Overall, horses with colic appear to have decreased diversity and changes in major phyla that compromise the healthy horse fecal microbiome.

Daly and coworkers[64] examined the fecal microbiome in three groups of horses: healthy horses under two dietary conditions (hay and hay plus concentrate) and horses with a large colon obstruction. Healthy horses consuming hay plus concentrate and those with colonic obstruction had an increased abundance of the *Bacillus-Lactobacillus-Streptococcus* families from the phyla Firmicutes, class Bacilli. These bacteria proliferate in starch-rich environments and produce lactate. Interestingly, elevations in the *Bacillus-Lactobacillus-Streptococcus* families are also found in oligofructose

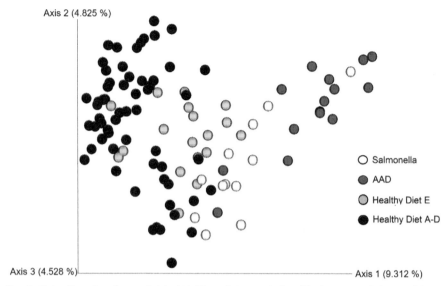

Fig. 5. Beta diversity of unweighted UniFrac distances in healthy horses and those with colitis caused by antimicrobials (antimicrobial-associated diarrhea, AAD) and salmonellosis (SAL). There is distinct clustering of horses with AAD (*red*) and salmonellosis (*yellow*) from healthy horses on Diets A–D (*royal blue*) and Diet E (*light blue*). There is statistically significant but less distinct separation of the two types of colitis horses from each other (AAD vs *Salmonella*, ANOSIM, analysis of similarities, $R = .226$, $P < .001$) and healthy horses on Diets A–D from those on Diet E (ANOSIM, $R = .287$, $P < .001$). (*From* Arnold, CE, Pilla, R, Chaffin, MK, et al. The effects of signalment, diet, geographic location, season, and colitis associated with antimicrobial use or Salmonella infection on the fecal microbiome of horses. J Vet Intern Med. 2021; 35(5): 2437–2448. https://doi.org/10.1111/jvim.16206.)

models of laminitis and in clinical patients with colitis and laminitis.[34,61,65–69] Changes in the bacterial community composition in disease states such as colitis indicate that dysbiosis may also play a role in colic due to large colon obstruction.

Venable and colleagues[70] collected feces from nine horses with acute colic attributable to the large colon and obtained samples 30 to 90 days following colic resolution.[70] Using 454 pyrosequencing, they found differences in taxa between groups. Although a large number of unidentified taxa that were excluded from analysis (54%), the investigators found 19 unique taxa in horses recovering from colic. Post-colic samples had a higher abundance of Firmicutes and a lower abundance of Bacteroidetes.

Weese and coworkers[49] performed a longitudinal, case-controlled study of prepartum and postpartum mares in central Kentucky. Feces were collected prospectively prepartum and postpartum and subsequently mares were categorized as those that developed colic ($n = 13$) and those that did not develop colic (control, $n = 13$). Eleven percent of pregnant mares developed colic in the postpartum period. Pregnant mares that developed colic had a higher abundance of Proteobacteria and lower abundance of Firmicutes. Mares that developed a large colon volvulus, the most severe form of colic, had significantly higher abundances of Proteobacteria compared with control mares. Postpartum mares that did not colic had a higher abundance of Lachnospiraceae and Ruminococcaceae from the class Clostridia compared with mares that developed a large colon volvulus.

Stewart and coworkers[71] performed a prospective clinical study comparing the fecal microbiome of horse with colic to that of healthy horses presenting for elective surgery. Horses with colic had decreased richness and diversity compared to horses without GI disease. Horses with colic had taxonomy changes at the phylum level affecting Firmicutes, Bacteroidetes, Spirochaetes, Fibrobacteres, Actinobacteria, and Proteobacteria compared with horses admitted for elective surgery.

Although these studies seem to implicate a role for dysbiosis in the microbiome of horses with colic, this relationship is purely associative at this point in time. Future studies using larger numbers of horses with clearly defined types of colic and more standard sequencing approaches will be needed to further define the role of the microbiome in colic.

Colitis

In human and companion animals, colitis has been associated with changes in the fecal microbiome. These changes are generally associated with inflammatory conditions such as ulcerative colitis, inflammatory bowel disease or Crohn's disease in humans,[17] or acute and chronic enteropathies in cats and dogs.[18–20] As with other species, horses develop colitis from multiple etiologies such as infectious diseases (*Salmonella, Clostridia,* and *Lawsonia*), antibiotic use, parasitic infestations, non-steroidal anti-inflammatory (NSAID) drugs, and undifferentiated or unknown causes. Although the effect on the fecal microbiome from each type of colitis has not yet been characterized in a large group of horses, studies have demonstrated that dysbiosis occurs in horses with colitis. Investigators have found that colitis decreases alpha diversity indices in the fecal microbiome, affecting both richness and evenness.[38,43,69,72] Costa and colleagues[38] found decreases in alpha diversity metrics in horses with undifferentiated colitis, whereas Arnold and colleagues[43] found similar trends with colitis caused by antimicrobial use and *Salmonella*. An example of this is shown in **Fig. 6**, where the ASVs of healthy horses were compared with those with antimicrobial-associated diarrhea (AAD) and *Salmonella* colitis.

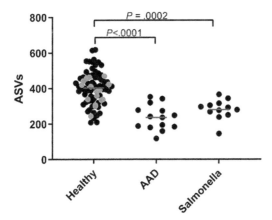

Fig. 6. Horses with antimicrobial-associated diarrhea (AAD) or salmonellosis had decreased diversity compared with two populations of healthy control horses (*black sphere,* low-concentrate diet; *blue sphere,* high-concentrate diet). (*From* Arnold, CE, Pilla, R, Chaffin, MK, et al. The effects of signalment, diet, geographic location, season, and colitis associated with antimicrobial use or Salmonella infection on the fecal microbiome of horses. J Vet Intern Med. 2021; 35(5): 2437–2448. https://doi.org/10.1111/jvim.16206.)

Horses with colitis also appear to have differences in beta diversity. Significant differences in beta diversity have been found in studies with horses with undifferentiated colitis,[38] AAD, and *Salmonella*[43] and colitis due to multiple etiologies.[69] In a study comparing 36 healthy horses to 55 diarrheic horse from multiple causes (*Neorickettsia*, *Clostridium difficile*, *Salmonella*, coronavirus, and undifferentiated),[69] there was distinct clustering between the two groups indicating differences in bacterial community composition (**Fig. 7**).

Similarly to changes in alpha and beta diversity, horses with colitis also demonstrate changes in taxonomy. In horses with undifferentiated colitis,[38] the phyla Bacteroidetes and Fusobacteria were increased in abundance, whereas Firmicutes (particularly Lachnospiraceae and Ruminococcaceae) were reduced compared with controls. When comparing horses with AAD and *Salmonella*, similar changes were found (**Fig. 8**).[43] All horses with colitis had increases in Bacteroidetes compared with healthy controls. Horses with AAD had increases in Proteobacteria and decreases in Verrucomicrobia. Horses with salmonellosis had decreases in Actinobacteria and Firmicutes compared with control horses. Similar changes were found by Ayoub and colleagues[69] and McKinney and colleagues[48] in which Enterobacteriaceae (phylum Proteobacteria) and *Lactobacillus* and *Streptococcus* (order Bacilli, phylum Firmicutes) were more abundant in horses with colitis and Ruminococcus and Lachnospiraceae from the phylum Firmicutes were decreased.

Antibiotics' effect on the microbiome

Antimicrobials can have a marked effect on the GI microbiome by reducing diversity and altering the bacterial community composition of the microbiome, even when animals remain healthy and maintain normal fecal consistency. This effect has been demonstrated with commonly used antimicrobials, such as penicillin, trimethoprim sulfa, ceftiofur, enrofloxacin, and metronidazole.[39,41,73–75] Although all antibiotics

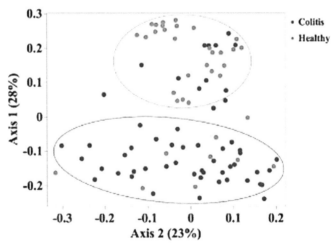

Fig. 7. Principal coordinate analysis (PCoA) based on Jaccard index analysis of the bacterial 16S rRNA gene sequence data for fecal samples collected from healthy horses (*n* = 36, *green*) and horses with colitis (*n* = 55, *red*). Although there is some overlap between red (colitis) and green (healthy) spheres, most of the spheres are spatially-separated by color indicating that they have a distinct bacterial composition. (*From* Ayoub C, Arroyo LG, MacNicol JL, et al. Fecal microbiota of horses with colitis and its association with laminitis and survival during hospitalization. *J Vet Intern Med* 2022, with permission.)

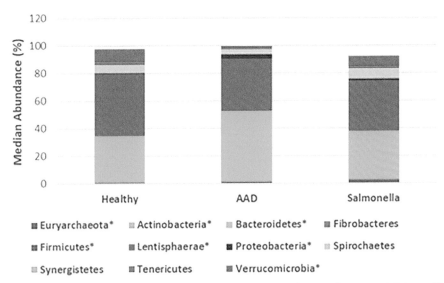

Fig. 8. The abundances of each phyla in healthy horses and those with AAD and *Salmonella* colitis are displayed in histograms. Phyla marked with an asterisk are significantly different across groups. (*From* Arnold, CE, Pilla, R, Chaffin, MK, et al. The effects of signalment, diet, geographic location, season, and colitis associated with antimicrobial use or Salmonella infection on the fecal microbiome of horses. J Vet Intern Med. 2021; 35(5): 2437–2448. https://doi.org/10.1111/jvim.16206.)

have the potential to cause diarrhea, some antimicrobial agents have been associated with an even higher risk because of the high drug concentrations in the intestinal lumen due to poor enteral absorption, biliary excretion, or enterohepatic recycling.[76] Mechanisms by which antimicrobials induce diarrhea include secondary functional metabolic changes and a decrease in the abundance of commensal bacteria leading to overgrowth and colonization by enteric pathogens.[77] To date, all antimicrobials used in horses have reported diarrhea in some patients.[39,78]

Most studies using NGS methods to evaluate the effects of antimicrobials on the fecal microbiome of healthy horses report that antimicrobials reduce the richness and evenness of the microbiome.[39,41,79] Usually, the maximal effect on diversity is seen on Day 3 to 5, with recovery often occurring after 30 days.[39,41,80] Costa and colleagues[41] compared procaine penicillin G, ceftiofur, trimethoprim sulfamethoxazole (TMS) and a saline control. In this study, TMS has the most dramatic effect on the microbiome, with the phyla Verrucomicrobia significantly reduced. This result was duplicated by Arnold and colleagues[81] by giving metronidazole orally. Liepman and colleagues[79] examined the effects of ceftiofur, enrofloxacin, and oxytetracycline against an untreated control group. Ceftiofur and enrofloxacin had the most significant effect, decreasing the abundance of Fibrobacteres and increasing Clostridial groups such as Lachnospiraceae.

In a matched case-controlled study, Arnold and colleagues[81] compared the fecal bacterial microbiota of horses that developed AAD with those that did not develop AAD controlling for drug, route of administration, dose rate, and days of administration. An untreated control group was included for comparison. Horses given antimicrobials had decreased fecal bacterial diversity compared with controls, but horses that developed AAD were not different from those given antimicrobials that did not develop diarrhea (**Fig. 9**). Horses that developed AAD had significant differences in major phyla including Bacteroidetes, Fibrobacteres, and Verrucomicrobia. The

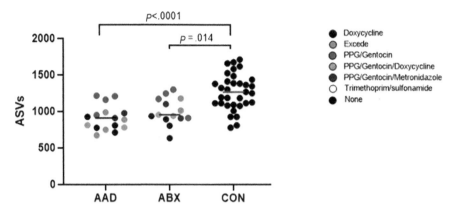

Fig. 9. Alpha diversity metrics of horses with antimicrobial-associated diarrhea (AAD), antibiotic control horses (ABX), and control horses (CON). AAD and ABX horses show a decrease in the number of species compared with CON horses but showed no significant difference between each other. Antibiotic use is denoted by color: doxycycline (*blue*), ceftiofur (*green*), procaine penicillin G/gentamycin (*red*), procaine penicillin G/gentamycin/doxycycline (*orange*), procaine penicillin G/gentamycin/metronidazole (*purple*), trimethoprim sulfonamide (*yellow*), and none (*black*).

depletion of Verrucomicrobia by antibiotics in horses with AAD may be an important finding in regard to the development of AAD. Verrucomicrobia is thought to play a role in the barrier function of the mucin layer at the colonic epithelial cell-lumen interface. Potentially, the disruption of barrier function could lead to the absorption of endotoxin and development of the systemic inflammatory response syndrome, commonly seen in equine patients with colitis.

SUMMARY

The microbiome of the horse's hindgut has an important role in the health of the horse. Changes in the microbial community in the hindgut due to GI disease such as colic, colitis, or the administration of antimicrobials result in dysbiosis. Key findings to date include a decrease in the diversity of species and changes in the bacterial community composition. Phyla consistently affected by GI disease in multiple studies have included Bacteroidetes, Firmicutes, and Verrucomicrobia. This likely reflects their important functional roles in GI health. Further studies using large numbers of horses with well-defined disease processes that use consistent methods of sample processing and sequencing will help eliminate bias related to methodology. Finally, the establishment of reference ranges of taxa important in states of health and disease will provide a framework in which to evaluate the microbiome.

DISCLOSURE

The authors have no disclosures.

REFERENCES

1. Curtis L, Burford JH, England GC, et al. Risk factors for acute abdominal pain (colic) in the adult horse: A scoping review of risk factors, and a systematic review of the effect of management-related changes. PLoS One 2019;14:e0219307.

2. Cohen ND, Matejka PL, Honnas CM, et al. Case-control study of the association between various management factors and development of colic in horses. Texas Equine Colic Study Group. J Am Vet Med Assoc 1995;206:667–73.
3. Cohen ND, Gibbs PG, Woods AM. Dietary and other management factors associated with colic in horses. J Am Vet Med Assoc 1999;215:53–60.
4. Cohen ND, Peloso JG. Risk factors for history of previous colic and for chronic, intermittent colic in a population of horses. J Am Vet Med Assoc 1996;208:697–703.
5. Hudson JM, Cohen ND, Gibbs PG, et al. Feeding practices associated with colic in horses. J Am Vet Med Assoc 2001;219:1419–25.
6. Hillyer MH, Taylor FGR, Proudman CJ, et al. Case control study to identify risk factors for simple colonic obstruction and distension colic in horses. Equine Vet J 2002;34:455–63.
7. Suthers JM, Pinchbeck GL, Proudman CJ, et al. Risk factors for large colon volvulus in the UK. Equine Vet J 2013;45:558–63.
8. Durham AE. The Role of Nutrition in Colic. Vet Clin N Am Equine Pract 2009;25:67–78.
9. Krunkosky TMJC, Moore JN. Gross and Microscopic Anatomy of the Equine Gastrointestinal Tract. In: Blikslager ATWN, Moore JN, Mair TS, editors. The equine acute abdomen. 3rd edition. Hoboken, New Jersey, USA: Wiley Blackwell; 2017. p. 3–18.
10. Incidence of colic in US horses In: systems NAHM. Fort Collins, CO: USDA APHIS; 1998. p. 1–2.
11. Incidence of colic in US horses In: system NAHM. Fot Collins, CO: USDA APHIS; 2001.
12. Equine managment and select equine health conditions in the United States, 2015. National animal health monitoring system. Fort Collins, CO: USDA; 2015. p. 1–171.
13. Bäckhed F, Ley RE, Sonnenburg JL, et al. Host-Bacterial Mutualism in the Human Intestine. Science 2005;307:1915–20.
14. Neish AS. Microbes in gastrointestinal health and disease. Gastroenterology 2009;136:65–80.
15. Lynch SV, Pedersen O. The Human Intestinal Microbiome in Health and Disease. N Engl J Med 2016;375:2369–79.
16. Pilla R, Suchodolski JS. The Role of the Canine Gut Microbiome and Metabolome in Health and Gastrointestinal Disease. Front Vet Sci 2020;6:498.
17. Buford TW. (Dis)Trust your gut: the gut microbiome in age-related inflammation, health, and disease. Microbiome 2017;5:80.
18. Honneffer JB, Minamoto Y, Suchodolski JS. Microbiota alterations in acute and chronic gastrointestinal inflammation of cats and dogs. World J Gastroenterol 2014;20:16489–97.
19. Suchodolski JS. Diagnosis and interpretation of intestinal dysbiosis in dogs and cats. Vet J 2016;215:30–7.
20. AlShawaqfeh MK, Wajid B, Minamoto Y, et al. A dysbiosis index to assess microbial changes in fecal samples of dogs with chronic inflammatory enteropathy. FEMS Microbiol Ecol 2017;93:fix136.
21. Stewart EJ. Growing Unculturable Bacteria. J Bacteriol 2012;194:4151–60.
22. Nichols D, Cahoon N, Trakhtenberg EM, et al. Use of Ichip for High-Throughput *In Situ* Cultivation of "Uncultivable" Microbial Species. Appl Environ Microbiol 2010;76:2445–50.

23. Ranjan R, Rani A, Metwally A, et al. Analysis of the microbiome: Advantages of whole genome shotgun versus 16S amplicon sequencing. Biochem Biophys Res Commun 2016;469:967–77.

24. Leo Lahti SS, Tuomas Borman and Felix GM Ernst. Orchestrating Microbiome Analysis. Available at: https://github.com.microbiom/OMA, 2022.

25. Hang I, Rinttila T, Zentek J, et al. Effect of high contents of dietary animal-derived protein or carbohydrates on canine faecal microbiota. BMC Vet Res 2012;8:90.

26. Andersson AF, Lindberg M, Jakobsson H, et al. Comparative analysis of human gut microbiota by barcoded pyrosequencing. PLoS One 2008;3:e2836.

27. Frey JC, Pell AN, Berthiaume R, et al. Comparative studies of microbial populations in the rumen, duodenum, ileum and faeces of lactating dairy cows. J Appl Microbiol 2010;108:1982–93.

28. Suchodolski JS, Ruaux CG, Steiner JM, et al. Assessment of the qualitative variation in bacterial microflora among compartments of the intestinal tract of dogs by use of a molecular fingerprinting technique. Am J Vet Res 2005;66:1556–62.

29. Dougal K, Harris PA, Edwards A, et al. A comparison of the microbiome and the metabolome of different regions of the equine hindgut. FEMS Microbiol Ecol 2012;82:642–52.

30. Costa MC, Silva G, Ramos RV, et al. Characterization and comparison of the bacterial microbiota in different gastrointestinal tract compartments in horses. Vet J 2015;205:74–80.

31. Ericsson AC, Johnson PJ, Lopes MA, et al. A Microbiological Map of the Healthy Equine Gastrointestinal Tract. PLoS One 2016;11:e0166523.

32. Grimm P, Philippeau C, Julliand V. Faecal parameters as biomarkers of the equine hindgut microbial ecosystem under dietary change. Animal 2017;11:1136–45.

33. Shade A, Handelsman J. Beyond the Venn diagram: the hunt for a core microbiome. Environ Microbiol 2012;14:4–12.

34. Al Jassim RA, Andrews FM. The bacterial community of the horse gastrointestinal tract and its relation to fermentative acidosis, laminitis, colic, and stomach ulcers. Vet Clin N Am Equine Pract 2009;25:199–215.

35. Zhao Y, Li B, Bai D, et al. Comparison of Fecal Microbiota of Mongolian and Thoroughbred Horses by High-throughput Sequencing of the V4 Region of the 16S rRNA Gene. Asian-Australas J Anim Sci 2016;29:1345–52.

36. Costa MC, Weese JS. Understanding the Intestinal Microbiome in Health and Disease. Vet Clin N Am Equine Pract 2018;34(1):1–12.

37. O' Donnell MM, Harris HMB, Jeffery IB, et al. The core faecal bacterial microbiome of Irish Thoroughbred racehorses. Lett Appl Microbiol 2013;57:492–501.

38. Costa MC, Arroyo LG, Allen-Vercoe E, et al. Comparison of the fecal microbiota of healthy horses and horses with colitis by high throughput sequencing of the V3-V5 region of the 16S rRNA gene. PLoS One 2012;7:e41484.

39. Arnold CE, Isaiah A, Pilla R, et al. The cecal and fecal microbiomes and metabolomes of horses before and after metronidazole administration. PLoS One 2020; 15:e0232905.

40. Biddle A, Stewart L, Blanchard J, et al. Untangling the Genetic Basis of Fibrolytic Specialization by Lachnospiraceae and Ruminococcaceae in Diverse Gut Communities. Diversity 2013;5:627–40.

41. Costa MC, Stampfli HR, Arroyo LG, et al. Changes in the equine fecal microbiota associated with the use of systemic antimicrobial drugs. BMC Vet Res 2015; 11:19.

42. Dougal K, de la Fuente G, Harris PA, et al. Characterisation of the faecal bacterial community in adult and elderly horses fed a high fibre, high oil or high starch diet using 454 pyrosequencing. PLoS One 2014;9:e87424.

43. Arnold CE, Pilla R, Chaffin MK, et al. The effects of signalment, diet, geographic location, season, and colitis associated with antimicrobial use or Salmonella infection on the fecal microbiome of horses. J Vet Intern Med 2021;35:2437–48.

44. Jugan MC. Effects of akkermansia muciniphila supplementation on markers of intestinal permeability in dogs following antibiotic treatment. Columbus, OH: The Ohio State University; 2017.

45. Macchione I, Lopetuso L, Ianiro G, et al. Akkermansia muciniphila: key player in metabolic and gastrointestinal disorders. Eur Rev Med Pharmacol Sci 2019;23: 8075–83.

46. Di Pietro R, Arroyo LG, Leclere M, et al. Species-Level Gut Microbiota Analysis after Antibiotic-Induced Dysbiosis in Horses. Animals (Basel) 2021;11(10):2859.

47. Massacci FR, Clark A, Ruet A, et al. Inter-breed diversity and temporal dynamics of the faecal microbiota in healthy horses. Journal of animal breeding and genetics = Zeitschrift fur Tierzuchtung und Zuchtungsbiologie 2020;137:103–20.

48. McKinney CA, Oliveira BCM, Bedenice D, et al. The fecal microbiota of healthy donor horses and geriatric recipients undergoing fecal microbial transplantation for the treatment of diarrhea. PLoS One 2020;15:e0230148.

49. Weese JS, Holcombe SJ, Embertson RM, et al. Changes in the faecal microbiota of mares precede the development of post partum colic. Equine Vet J 2015;47: 641–9.

50. Faubladier C, Chaucheyras-Durand F, da Veiga L, et al. Effect of transportation on fecal bacterial communities and fermentative activities in horses: impact of Saccharomyces cerevisiae CNCM I-1077 supplementation. J Anim Sci 2013; 91:1736–44.

51. Almeida ML, Feringer WHJ, Carvalho JR, et al. Intense Exercise and Aerobic Conditioning Associated with Chromium or L-Carnitine Supplementation Modified the Fecal Microbiota of Fillies. PLoS One 2016;11:e0167108.

52. Janabi AHD, Biddle AS, Klein D, et al. Exercise training-induced changes in the gut microbiota of Standardbred racehorses. Comp Exerc Physiol 2016;12: 119–30.

53. Janabi AHD, Biddle AS, Klein DJ, et al. The effects of acute strenuous exercise on the faecal microbiota in Standardbred racehorses. Comp Exerc Physiol 2017;13: 13–24.

54. Schoster A, Mosing M, Jalali M, et al. Effects of transport, fasting and anaesthesia on the faecal microbiota of healthy adult horses. Equine Vet J 2016;48:595–602.

55. Kuhn M, Guschlbauer M, Feige K, et al. Feed restriction enhances the depressive effects of erythromycin on equine hindgut microbial metabolism in vitro. Berl Munch Tierarztl Wochenschr 2012;125:351–8.

56. Salem SE, Maddox TW, Berg A, et al. Variation in faecal microbiota in a group of horses managed at pasture over a 12-month period. Sci Rep 2018;8:8510.

57. Metcalf JL, Song SJ, Morton JT, et al. Evaluating the impact of domestication and captivity on the horse gut microbiome. Sci Rep 2017;7:15497.

58. Garber A, Hastie P, McGuinness D, et al. Abrupt dietary changes between grass and hay alter faecal microbiota of ponies. PLoS One 2020;15:e0237869.

59. Collinet A, Grimm P, Julliand S, et al. Sequential Modulation of the Equine Fecal Microbiota and Fibrolytic Capacity Following Two Consecutive Abrupt Dietary Changes and Bacterial Supplementation. Animals 2021;11:1278.

60. Willing B, Voros A, Roos S, et al. Changes in faecal bacteria associated with concentrate and forage-only diets fed to horses in training. Equine Vet J 2009; 41:908–14.

61. Warzecha CM, Coverdale JA, Janecka JE, et al. Influence of short-term dietary starch inclusion on the equine cecal microbiome. J Anim Sci 2017;95:5077–90.

62. Rothschild D, Weissbrod O, Barkan E, et al. Environment dominates over host genetics in shaping human gut microbiota. Nature 2018;555:210–5.

63. Kaiser-Thom S, Hilty M, Gerber V. Effects of hypersensitivity disorders and environmental factors on the equine intestinal microbiota. Vet Q 2020;40:97–107.

64. Daly K, Proudman CJ, Duncan SH, et al. Alterations in microbiota and fermentation products in equine large intestine in response to dietary variation and intestinal disease. Br J Nutr 2012;107:989–95.

65. Jevit M. Microflora of the equine gut and its ramifications on the development of laminitis; A comparison of fecal and cecal diversity and Illumina and Roche 454 sequencers *Bayer School of Natural and Environmental Science*. Pittsburgh, PA: Duquesne University; 2016. p. 1–110.

66. Milinovich GJ, Trott DJ, Burrell PC, et al. Changes in equine hindgut bacterial populations during oligofructose-induced laminitis. Environ Microbiol 2006;8: 885–98.

67. Moreau MM, Eades SC, Reinemeyer CR, et al. Illumina sequencing of the V4 hypervariable region 16S rRNA gene reveals extensive changes in bacterial communities in the cecum following carbohydrate oral infusion and development of early-stage acute laminitis in the horse. Vet Microbiol 2014;168:436–41.

68. Steelman SM, Chowdhary BP, Dowd S, et al. Pyrosequencing of 16S rRNA genes in fecal samples reveals high diversity of hindgut microflora in horses and potential links to chronic laminitis. BMC Vet Res 2012;8:231.

69. Ayoub C, Arroyo LG, MacNicol JL, et al. Fecal microbiota of horses with colitis and its association with laminitis and survival during hospitalization. J Vet Intern Med 2022;36(6):2213–23.

70. Venable EB, Kerley MS, Raub R. Assessment of equine fecal microbial profiles during and after a colic episode using pyrosequencing. J Equine Vet Sci 2013; 33:347–8.

71. Stewart HL, Southwood LL, Indugu N, et al. Differences in the equine faecal microbiota between horses presenting to a tertiary referral hospital for colic compared to an elective surgical procedure. Equine Vet J 2019;51(3):336–42.

72. Arroyo LG, Rossi L, Santos BP, et al. Luminal and Mucosal Microbiota of the Cecum and Large Colon of Healthy and Diarrheic Horses. Animals 2020;10:1403.

73. Gronvold AM, L'Abee-Lund TM, Strand E, et al. Fecal microbiota of horses in the clinical setting: potential effects of penicillin and general anesthesia. Vet Microbiol 2010;145:366–72.

74. Harlow BE, Lawrence LM, Flythe MD. Diarrhea-associated pathogens, lactobacilli and cellulolytic bacteria in equine feces: responses to antibiotic challenge. Vet Microbiol 2013;166:225–32.

75. Harlow BE. Changes to the Equine Hindgut Micrflora in Response to Antibiotic Challenge. In: Animal and food science. Lexington, KY: University of Kentucky; 2012. p. 244.

76. Scott Weese J, Baptiste KE, Baverud V, Toutain P-L. Guidelines for antimicrobial use in horses: chapter 10. In: Guardabassi L, Jensen LB, Kruse H, editors, editors. Guide to antimicrobial use in animals. Blackwell Publishing; 2008. p. 161–82.

77. Willing BP, Russell SL, Finlay BB. Shifting the balance: antibiotic effects on host–microbiota mutualism. Nat Rev Microbiol 2011;9:233–43.

78. McGorum BC, Pirie RS. Antimicrobial associated diarrhoea in the horse. Part 2: Which antimicrobials are associated with AAD in the horse? Equine Vet Educ 2010;22:43–50.
79. Liepman RS, Swink JM, Habing GG, et al. Effects of intravenous antimicrobial drugs on the equine fecal microbiome. Animals (Basel) 2022;12.
80. Liepman RS. Alterations in the fecal microbiome of healthy horses in response to antibiotic treatment. Columbus, OH: The Ohio State University; 2015.
81. Arnold C, Pilla R, Chaffin K, et al. Alterations in the fecal microbiome and metabolome of horses with antimicrobial-associated diarrhea compared to antibiotic-treated and non-treated healthy case controls. Animals 2021;11:1807.

Recurrent Colic
Diagnosis, Management, and Expectations

Tim Mair, BVSc, PhD, DEIM, DESTS, DipECEIM, AssocECVDI, FRCVS*,
Ceri Sherlock, BVetMed, MS, MVetMed, DACVS-LA, DECVS-LA, DipECVDI-LA,
MRCVS

KEYWORDS

- Recurrent colic • Spasmodic colic • Intestinal obstruction
- Inflammatory bowel disease • Gastric ulceration • Abdominal adhesions
- False colic

KEY POINTS

- Many cases of recurrent colic are mild and self-limiting with non-specific findings on clinical examination.
- Diet, access to pasture, dental health, and gastric ulceration may be important factors that predispose individual horses to recurrent colic.
- Recurrent bouts of colic that are becoming more frequent or more severe suggest the presence of a serious underlying condition such as partial intestinal obstruction, inflammatory bowel disease, or intestinal neoplasia.
- Abdominal adhesions are common causes of recurrent colic following exploratory laparotomy; adhesiolysis is associated with a high rate of repeated adhesion formation.
- Non-gastrointestinal diseases should be considered as potential causes of recurrent pain ("false colics").

INTRODUCTION/DEFINITIONS

The term *recurrent colic* is used to describe repeated episodes of abdominal discomfort over weeks to years with normal periods in between. Although recurrent colic is a common clinical scenario, it can be frustrating and difficult to investigate, and frequently poses a diagnostic dilemma.[1–3] As a large majority of the diseases associated with recurrent colic are mild, have non-specific clinical findings, and respond to analgesics, the precise cause often goes undiagnosed.[4]

Risk factors for intermittent colic related to history, signalment, diet, and environment include the following: previous abdominal surgery, consuming coastal grass hay, being more than 8 years of age, being of the Arabian breed, being a gelding, having a recent change in diet, dental disease, cribbing/wind-sucking and weaving

CVS Ltd, Bell Equine Veterinary Clinic, Mereworth, Maidstone, Kent, ME18 5GS, UK
* Corresponding author.
E-mail address: tim.mair@btinternet.com

Vet Clin Equine 39 (2023) 399–417
https://doi.org/10.1016/j.cveq.2023.03.014
0749-0739/23/© 2023 Elsevier Inc. All rights reserved.

behavior, and living in an environment with a high density of horses.[5,6] In contrast, there is a reduced risk for recurrent colic associated with increasing time at pasture.[4,7]

Recurrent or intermittent colic can be classified into three categories: primary recurrent colic, recurrent colic after surgery, and recurrence of false colic.[6]

PRIMARY RECURRENT COLIC

Many studies have shown that horses with a history of colic are more likely to suffer further episodes of colic.[8–11] In one study of 127 horses diagnosed with medical colic in the United Kingdom, the recurrence rate in the following 12 months was 50 colic events/100 horse years at risk. A multivariable logistic regression model showed that horses who had a known dental problem or that crib-bite/windsuck were at increased risk of recurrence during the year following a colic event.[4]

Most repeat episodes of non-specific or gas/spasmodic colic are mild and self-limiting, and the results of clinical examinations are often unremarkable. Differentiating these cases from more serious diseases can be difficult, but repeated evaluations, including gastroscopy, dental examination, transrectal palpation, abdominal ultrasonography, abdominal paracentesis, and blood analyses are warranted to identify underlying conditions, especially if the episodes of colic are becoming more frequent or more severe. Additionally, there may be a place for cross-sectional imaging of the abdomen of small equids[12] with the more widespread availability of large-bore computed tomography machines (**Fig. 1**). Ultimately, exploratory laparotomy or laparoscopy may be required to identify physical abnormalities that could cause partial intestinal obstruction or to allow bowel wall biopsies to be obtained.

In one retrospective study,[13] the clinical features of 58 horses presenting with recurrent colic examined over 5 years were reviewed. The horses were categorized into three groups based on the history of colic episodes. Recurrent transient colic (*Group 1*) was characterized by three or more episodes of transient colic (of apparently similar type) occurring within 1 month. This group included 15 horses, and it had a high mortality rate (53%). It included three horses with lymphoma, two with intussusceptions,

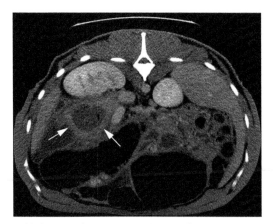

Fig. 1. Transverse multiplanar reformation CT image (post intravenous contrast) of the abdomen of a 10-year-old female miniature horse with a history of recurrent colic over a 2-month period. There is a large cystic mass with a thick mildly enhancing rim and hypoattenuating center with gas pockets in the right dorsal abdomen ventral to the right kidney and to the right of the portal vein (*arrows*). Transcutaneous biopsy confirmed chronic pancreatitis.

two with thromboembolic disease/verminous arteritis, two with partial ileal obstructions, and 1 case each of colitis, mesenteric hemorrhage, and ovulation pain; three cases remained undiagnosed. Recurrent transient colic (*Group 2*) was characterized by three or more episodes of transient colic occurring within 1 year. This group comprised 27 horses and had a mortality rate of 4%. Nine of these horses were diagnosed with spasmodic colic, two had thromboembolic disease, and there was one case each of lymphoma, colonic impactions, intestinal adhesions, and ileal muscular hypertrophy; 12 cases remained undiagnosed. Recurrent prolonged colic (*Group 3*) was characterized by three or more episodes of prolonged colic occurring within 1 year and included 16 horses with a mortality rate of 31%. This included three cases of recurrent colonic impaction and two cases each of lymphoma, thromboembolic disease, partial ileal obstructions, and intestinal adhesions, and one case each of intussusception, colitis, equine grass sickness, and gastric ulceration; one case remained undiagnosed. This study involved horses referred to a UK veterinary teaching hospital and may not be representative of cases of recurrent colic seen in first-opinion veterinary practice. However, the results suggest that horses presenting with very frequent bouts of recurrent colic are likely to have more serious diseases and a higher mortality rate, compared to horses presenting with less frequent bouts of transient colic, which are more likely to have recurrent non-specific, "spasmodic" colic (or remain undiagnosed). Horses with recurrent bouts of prolonged colic are more likely to have motility issues (resulting in repeated colonic impactions for example) or partial intestinal obstruction. Intestinal dysmotility leading to recurrent colic, including colic due to impactions, can be caused by alterations in the neurons in the myenteric plexus, including ganglionitis or a reduction in the number of ganglia; such changes have been identified in the large colon and cecum after prolonged obstruction or volvulus.[14–19] A reduction in the number of enteric ganglia is also a feature of equine grass sickness; horses with the chronic form of this disease that survive may be prone to recurrent colic associated with chronic intestinal dilatation and hypertrophy of the intestinal walls (**Figs. 2** and **3**). Horses with chronic equine chronic grass sickness typically show other clinical signs as well as colic (severe weight loss, base narrow stance, weakness and toe dragging, ptosis, persistent tachycardia, muscle tremors, patchy sweating, rhinitis sicca); however, in animals which survive these other signs may partially or completely resolve, but the horse may still be affected by recurrent bouts of abdominal pain.

Alterations in the intestinal muscle can also be detected in some other horses with recurrent colic.[20] Diagnosis of these pathologies requires full-thickness intestinal biopsies obtained via exploratory laparotomy. However, the strength of an association, if any, between changes in the enteric nervous system or smooth muscle and recurrent colic episodes remains to be determined.[6]

Inflammatory Bowel Disease

Inflammatory bowel diseases (IBD) have been associated with a variety of different clinical presentations including lethargy, diarrhea, weight loss (despite good appetite), ventral edema, and recurrent colic.[21] Several different types of IBD are histopathologically distinguishable: granulomatous enteritis, multisystemic eosinophilic epitheliotropic disease, lymphocytic-plasmacytic enterocolitis, diffuse eosinophilic enterocolitis, and proliferative enteritis.[21–24] Diagnosis of IBD ultimately requires histopathological examination of full-thickness intestinal tissue samples/biopsies, which are best obtained by exploratory laparotomy (performed under general anesthesia or standing[25]), but less invasive mucosal pinch biopsies of the rectum or duodenum (obtained via gastroduodenoscopy) that can be easily harvested in standing horses

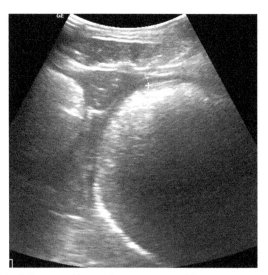

Fig. 2. Transabdominal ultrasound image from a 12-year-old Connemara mare with a history of recurrent colic. The mare was diagnosed with chronic equine grass sickness 3 years previously. Ultrasonography on numerous occasions revealed multiple loops of dilated and thickened small intestines. The thickness of the small intestinal wall measured between 5 and 8 mm.

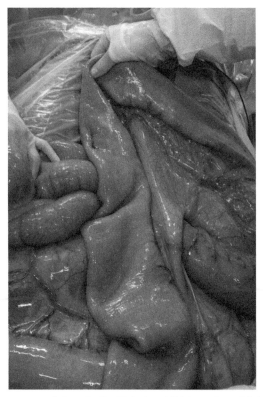

Fig. 3. Surgical appearance of chronically dilated and thickened small intestinal loops in the horse described in **Fig. 3**.

may provide a diagnosis in some cases[26]; however, the sensitivity of duodenal and rectal pinch biopsies to diagnose IBD is low. Furthermore, the histopathological interpretation of enteric biopsies is problematic, with only limited data on the variations in inflammatory cell populations in the mucosa and submucosa of normal horses; there is a need for better standardization of enteral biopsy procedures and the histopathological scoring of biopsies.[21] Other diagnostic techniques that can provide supportive information include serum biochemistry (hypoproteinemia and hypoalbuminemia), oral glucose tolerance test or xylose absorption test (reduced absorption), and abdominal ultrasonography (intestinal wall thickening) (**Figs. 4** and **5**). Enlargement of the cecal lymph nodes may also be appreciated in some cases of IBD or neoplasia (**Fig. 6**). Stewart and colleagues[27] reported the histopathological findings of 66 horses which were presented for recurrent colic and had intestinal biopsies obtained. The results indicated that a high proportion (55%) of horses with recurrent colic had a form of inflammatory gastrointestinal disease. The use of a rectal biopsy alone to obtain biopsy specimens was more likely to result in no histologic diagnosis in this study. Treatment of horses with IBD with corticosteroids (dexamethasone or prednisolone) can be helpful in some cases, but the response is variable.[27] The long-term prognosis is generally better if the horse shows a good initial response to corticosteroid treatment.[28]

Gastric Ulceration

Equine gastric ulcer syndrome (EGUS) is the most common disease of the equine stomach with a high prevalence of both squamous and glandular disease reported in various populations of horses.[29,30] Clinical signs of EGUS are varied, including recurrent colic, poor appetite, weight loss, hair coat changes, poor performance, behavioral changes, and pain on tightening of the girth.[31,32] As many clinically normal horses have evidence of EGUS, the clinical relevance can be difficult to ascertain with certainty, and there is only limited evidence that EGUS is an important cause of recurrent colic. Gastric ulcers were reported in 83% of horses with recurrent colic in one study of which 28% had colic attributable to gastric ulceration as documented by a response to acid-suppressive treatment.[33] In another study,[34] 3.5% of horses with

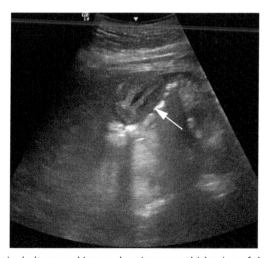

Fig. 4. Transabdominal ultrasound image showing gross thickening of the duodenal wall in a 15-year-old sports horse gelding with a history of recurrent colic and suspected inflammatory bowel disease. The duodenal wall measured 1.15 cm thick (*arrow*).

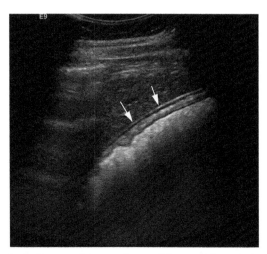

Fig. 5. Transabdominal ultrasound image from a 12-year-old sports horse mare with suspected inflammatory bowel disease showing thickening of the right dorsal colon wall adjacent to the liver (*arrows*).

squamous ulcers were reported to have exhibited colic over the preceding month. Despite the lack of conclusive evidence that EGUS causes colic, it should be considered as a differential diagnosis in any horse demonstrating clinical signs potentially referable to gastrointestinal discomfort.[35]

Gastroscopy is the most accurate way of diagnosing EGUS, although the use of a therapeutic trial is logical when gastroscopy is not available; a positive response to treatment increases the index of suspicion of EGUS. Likewise, a positive response to treatment supports the clinical relevance of mild lesions if the results of gastroscopy are equivocal.[35] There are two distinct forms of EGUS, namely equine squamous

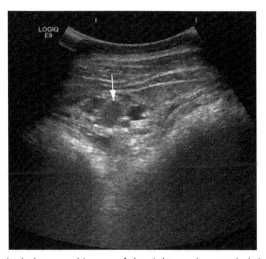

Fig. 6. Transabdominal ultrasound image of the right caudoventral abdomen of a 12-year-old sports horse mare with suspected inflammatory bowel disease showing enlargement of the cecal lymph nodes (*arrow*).

gastric ulcer syndrome (ESGUS) and equine glandular gastric ulcer syndrome (EGGUS). These are diagnosed by gastroscopy and are considered to be separate diseases requiring different treatments.[36,37] Acid-suppressive therapy (eg, omeprazole) is the most effective treatment of ESGUS (along with nutritional management) but is less effective as a stand-alone therapy for EGGUS. Instead, the use of adjunctive treatments for EGGUS is beneficial, in particular, sucralfate.[37] See Michelle Henry Barton and Gayle D. Hallowell article, "Current Topics in Medical Colic,": Current topics on medical colic.

Parasites

The strongyles, including both the large strongyles (*Strongylus vulgaris*) and the small strongyles (cyathostomins) have long been implicated as causes of colic.[38] Cranial mesenteric arteritis and thromboembolism resulting in intestinal ischemia and infarction associated with *S vulgaris* larval migration was commonly recognized as a cause of colic, including recurrent colic, in the years before the introduction of modern larvicidal anthelmintics. The incidence subsequently showed a dramatic decline in most countries. However, since the implementation of prescription-only anthelmintic treatment and a more selective anthelmintic treatment strategy in countries such as Sweden and Denmark, there has been an increase in *S. vulgaris* prevalence and an associated increase in reported cases of colic and peritonitis caused by this parasite.[39]

The cyathostomins (small redworms) are ubiquitous parasites of grazing horses. Although they are closely related to the large strongyles, their life cycle does not involve somatic migration. Anthelmintic resistance is common in cyathostomins with reports globally of increasing levels of resistance to all classes of anthelmintics. The small redworms have been associated with several clinical conditions, including weight loss, colic, and diarrhea (acute larval cyathostominosis is a severe form of colitis resulting in profuse diarrhea and profound weight loss, and has a high mortality rate, despite attempted treatment). Cyathostomins have a period of larval development in the large intestinal wall; thousands of larvae can accumulate, especially in young horses; these play an important role in the pathogenesis of acute larval cyathostominosis, and possibly colic. As the larval stages of the parasite do not produce eggs, a fecal examination cannot be used to determine the size of any larval parasite burden. An antibody-based blood test is available in some countries to detect and quantify intra-host infections with cyathostomins. The association between colic and cyathostomins is unclear. Some studies have suggested that high burdens of cyathostomins predispose horses to colic,[40] whereas others have suggested the opposite.[41]

Anoplocephala perfoliata is the most prevalent cestode parasite worldwide. Masses of *A perfoliata* attached near the ileocecal valve cause inflammation and ulceration of the cecal mucosa. These lesions have been associated with an increased incidence of ileocecal intussusceptions (**Figs. 7** and **8**), ileal impactions, cecal rupture, and spasmodic colic, including recurrent spasmodic colic.[42–44]

Congenital Intestinal Abnormalities

A variety of congenital gastrointestinal abnormalities have been reported in the horse.[45] Even though, by definition, congenital defects are present from birth, clinical signs in some cases may occur at any point during the lifetime of a horse. Examples include abdominal hernias (umbilical, inguinal, diaphragmatic), vitelline anomalies (mesodiverticular bands, Meckel's diverticulum) (**Fig. 9**), intestinal atresia, mesenteric anomalies, malformations, duplication cysts, and rotation deformity.

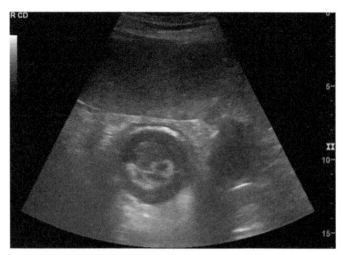

Fig. 7. Transabdominal ultrasound image from the right caudoventral abdomen of a 12-year-old Shetland pony mare with a history of several bouts of recurrent colic of increasing frequency and severity over the preceding 5 days. Note the "target" appearance consistent with intestinal intussusception.

Other Causes of Primary Recurrent Colic

There are numerous other potential causes of primary recurrent colic related to the gastrointestinal tract (**Box 1**), including repeated colon displacements,[46,47] sand enteropathy,[48] intestinal neoplasia[49] (**Figs. 10–13**), enterolithiasis,[50] pyloric obstructions,[51] abdominal abscesses,[52] enteritis,[53] muscular hypertrophy of the cecum[54] and ileum[55] (**Fig. 14**), and sessile (ie, non-pedunculated) lipomas (**Figs. 15** and **16**) or intestinal lipomatosis.[56]

Future colic episodes may be prevented when certain diseases are identified during the exploratory surgery. These include removal of sessile lipomas, mesenteric rents that can be closed, muscular hypertrophy amenable to surgical bypass, and large colon volvulus/displacement that can be prevented either by colopexy or colon

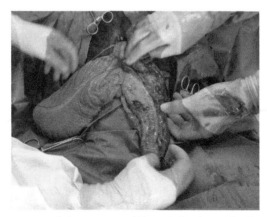

Fig. 8. Surgical appearance of the cecum and ileum following reduction of an intussusception in the pony described in **Fig. 7**.

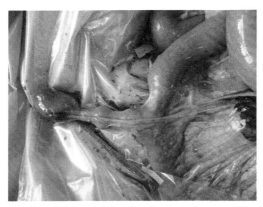

Fig. 9. Meckel's diverticulum in a 17-year-old sport horse mare with a history of recurrent colic of moderate severity before developing acute, severe colic associated with small intestinal volvulus involving the diverticulum.

Box 1.
Gastrointestinal causes of recurrent transient colic

Non-specific/"spasmodic" colic

Gas colic (tympany)

(Partial) intestinal obstruction
    Neoplasia, eg, non-strangulating sessile lipoma, lymphoma, gastrointestinal stromal tumor, leiomyoma, leiomyosarcoma, adenocarcinoma
    Muscular hypertrophy (ileum, cecum, large colon, jejunum)
    Intestinal diverticulae
    Intra-abdominal adhesions
    Intussusception
    Intestinal fibrosis
    Congenital abnormalities
    Mesenteric rent
    Abdominal hernias

Inflammatory bowel disease

Parasites
    Strongylus vulgaris
    Cyathostomins
    Tapeworm

Gastric impaction

Gastric ulceration and pyloric obstruction

Intestinal dysmotility
    Ganglionitis
    Reduced number of ganglia
    Intestinal muscle damage/fibrosis
    Equine grass sickness

Intestinal displacements

Cecal and colonic impactions

Sand impactions

Non-strangulating intestinal infarction/thromboembolic disease

Enterolithiasis

Intestinal lipomatosis

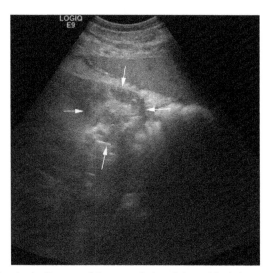

Fig. 10. Transabdominal ultrasound image of the right mid abdomen of a 30-year-old Warmblood gelding with a 1-month history of weight loss and recurrent colic, with the colic episodes becoming more frequent and more severe. There is irregular thickening of the small intestinal walls with heterogeneous echogenicity (*arrows*).

amputation and left dorsal displacement that can be prevented by ablation of the nephrosplenic space.[6]

Gut Microbiome and Nutritional Management

Recent investigations into the equine gut microbiome, the complex and diverse ecosystem composed primarily of bacteria, which cohabit with viruses, archaea, and fungi, support that horses with colic have an altered gut microbiome (dysbiosis).[57–60] However, it is uncertain if this dysbiosis is a cause or effect of the colic and further studies in horses with recurrent colic are needed.[61] See Carolyn E. Arnold and Rachel Pilla article, "What is the microbiota and what is its role in colic?,": What is the microbiota and what is its role in colic?

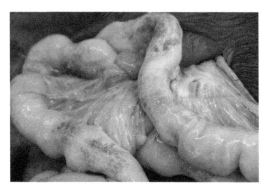

Fig. 11. Post-mortem appearance of the small intestine of the horse described in **Fig. 10**. There is marked thickening of the small intestinal walls. Histopathology confirmed intestinal adenocarcinoma.

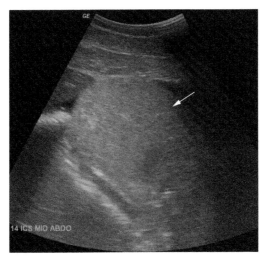

Fig. 12. Transabdominal ultrasound image of the right caudoventral abdomen of a 25-year-old Connemara gelding with a history of recurrent colic for approximately 6 months. A discrete large homogeneous spherical mass was identified in the mid-left abdomen (*arrow*).

Nutrition may play an important role in predisposing some horses to recurrent colic. For example, in a subpopulation of crib-biting/wind-sucking horses, colic risk was found to be higher in horses fed either hay or haylage compared to grass.[62] Although an association between feeding practices and disturbances in gastrointestinal function has long been hypothesized, the mechanisms linking diet with the development of intestinal dysfunction are poorly understood.[63,64] Several different management and nutritional changes are commonly employed in individual horses with recurrent colic in an attempt to reduce the incidence of colic.[65] Unfortunately, the evidence base for different nutritional strategies is very limited; nutritional management is often led by trial and error, and what ultimately is best tolerated by the patient.[65] A common

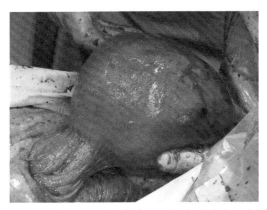

Fig. 13. Surgical appearance of an intraluminal mass in the left dorsal colon of the horse in **Fig. 12** The mass measured approximately 14 cm diameter and weighed 1.3 kg. Histopathological examination of the mass following surgical resection confirmed a leiomyoma. The horse made an uneventful recovery following surgery.

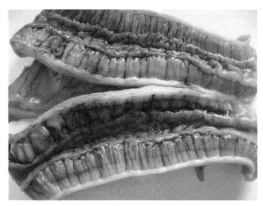

Fig. 14. Post-mortem appearance of ileal muscular hypertrophy from a 5-year-old Camargue pony mare with a history of recurrent colic.

approach is to recommend a strict exercise and feeding routine, turn the horse out to pasture as frequently as possible, decrease the quantity of concentrates in the diet as much as possible, provide free choice roughage and water, control parasites, provide routine dental care, and take steps to prevent the ingestion of sand.[6] In most horses, fiber and forage should form the mainstay of the diet (at least 2% of body weight), and ensuring optimum intake will also help to maintain colonic hydration. If a concentrate feed is required, a nut or pelleted form that can be soaked into a wet but not sloppy mash may be preferable. This can be mixed with some alfalfa/chaff, which will slow down the rate of intake and make sure that the food is being properly chewed. Adding a tablespoon of salt to the feed each day, as well as allowing ad-lib access to a salt block will ensure intake of sodium and chloride which will help to stimulate water

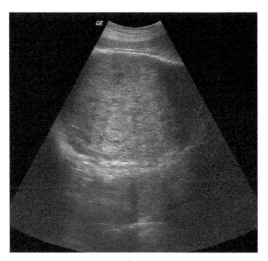

Fig. 15. Transabdominal ultrasound image of the right caudoventral abdomen of a 15-year-old Connemara gelding with a history of recurrent colic of increasing frequency for approximately 6 months. There is a large mass of homogeneous echogenicity in the right ventral abdomen.

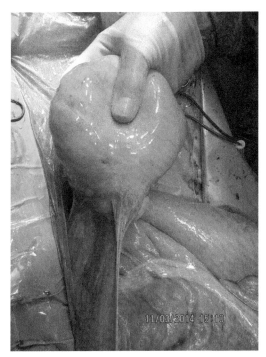

Fig. 16. Surgical appearance of a large lipoma in the horse described in **Fig. 15**. The lipoma measured 15 cm in diameter and was attached to the serosa of the right ventral colon.

intake and thus help to add fluid to the colon. Regular exercise is important to stimulate intestinal motility. Nutritional supplements including bran mash, pre- and probiotics, and special diets have not been scientifically proven to decrease or prevent colic.[66] If used, they should be part of the daily routine and considered when formulating energy intake in the diet.[6]

RECURRENT COLIC AFTER SURGERY

Horses which have undergone colic surgery are at an increased risk of developing recurrent colic, predominately due to intestinal scarring and adhesions from distention, ischemia, intestinal trauma, or contamination.[6,67] Many adhesions are likely to be clinically silent, but they can cause clinical problems when fibrinous adhesions mature into restrictive fibrous adhesions that compress or anatomically distort the intestine, narrowing the intestinal lumen and impeding the normal passage of ingesta[68] (**Fig. 17**). Adhesions may also result in intestinal incarceration, strangulation, or volvulus, resulting in severe, unrelenting abdominal pain. The true prevalence of abdominal adhesions following surgery is uncertain because many animals which suffer recurrent colic are managed medically or are euthanized without necropsy. However, it has been proposed that adhesions are the reason for euthanasia in 26% of cases following small intestinal resection and anastomosis.[69] In a retrospective study of 99 horses undergoing repeat laparotomy, an adhesion prevalence of 32% was determined, with no association between the site of lesion or resection at first surgery and subsequent adhesion formation.[70] Diagnosis is likely to require exploratory laparotomy, although transrectal palpation and abdominal ultrasonography may also be

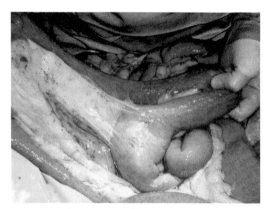

Fig. 17. Surgical appearance of intestinal adhesions in a 16-year-old Warmblood gelding which developed recurrent colic following colic surgery 3 years previously.

useful in raising the index of suspicion of abdominal adhesions in horses with a history of previous abdominal surgery. These examinations may reveal distended loops of small intestine. Adhesions are rarely demonstrable by ultrasonography unless the ventral abdominal wall is involved, and it is difficult to distinguish between fibrin, fibrous adhesions, and mesentery; however abnormal findings that are consistently seen on repeated evaluations should raise the index of suspicion. Chronic, partial obstruction can result in dilated, thickened intestine proximal to the obstruction, which may be palpable per rectum or identifiable ultrasonographically,[71] although surgery (including laparoscopic surgery) is usually required to confirm the diagnosis of adhesions.[72] Treatment of horses with mature adhesions is often unrewarding, costly, and associated with a poor prognosis for survival.[68] In less severe cases, recurrent colic associated with postoperative adhesions may be managed by feeding a low residue diet of complete pellet rations and grazing green grass.[68] More severe restrictive adhesions causing intestinal obstruction require repeat surgery or euthanasia. Surgical treatment aims to restore a functional intestinal lumen and removal of any devitalized intestine and may necessitate resection and anastomosis or bypass procedures. Adhesiolysis alone is associated with a high rate of repeated adhesion formation, although laparoscopic adhesiolysis of focal intestinal adhesions has been reported.[72,73] In general, the prognosis for horses requiring repeat laparotomy due to adhesions is poor. In a survey of equine surgeons, 91% reported a less than 50% success rate for the surgical treatment of horses with adhesions.[74] See Isabelle Kilcoyne article, "When Things Don't Go as Planned: Update On Complications and impact on outcome,": When things don't go as planned: update on complications and impact on outcome.

Recurrence of False Colic

Colic is neither a specific disease nor a diagnosis, but simply represents the behavioral manifestations of abdominal pain. Although it is generally associated with diseases of the gastrointestinal tract, conditions of other body systems can also cause pain that creates a behavior like colic. These clinical signs can be difficult to differentiate from pain due to gastrointestinal disease. These conditions are commonly referred to as "false colics".[75]

Differentiation between "true" and "false" colic depends on an accurate history and performing a careful physical examination, coupled where appropriate with further diagnostic procedures such as clinical pathology and diagnostic imaging. Horses exhibiting colic caused by disorders of systems other than the gastrointestinal tract will often show mild to moderate pain (eg, pawing the ground, lying in sternal or lateral recumbency for prolonged periods, or reluctance to move) or other additional signs, but rarely demonstrate signs of severe pain. However, distinguishing signs of mild to moderate abdominal pain from pain arising elsewhere can be challenging.

Diseases that have been associated with recurring "false colics" include ovulation pain,[76] granulosa cell tumors,[77] pregnancy,[78,79] uterine marbles,[80] testicular torsion,[81] urolithiasis,[82] cholelithiasis,[83] acute and chronic pancreatitis[84,85] (see **Fig. 1**), aortoiliac thrombosis,[86] aorto-pulmonary fistulation,[87] recurrent exertional rhabdomyolysis[88], and pheochromocytoma.

CLINICS CARE POINTS

- A detailed history of the frequency of recurrent colic episodes, as well as the signalment of the horse and details of other medical problems are important in the work-up of horses with recurrent colic.
- Physical examination, laboratory evaluations and abdominal ultrasonography are important components of the evaluation of these cases.
- Gastroscopy may be required to assess the stomach for EGUS.
- Exploratory laparotomy may be requred to confirm lesions such as intestinal adhesions and intestinal neoplasia, as well as allowing full thickness intestinal biopsies.

DISCLOSURE

No commercial or financial conflicts of interest. No funding.

REFERENCES

1. Beard WL, Freeman DE. Clinical case conference. J Am Vet Med Assoc 1994; 204:1165.
2. Schramme M. Investigation and management of recurrent colic in the horse. In Pract 1995;17:303–14.
3. Hart S, Southwood LL. The enigma of post operative recurrent colic: Challenges with diagnosis and management. Equine Vet J 2010;22:408–11.
4. Scantlebury CE, Archer DC, Proudman CJ, et al. Recurrent colic in the horse: Incidence and risk factors for recurrence in the general practice population. Equine Vet J 2011;43 S39:81–8.
5. Cohen ND, Peloso JG. Risk factors for history of previous colic and for chronic, intermittent colic in a population of horses. J Am Vet Med Assoc 1996;208: 697–703.
6. White NA. Investigations of chronic and recurrent colic. In: Blikslager AT, White NA, Moore JN, et al, editors. The equine acute abdomen. 3rd Edition. Hoboken, NJ: Wiley Blackwell; 2017. p. pp263–5.
7. Scantlebury CE, Archer DC, Proudman CJ, et al. Management and horse-level risk factors for recurrent colic in the UK general equine practice population. Equine Vet J 2015;47:202–6.
8. Reeves MJ, Salman MD, Smith G. Risk factors for equine acute abdominal disease (colic): results from a multi-centre case-control study. Prev Vet Med 1996; 26:285–301.

9. Tinker MK, White NA, Lessard P, et al. Prospective study of equine colic risk factors. Equine Vet J 1997;29:454–8.

10. Hillyer MH, Taylor FGR, Proudman CJ, et al. Case control study to identify risk factors for simple colonic obstruction and distension colic in horses. Equine Vet J 2002;34:455–63.

11. Tannahill VJ, Cardwell JM, Witte TH. Colic in the British military working horse population: a retrospective analysis. Vet Rec 2019;184:24.

12. Nakame Y, Ishihara A, Itoh M, et al. Displacement of the large colon in a horse with enterolithiasis due to changed positions observed by computed tomography. J Equine Sci 2018;29:9–13.

13. Hillyer MH, Mair TS. Recurrent colic in the mature horse: a retrospective review of 58 cases. Equine Vet J 1997;29:421–4.

14. Blake KR, Affolter VK, Lowenstine LJ, et al. Myenteric ganglionitis as a cause of recurrent colic in an adult horse. J Am Vet Med Assoc 2012;240:1494–500.

15. Schusser GE, White NA. Morphologic and quantitative evaluation of the myenteric plexuses and neurons in the large colon of horses. J Am Vet Med Assoc 1997;210:928–34.

16. Fintl C, Hudson NP, Mayhew IG, et al. Interstitial cells of Cajal (ICC) in equine colic: an immunohistochemical study of horses with obstructive disorders of the small and large intestines. Equine Vet J 2004;36:474–9.

17. Schusser GF, Scheidemann W, Huskamp B. Muscle thickness and neuron density in the caecum of horses with chronic recurrent caecal impaction. Equine Vet J 2000;32 S32:69–73.

18. Pavone S, Sforna M, Gialletti R, et al. Extensive myenteric ganglionitis in a case of equine chronic intestinal pseudo-obstruction associated with EHV-1 infection. J Comp Pathol 2013;148:289–93.

19. Ortolani F, Nannarone S, Sforna M, et al. Diagnostic and clinical course of small colon recurrent impaction associated with severe myenteric ganglionopathy in a mare. J Equine Vet Sci 2021;101:103453.

20. Mair TS, Sherlock CE, Fews D, et al. Idiopathic fibrosis of the tunica muscularis of the large intestine in five horses with colic. J Comp Pathol 2016;154:231–4.

21. Boshuizen B, Ploeg M, Dewulf J, et al. Inflammatory bowel disease (IBD) in horses: a retrospective study exploring the value of different diagnostic approaches. BMC Vet Res 2018;14:21.

22. Schumacher J, Edwards JF, Cohen ND. Chronic idiopathic inflammatory bowel diseases of the horse. J Vet Intern Med 2000;14:258–65.

23. Mair TS, Pearson GR, Divers T. Malabsorption syndromes in the horse. Equine Vet Educ 2006;18:299–308.

24. Kalck KA. Inflammatory bowel disease in horses. Vet Clin N Am Equine Pract 2009;25:303–15.

25. Coomer R, McKane S, Roberts V, et al. Small intestinal biopsy and resection in standing sedated horses. Equine Vet Educ 2016;28:636–40.

26. Divers TJ, Pelligrini-Masini A, McDonough S. Diagnosis of inflammatory bowel disease in a hackney pony by gastroduodenal endoscopy and biopsy and successful treatment with corticosteroids. Equine Vet Educ 2006;18:284–7.

27. Stewart HL, Engiles JB, Stefanovski D, et al. Clinical and intestinal histologic features of horses treated for recurrent colic: 66 cases (2006-2015). J Am Vet Med Assoc 2018;252:1279–88.

28. Kaikkonen R, Niinisto K, Sykes B, et al. Diagnostic evaluation and short-term outcome as indicators of long-term prognosis in horses with findings suggestive

of inflammatory bowel disease treated with corticosteroids and anthelmintics. Acta Vet Scand 2014;56:35.

29. Luthersson N, Nielsen KH, Harris P, et al. The prevalence and anatomical distribution of equine gastric ulceration syndrome (EGUS) in 201 horses in Denmark. Equine Vet J 2009;41:619–24.

30. Tamzali Y, Marguet C, Priymenko N, et al. Prevalence of gastric ulcer syndrome in high-level endurance horses. Equine Vet J 2011;43:141–4.

31. Murray MJ, Grodinsky C, Anderson CW, et al. Gastric ulcers in horses: a comparison of endoscopic findings in horses with and without clinical signs. Equine Vet J 1989;21 S7:68–72.

32. Hepburn R. Gastric ulceration in horses. In Pract 2011;33:116–24.

33. Murray MJ. Gastric ulceration in horses: 91 cases (1987– 1990). J Am Vet Med Assoc 1992;201:117–20.

34. Vatistas NJ, Snyder JR, Carlson G, et al. Cross-sectional study of gastric ulcers of the squamous mucosa in Thoroughbred racehorses. Equine Vet J 1999;31 S29:34–9.

35. Sykes BW, Jokisalo JM. Rethinking equine gastric ulcer syndrome: Part 1 – Terminology, clinical signs and diagnosis. Equine Vet Educ 2014;26:543–7.

36. Sykes BW, Jokisalo JM. Rethinking equine gastric ulcer syndrome: Part 2 – Equine squamous gastric ulcer syndrome (ESGUS). Equine Vet Educ 2015a; 27:264–8.

37. Sykes BW, Jokisalo JM. Rethinking equine gastric ulcer syndrome: Part 3 – Equine glandular gastric ulcer syndrome (EGGUS) Equine. Vet Educ 2015b;27: 372–5.

38. Reinemeyer CR, Nielsen MK. Parasitism and colic. Vet Clin N Am Equine Pract 2009;25:233–45.

39. Hedberg-Alm Y, Tydén E, Tamminen L-M, et al. Clinical features and treatment response to differentiate idiopathic peritonitis from non-strangulating intestinal infarction of the pelvic flexure associated with *Strongylus vulgaris* infection in the horse. BMC Vet Res 2022;18:149.

40. Uhlinger C. Effects of three anthelmintic schedules on the incidence of colic in horses. Equine Vet J 1990;22:251–4.

41. Stancampiano L, Usai F, Marigo A, et al. Are small strongyles (Cyathostominae) involved in horse colic occurrence? Vet Parasitol 2017;247:33–6.

42. Owen R, Jagger DW, Quan-Taylor R. Caecal intussusceptions in horses and the significance of Anoplocephala perfoliata. Vet Rec 1989;124:34–7.

43. Proudman C, Edwards G. Are tapeworms associated with equine colic? A case control study. Equine Vet J 1993;25:224–6.

44. Proudman CJ, French NP, Trees AJ. Tapeworm infection is a significant risk factor for spasmodic colic and ileal impaction colic in the horse. Equine Vet J 1988;30: 194–9.

45. Epstein K. Congenital cause of gastrointestinal disease. Equine Vet Educ 2014; 26:345–6.

46. Baird AN, Cohen ND, Taylor TS, et al. Renosplenic entrapment of the large colon in horses: 57 cases (1983–1988). J Am Vet Med Assoc 1991;198:1423–6.

47. Farstvedt E, Hendrickson D. Laparoscopic closure of the nephrosplenic space for prevention of recurrent nephrosplenic entrapment of the ascending colon. Vet Surg 2005;34:642–5.

48. Loschelder J, Gehlen H. Sand colic in the horse - review and case examples. Pferdeheilkunde 2017;33:591–6.

49. Spanton JA, Smith LJ, Sherlock CE, et al. A review of 34 cases. Equine Vet Educ 2000;32:155–65.
50. Hassel DM, Langer DL, Snyder JR, et al. Evaluation of enterolithiasis in equids: 900 cases (1973–1996). J Am Vet Med Assoc 1999;214:233–7.
51. Bezdekova B, Wohlsein P, Venner M. Chronic severe pyloric lesions in horses: 47 cases. Equine Vet J 2020;52:200–4.
52. Mair TS, Sherlock CE. Surgical drainage and post operative lavage of large abdominal abscesses in six mature horses. Equine Vet J 2011;43 S39:123–7.
53. Barclay WP, Mccracken RJ, Phillips TN, et al. Chronic nongranulomatous enteritis in seven horses. J Am Vet Med Assoc 1987;190:684–6.
54. Huskamp B, Scheidemann W. Diagnosis and treatment of chronic recurrent caecal impaction. Equine Vet J 2000;S32:65–8.
55. Chaffin MK, Fuenteabla IC, Schumacher J, et al. Idiopathic muscular hypertrophy of the equine small intestine: 11 cases (1980–1991). Equine Vet J 1992;24:372–8.
56. Horstmeier C, Gerlach K, Mottl A, et al. Intestinal lipomatosis as a cause of colic in two horses. Pferdeheilkunde 2019;35:321–5.
57. Costa MC, Weese JS. Understanding the intestinal microbiome in health and disease. Vet Clin N Am Equine Pract 2018;34:1–12.
58. Blikslager AT. Colic prevention to avoid colic surgery: a surgeon's perspective. J Equine Vet Sci 2019;76:1–5.
59. Salem SE, Maddox TW, Berg A, et al. D.C. Variation in faecal microbiota in a group of horses managed at pasture over a 12-month period. Sci Rep 2018;8: e8510.
60. Salem S, Hough R, Probert C, et al. A longitudinal study of the faecal microbiome and metabolome of periparturient mares. PeerJ 2019;7:e6687.
61. Lara F, Castro C, Thomson P. Changes in the gut microbiome and colic in horses: are they causes or consequences? Open Vet J 2022;12:242–9.
62. Escalona EE, Okell CN, Archer DC. Prevalence and risk factors for colic in horses that display crib-biting behaviour. BMC Vet Res 2014;10(Suppl.1):53–60.
63. Clarke LL, Roberts MC, Argenzio RA. Feeding and digestive problems in horses. Physiologic responses to a concentrated meal. Vet Clin N Am Equine Pract 1990; 6:433–50.
64. Geor RJ, Harris PA. How to minimize gastrointestinal disease associated with carbohydrate nutrition in horses. Proc Am Ass Equine Practnr 2007;53:178–85.
65. House AM, Warren LK. Nutritional management of recurrent colic and colonic impactions Equine. Vet Educ 2016;28:167–72.
66. Schoster A, Weese JS, Guardabassi L. Probiotic use in horses – What is the evidence for their clinical efficacy? J Vet Intern Med 2014;28:1640–52.
67. JPAMvan L, Visser EMS, deMik-Van Mourik M, et al. Colic surgery in horses: a retrospective study into short- and long-term survival rate, complications and rehabilitation toward sporting activity. J Equine Vet Sci 2020;90:103012.
68. Mueller PO. Pathophysiology, prevention, and treatment of adhesions. In: Blikslager AT, White NA, Moore JN, et al, editors. The equine acute abdomen. 3rd Edition. Hoboken, NJ: Wiley Blackwell; 2017. p. pp153–65.
69. Macdonald M, Pascoe J, Stover S. Survival after small intestine resection and anastomosis in horses. Vet Surg 1989;18:415–23.
70. Gorvy DA, Edwards GB, Proudman CJ. Intra-abdominal adhesions in horses: a retrospective evaluation of repeat laparotomy in 99 horses with acute gastrointestinal disease. Vet J 2008;175:194–201.
71. Scharner D, Rotting A, Gerlach K, et al. Ultrasonagraphy of the abdomen in the horse with colic. Clin Tech Equine Pract 2002;1:118–24.

72. Rocken M, Schamer D, Gerlach K, et al. Laparoscopic evaluation of type and incidence of abdominal adhesions in horses with chronic colic and experiences with laparoscopic adhesiolysis. Pferdeheilkunde 2002;18:574–8.

73. Boure LP, Pearce SG, Kerr CL, et al. Evaluation of laparoscopic adhesiolysis for the treatment of experimentally induced adhesions in pony foals. Am J Vet Res 2002;63:289.

74. Southwood LL, Baxter GM, Hutchison JM, et al. Survey of diplomates of the American College of Veterinary Surgeons regarding postoperative intra- abdominal adhesion formation in horses undergoing abdominal surgery. J Am Vet Med Assoc 1997;211:1573–6.

75. Mair TS. Colic from alternative systems: "false colics". In: Blikslager AT, White NA, Moore JN, et al, editors. The equine acute abdomen. 3rd Edition. Hoboken, NJ: Wiley Blackwell; 2017. p. pp831–42.

76. Schweizer CM. Causes of colic associated with reproduction and the reproductive tract in the brood mare. In: Mair T, Divers T, Ducharme N, editors. Manual of equine gastroenterology. London: W.B. Saunders; 2002. p. pp351–61.

77. Sherlock CE, Lott-Ellis K, Bergren A, et al. Granulosa cell tumours in the mare: a review of 52 cases. Equine Vet Educ 2016;28:75–82.

78. Frazer GS. Postpartum complications in the mare: Part 1. Conditions affecting the uterus. Equine Vet Educ Manual 2002;5:41–9.

79. Douglas HF, Stefanovski D, Southwood LL. Outcomes of pregnant broodmares treated for colic at a tertiary care facility. Vet Surg 2021;50:1579–91.

80. Freeman CE, Lyle SK. Chronic intermittent colic in a mare attributed to uterine marbles. Equine Vet Educ 2015;26:469–73.

81. Varner DD, Schumacher J. Diseases of the spermatic cord. In: Colahan PT, Mayhew IG, Merritt AM, et al, editors. Equine medicine and surgery. 5th edn. St. Louis: Mosby; 1999. p. pp1054–7.

82. Laverty S, Pascoe JR, Ling GV, et al. Urolithiasis in 68 horses. Vet Surg 1992;21: 56–62.

83. Ryu SH, Bak UB, Lee CW, et al. Cholelithiasis associated with recurrent colic in a Thoroughbred mare. J Vet Sci 2004;5:79–82.

84. Leipig M, Abenthum K, Wollanke B, et al. Chronic pancreatitis with acinar-ductal metaplasia and ductal dysplasia in a horse. J Comp Pathol 2015;153:131–4.

85. Lack AC, Crabtree NE, Won WW, et al. Clinical pathology and ultrasonographic findings from a warmblood gelding with primary, severe, acute pancreatitis. Equine Vet Educ 2020;33:454.

86. Maxie M, Physick-Sheard P. Aortic–iliac thrombosis in horses. Vet Pathol 1985;22: 238–49.

87. Ploeg M, Saey V, de Bruijn CM, et al. Aortic rupture and aorto-pulmonary fistulation in the Friesian horse: characterisation of the clinical and gross post mortem findings in 24 cases. Equine Vet J 2013;45:101–6.

88. Valberg SJ. Muscle conditions affecting sport horses. Vet Clin N Am Equine Pract 2018;34:253–76.

Moving?

Make sure your subscription moves with you!

To notify us of your new address, find your **Clinics Account Number** (located on your mailing label above your name), and contact customer service at:

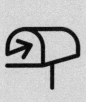

Email: journalscustomerservice-usa@elsevier.com

800-654-2452 (subscribers in the U.S. & Canada)
314-447-8871 (subscribers outside of the U.S. & Canada)

Fax number: 314-447-8029

Elsevier Health Sciences Division
Subscription Customer Service
3251 Riverport Lane
Maryland Heights, MO 63043

*To ensure uninterrupted delivery of your subscription, please notify us at least 4 weeks in advance of move.

Printed and bound by CPI Group (UK) Ltd, Croydon, CR0 4YY

03/10/2024

01040466-0004